Chronic Obstructive Pulmonary Disease

Editors

GERARD J. CRINER
BARTOLOME R. CELLI

CLINICS IN CHEST MEDICINE

www.chestmed.theclinics.com

September 2020 • Volume 41 • Number 3

ELSEVIER

1600 John F. Kennedy Boulevard • Suite 1800 • Philadelphia, Pennsylvania, 19103-2899

http://www.theclinics.com

CLINICS IN CHEST MEDICINE Volume 41, Number 3
September 2020 ISSN 0272-5231, ISBN-13: 978-0-323-68304-3

Editor: Colleen Dietzler
Developmental Editor: Casey Potter

Clinics in Chest Medicine (ISSN 0272-5231) is published quarterly by Elsevier Inc., 360 Park Avenue South, New York, NY 10010-1710. Months of issue are March, June, September, and December. Periodicals postage paid at New York, NY and additional mailing offices. Subscription prices are $388.00 per year (domestic individuals), $766.00 per year (domestic institutions), $100.00 per year (domestic students/residents), $423.00 per year (Canadian individuals), $952.00 per year (Canadian institutions), $484.00 per year (international individuals), $952.00 per year (international institutions), $100.00 per year (Canadian Students), and $230.00 per year (International Students). International air speed delivery is included in all Clinics subscription prices. All prices are subject to change without notice. **POSTMASTER:** Send address changes to Clinics in Chest Medicine, Elsevier Health Sciences Division, Subscription Customer Service, 3251 Riverport Lane, Maryland Heights, MO 63043. **Customer Service: Telephone: 1-800-654-2452** (U.S. and Canada); **1-314-447-8871** (outside U.S. and Canada). **Fax: 1-314-447-8029. E-mail: journalscustomerservice-usa@elsevier.com (for print support); journalsonlinesupport-usa@elsevier.com (for online support).**

Reprints. For copies of 100 or more of articles in this publication, please contact the Commercial Reprints Department, Elsevier Inc., 360 Park Avenue South, New York, NY 10010-1710. Tel.: 212-633-3874; Fax: 212-633-3820; E-mail: reprints@elsevier.com.

Clinics in Chest Medicine is covered in *MEDLINE/PubMed (Index Medicus), Current Contents/Clinical Medicine, EMBASE/ Excerpta Medica, Science Citation Index,* and *ISI/BIOMED.*

Contributors

EDITORS

BARTOLOME R. CELLI, MD
Professor of Medicine, Pulmonary and Critical Care Division, Brigham and Women's Hospital, Harvard Medical School, Boston, Massachusetts, USA

GERARD J. CRINER, MD
Professor and Founding Chair, Department of Thoracic Medicine and Surgery, Lewis Katz School of Medicine at Temple University, Philadelphia, Pennsylvania, USA

AUTHORS

ALVAR AGUSTI, MD, PhD
Respiratory Institute, Hospital Clinic, University of Barcelona, Institut d'Investigacio August Pi I Sunyer (IDIBAPS), Barcelona, Spain; Centro de Investigación Biomédica en Red (CIBER) Enfermedades Respiratorias, Instituto de Salud Carlos III, Madrid, Spain

PETER ALTER, MD
Department of Internal Medicine, Pulmonary and Critical Care Medicine, University Medical Center Giessen and Marburg, Philipps-Universität Marburg (UMR), Member of the German Center for Lung Research (DZL), Marburg, Germany

JEAN BOURBEAU, MD, MSC, FRCPC
Respiratory Epidemiology and Clinical Research Unit, Montreal Chest Institute, McGill University Health Centre, Research Institute of the McGill University Health Centre, McGill University, Montréal, Québec, Canada

BARTOLOME R. CELLI, MD
Professor of Medicine Pulmonary and Critical Care Division, Brigham and Women's Hospital, Harvard Medical School, Boston, Massachusetts, USA

GERARD J. CRINER, MD
Professor and Founding Chair, Department of Thoracic Medicine and Surgery, Lewis Katz School of Medicine at Temple University, Philadelphia, Pennsylvania, USA

AYHAM DAHER, MD
Department of Pneumology and Intensive Care Medicine, University Hospital Aachen, Aachen, Germany

MIGUEL DIVO, MD, MPH
Instructor in Medicine, Pulmonary and Critical Care Division, Brigham and Women's Hospital, Harvard Medical School, Boston, Massachusetts, USA

MARK T. DRANSFIELD, MD
Division of Pulmonary, Allergy and Critical Care Medicine, Lung Health Center, The University of Alabama at Birmingham, Birmingham, Alabama, USA

MICHAEL DREHER, MD
Department of Pneumology and Intensive Care Medicine, University Hospital Aachen, Aachen, Germany

SEAN DUFFY, MD
Assistant Professor, Department of Thoracic Medicine and Surgery, Lewis Katz School of Medicine at Temple University, Philadelphia, Pennsylvania, USA

LEONARDO M. FABBRI, MD
Section of Respiratory Diseases, Department of Morphology, Surgery and Experimental Medicine, University of Ferrara, Ferrara, Italy

ROSA FANER, PhD
Institut d'Investigacio August Pi I Sunyer
(IDIBAPS), Barcelona, Spain; Centro de
Investigación Biomédica en Red (CIBER)
Enfermedades Respiratorias, Instituto de
Salud Carlos III, Madrid, Spain

SEBASTIEN GAGNON, MD
Respiratory Epidemiology and Clinical
Research Unit, Montreal Chest Institute, McGill
University Health Centre, Montréal, Québec,
Canada; Department of Medicine, Division of
Respiratory Medicine, CHU de Québec,
Québec, Canada

MEILAN K. HAN, MD, MS
Associate Professor of Medicine, Division of
Pulmonary and Critical Care Medicine,
University of Michigan School of Medicine, Ann
Arbor, Michigan, USA

**DAVID M.G. HALPIN, MB BS, MA, DPhil,
FRCP, FERS**
University of Exeter Medical School, College of
Medicine and Health, University of Exeter,
Exeter, United Kingdom

RAJESH KUNADHARAJU, MD
Division of Pulmonary/Critical Care and Sleep
Medicine, Department of Medicine, Jacobs
School of Medicine and Biomedical Sciences,
University at Buffalo, SUNY, Buffalo, New York,
USA

NATHANIEL MARCHETTI, DO
Professor, Department of Thoracic Medicine
and Surgery, Lewis Katz School of Medicine at
Temple University, Philadelphia, Pennsylvania,
USA

FERNANDO J. MARTINEZ, MD, MS
Chief, Division of Pulmonary and Critical
Care Medicine, Internal Medicine, Weill
Cornell Medicine, New York, New York,
USA

ALEXANDER G. MATHIOUDAKIS, MD
Division of Infection, Immunity and Respiratory
Medicine, School of Biological Sciences, The
University of Manchester, Manchester
Academic Health Science Centre, North West
Lung Centre, Wythenshawe Hospital,
Manchester University NHS Foundation Trust,
Manchester, United Kingdom

KATHRYN M. MILNE, MD FRCP(C)
Division of Respiratory Medicine, Department
of Medicine, Kingston Health Science Center,
Queen's University, Kingston, Ontario,
Canada; Clinician Investigator Program,
Department of Medicine, University of British
Columbia, Vancouver, British Columbia,
Canada

**STEPHEN MILNE, BBiomedSc, MBBS,
FRACP, PhD**
Division of Respiratory Medicine, Centre for
Heart Lung Innovation, St Paul's Hospital,
University of British Columbia, Vancouver,
British Columbia, Canada; Faculty of Medicine
and Health, University of Sydney,
Camperdown, New South Wales, Australia

TAKUDZWA MKOROMBINDO, MD
Division of Pulmonary, Allergy and Critical Care
Medicine

MARIA MONTES DE OCA, MD, PhD
Servicio de Neumonología, Hospital
Universitario de Caracas, Facultad de
Medicina, Universidad Central de Venezuela,
Centro Médico de Caracas, Caracas,
Venezuela

LUCA MORANDI, MD
Section of Respiratory Diseases, Department
of Morphology, Surgery and Experimental
Medicine, University of Ferrara, Ferrara, Italy

**J. ALBERTO NEDER, MD, PhD, FRCP(C),
FERS**
Division of Respiratory Medicine, Department
of Medicine, Kingston Health Science Center,
Queen's University, Kingston, Ontario, Canada

**DENIS E. O'DONNELL, MD, FRCP(I),
FRCP(C), FERS**
Division of Respiratory Medicine, Department
of Medicine, Kingston Health Science Center,
Queen's University, Kingston, Ontario, Canada

JUAN PABLO DE-TORRES, MD, PhD
Division of Respiratory Medicine, Department
of Medicine, Kingston Health Science Center,
Queen's University, Kingston, Ontario, Canada

ALBERTO PAPI, MD
Section of Respiratory Diseases, Department
of Morphology, Surgery and Experimental
Medicine, University of Ferrara, Ferrara, Italy

CARRIE L. PISTENMAA, MD
Division of Pulmonary and Critical Care, Brigham and Women's Hospital, Instructor of Medicine, Harvard Medical School, Boston, Massachusetts, USA

ANDREW I. RITCHIE, MBChB
National Heart and Lung Institute, Imperial College, London, United Kingdom

NICOLAS ROCHE, MD, PhD, FERS
Respiratory Medicine, Pneumologie et Soins Intensifs Respiratoires, APHP Centre, Cochin Hospital, Université de Paris (Descartes), Institut Cochin (UMR 1016), Paris, France

BRYAN ROSS, MD, MSC, FRCPC
Respiratory Epidemiology and Clinical Research Unit, Montreal Chest Institute, McGill University Health Centre, Montréal, Québec, Canada

LISA RUVUNA, MD
Resident, Department of Internal Medicine, University of New Mexico School of Medicine, Albuquerque, New Mexico, USA

SANJAY SETHI, MD
Division of Pulmonary/Critical Care and Sleep Medicine, Department of Medicine, Jacobs School of Medicine and Biomedical Sciences, University at Buffalo, SUNY, Buffalo, New York, USA

DON D. SIN, MD, MPH, FRCP(C)
Division of Respiratory Medicine, Centre for Heart Lung Innovation, St Paul's Hospital, University of British Columbia, Vancouver, British Columbia, Canada

DAVE SINGH, PhD
Division of Infection, Immunity and Respiratory Medicine, School of Biological Sciences, The University of Manchester, Manchester

Academic Health Science Centre, North West Lung Centre, Wythenshawe Hospital, Manchester University NHS Foundation Trust, Medicines Evaluation Unit, Manchester, United Kingdom

AKSHAY SOOD, MD, MPH
Professor, Department of Internal Medicine, University of New Mexico School of Medicine, Albuquerque, New Mexico, USA

CHARLIE STRANGE, MD
Professor, Division of Pulmonary, Critical Care, Allergy and Sleep Medicine, Medical University of South Carolina, Charleston, South Carolina, USA

JØRGEN VESTBO, DMSc
Division of Infection, Immunity and Respiratory Medicine, School of Biological Sciences, The University of Manchester, Manchester Academic Health Science Centre, North West Lung Centre, Wythenshawe Hospital, Manchester University NHS Foundation Trust, Manchester, United Kingdom

CLAUS F. VOGELMEIER, MD
Department of Internal Medicine, Pulmonary and Critical Care Medicine, University Medical Center Giessen and Marburg, Philipps-Universität Marburg (UMR), Member of the German Center for Lung Research (DZL), Marburg, Germany

GEORGE R. WASHKO, MD, MSc
Division of Pulmonary and Critical Care, Brigham and Women's Hospital, Associate Professor of Medicine Harvard Medical School, Boston, Massachusetts, USA

JADWIGA A. WEDZICHA, PhD
Professor, National Heart and Lung Institute, Imperial College, London, United Kingdom

Contents

Section I: COPD Pathogenesis and Risk Factors

Chronic obstructive pulmonary disease (COPD) has been traditionally considered a self-inflicted disease caused by tobacco smoking. Current available evidence, however, indicates that the pathogenesis of COPD needs to consider the dynamic and cumulative nature of a series of environment (including smoking plus other exposures)-host interactions that eventually determine lung development, maintenance, repair, and aging. By doing so, these factors modulate the trajectory of lung function of the individual through life and the odds of developing COPD through different routes, which likely represent different forms of the disease that require different preventive and therapeutic strategies.

 Video content accompanies this article at http://www.chestmed.theclinics.com.

Chronic obstructive pulmonary disease (COPD) affects about 300 million people worldwide, resulting in approximately 64 million disability-adjusted life years. Household air pollution affects almost 3 billion people worldwide and is a major risk factor for COPD. An estimated 25% to 45% of patients with COPD worldwide have never smoked. Fourteen percent of the overall COPD burden is attributable to occupational exposures. Rural populations are at higher risk for COPD than urban residents. African American never-smokers have a disproportionately high prevalence and Hispanic people have a low prevalence of COPD.

Although smoking results in lung pathology in many, still not all smokers develop chronic obstructive pulmonary disease (COPD). Roughly a quarter of patients with COPD have never smoked. An understanding of both host and environmental factors beyond smoking that contribute to disease development remain critical to understanding disease prevention and ultimately effectively intervene. In this article, we summarize host factors, including genetics and gender, as well as early-life events that contribute to the development of COPD.

Alpha-1 antitrypsin deficiency (AATD) was the first genetic risk factor for chronic obstructive pulmonary disease (COPD) described. In the more than 50 years since its description, the disease continues to provide insights into more common forms of COPD. Although AATD is caused by a single genetic variant, the clinical manifestations of disease include panacinar emphysema, airway hyperresponsiveness, and bronchiectasis. With improved molecular understanding of the mechanisms of disease pathogenesis and progression, new therapies in addition to intravenous augmentation therapy are on the horizon.

Section II: Diagnosis and Assessment of COPD

J. Alberto Neder, Juan Pablo de-Torres, Kathryn M. Milne, and Denis E. O'Donnell

Lung function testing has undisputed value in the comprehensive assessment and individualized management of chronic obstructive pulmonary disease, a pathologic condition in which a functional abnormality, poorly reversible expiratory airway obstruction, is at the core of its definition. After an overview of the physiologic underpinnings of the disease, the authors outline the role of lung function testing in this disease, including diagnosis, assessment of severity, and indication for and responses to pharmacologic and nonpharmacologic interventions. They discuss the current controversies surrounding test interpretation with these purposes in mind and provide balanced recommendations to optimize their usefulness in different clinical scenarios.

Claus F. Vogelmeier and Peter Alter

Evaluating symptoms is a central part of the chronic obstructive pulmonary disease (COPD) assessment system as suggested by the Global Initiative for Chronic Obstructive Lung Disease (GOLD). Considering the pros and cons of all currently available tests, GOLD suggests using primarily the modified Medical Research Council dyspnea scale or the COPD Assessment Test. Based on the test results, patients are categorized as having a low or high level of symptoms. This level then becomes one of the 2 dimensions of the ABCD grading system, which was designed to match the best initial treatment option to the individual patient's needs.

Carrie L. Pistenmaa and George R. Washko

Computerized tomography in chronic obstructive pulmonary disease (COPD) has been the subject of intense interest in the research and clinical community. Methods have been developed to objectively detect and quantify processes affecting the lung parenchyma, airways and vasculature, as well as extrapulmonary manifestations of the noxious effects of chronic inhalational exposures, such as tobacco smoke. This article provides a brief overview of image-based advances in COPD research and then discusses how these advances have translated to clinical care, finishing with a brief description of a path forward for the convergence of research and care at the bedside.

Stephen Milne and Don D. Sin

Chronic obstructive pulmonary disease (COPD) is a highly heterogeneous disease with limited adequate treatments. Biomarkers—which may relate to disease susceptibility, diagnosis, prognosis, or treatment response—are ideally suited to dissecting such a complex disease and form a critical component of the precision medicine paradigm. Not all potential candidates, however, make good biomarkers. To date, only plasma fibrinogen has been approved by regulatory bodies as a biomarker of exacerbation risk for clinical trial enrichment. This review outlines some of the challenges of biomarker research in COPD and highlights novel and promising biomarker candidates.

The term asthma chronic obstructive pulmonary disease (COPD) overlap (ACO) has been popularized to describe people who simultaneously have features of both diseases. Analysis of the basis of disease classification and comparison of the clinical, pathophysiological, and therapeutic features of asthma and COPD concludes that it is not useful to use the term ACO. Rather, it is important to make the individual diagnoses, recognizing that both diseases may coexist. If a concurrent diagnosis of COPD is suspected in people with asthma, pharmacotherapy should primarily follow asthma guidelines, but pharmacologic and nonpharmacologic approaches also may be needed for COPD.

Chronic obstructive pulmonary disease (COPD) is a complex disease manifested primarily as airflow limitation that is partially reversible as confirmed by spirometry. COPD patients frequently develop systemic manifestations, such as skeletal muscle wasting and cachexia. COPD patients often develop other comorbid diseases, such as ischemic heart disease, heart failure, osteoporosis, anemia, lung cancer, and depression. Comorbidities complicate management of COPD and need to be evaluated because detection and treatment have important consequences. Novel approaches aimed at integrating the multiple morbidities seen in COPD and other chronic diseases will provide new avenues of research and allow developing more comprehensive and effective therapeutic approaches.

Section III: Exacerbations

Acute exacerbations of chronic obstructive pulmonary disease (AECOPD) are episodes of symptom worsening which have significant adverse consequences for patients. Exacerbations are highly heterogeneous events associated with increased airway and systemic inflammation and physiological changes. The frequency of exacerbations is associated with accelerated lung function decline, quality of life impairment and increased mortality. They are triggered predominantly by respiratory viruses and bacteria, which infect the lower airway and increase airway inflammation. A proportion of patients appear to be more susceptible to exacerbations, with poorer quality of life and more aggressive disease progression than those who have infrequent exacerbations. Exacerbations also contribute significantly to healthcare expenditure. Prevention and mitigation of exacerbations are therefore key goals of COPD management.

Management of a chronic obstructive pulmonary disease (COPD) exacerbation begins with an accurate diagnosis. Although more than 80% of exacerbations are managed on an outpatient basis, hospitalization is all too common and associated with considerable health care costs and mortality. Irrespective of the site of treatment, the treatment modalities are the same. Noninvasive ventilation has greatly decreased the mortality in exacerbations that require ventilatory support. Across the range of exacerbation severity, treatment failure and relapses are frequent, and should be carefully evaluated. New therapeutic options to address infection and inflammation in COPD are needed to improve the outcome of exacerbations.

Governments could help prevent chronic obstructive pulmonary disease (COPD) by reducing smoking rates; for example, through tobacco sale restriction, increasing tobacco prices, reducing nicotine content, and banning smoking in public areas and workplaces. Smoking cessation in general, and in particular among patients with COPD, could be achieved through specific programs, including behavior modification and the use of nicotine replacement therapy, bupropion, or varenicline. Prevention and/or slowed COPD progression could be achieved by occupational exposure prevention; improved indoor/outdoor air quality; reduced cooking and heating pollutants; use of better stoves and chimneys, and alternative energy sources; and influenza and pneumococcal vaccination.

Section IV: Pharmacologic Therapy in COPD

Long-acting bronchodilators represent the mainstay of maintenance treatment of chronic obstructive pulmonary disease (COPD). This state-of-the-art review summarizes currently available data on the safety, efficacy, and clinical effectiveness of long-acting bronchodilators and describes their role in the management of COPD, as defined by current national and international guidelines. Data from extensive clinical trials and real-life studies have demonstrated that long-acting beta-2 agonists and long-acting muscarinic antagonists can safely reduce the frequency of exacerbations, alleviate symptoms, and improve quality of life, exercise tolerance, and lung function of patients with COPD. They are recommended as first-line maintenance treatment of COPD.

Inhaled corticosteroids (ICSs), when used in combination with long-acting bronchodilators, reduce the risk of exacerbations and improve health-related quality of life in patients with chronic obstructive pulmonary disease (COPD) compared with bronchodilator or ICS therapy alone. Potential side effects of ICSs include adverse effects on glycemic control, bone density, cataract formation, skin changes, oral candidiasis, and pulmonary infections. Pneumonia is observed at increased rates in COPD patients, in particular those with greater airflow limitation, low body mass index, advanced age, and male gender, and ICSs may increase this risk. Risk assessment is essential in selecting appropriate patients for ICS-containing therapy.

Inhaled therapy remains the cornerstone of chronic obstructive pulmonary disease pharmacologic care, but some systemic treatments can be of help when the burden of the disease remains high. Azithromycin, phosphodiesterase-4 inhibitors, and mucoactive agents can be used in such situations. The major difficulty remains in the identification of the optimal target populations. Another difficulty is to determine how these treatments should be positioned in the global treatment algorithm. For instance, should they be prescribed in addition to other antiinflammatory agents or should they replace them in some cases? Research is ongoing to identify new therapeutic targets.

Section V: Non-pharmacological Therapy in COPD

More than one-third of patients with chronic obstructive pulmonary disease (COPD) continue to smoke cigarettes despite knowing they have the disease. This behavior has a negative impact on prognosis and progression, as repeated injury enhances the pathobiological mechanisms responsible for the disease. A combination of counseling plus pharmacotherapy is the most effective cessation treatment of smokers with COPD, and varenicline seems to be the most effective pharmacologic intervention. Preventing exacerbations in patients with COPD is a major goal of treatment, and vaccination against influenza and pneumococcus is an effective preventive strategy to achieve this goal.

Pulmonary rehabilitation (PR) is an essential intervention in the management of patients with chronic obstructive pulmonary disease. To guide health care professionals in the implementation and evaluation of a PR program, this article discusses the current key concepts regarding exercise testing, prescription, and training, as well as self-management intervention as essential parts of PR and post-rehabilitation maintenance. Moreover, new approaches (alternative forms of organization and delivery, tele-rehabilitation, exercise adjuncts) and unique with challenges situations (patients experiencing acute exacerbations, advanced disease) are thoroughly reviewed. Finally, validated point-of-care resources and online tools are provided.

Both hypoxemic and hypercapnic respiratory failure occur in patients with progressive chronic obstructive pulmonary disease (COPD). The presence of respiratory

CLINICS IN CHEST MEDICINE

THE CLINICS ARE AVAILABLE ONLINE!
Access your subscription at:
www.theclinics.com

CLINICS IN CHEST MEDICINE

Preface

Chronic Obstructive Pulmonary Disease in the Twenty-First Century

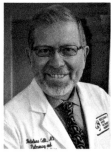 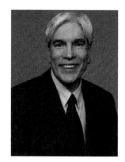

Bartolome R. Celli, MD Gerard J. Criner, MD

Editors

In 1819, over 200 years ago Rene Laennec published his treatise, *"De l'Auscultation Mediate ou Traite du Diagnostic des Maladies des Poumons et du Coeur,"* which was translated into English in 1821.[1] Besides describing for the first time the stethoscope, he touched upon several diseases of the chest, including the pathologic dilation of alveoli, an entity that he first named emphysema. In relation to what we today know as chronic obstructive pulmonary disease (COPD), he prophetically stated:

The disease can begin in infancy and continue for many years. More often cough with mucous catarrh, worsens in the winter and in the mornings. It is often accompanied by difficult respiration, which might end fatally with 'suffocative catarrh.' Once present, dyspnea is constant, worsened by anxiety and exercise and additionally by acute catarrh.

In these 4 lines, he made a complete summary of the origin, clinical presentation, and course of what we know as COPD today. In this issue of *Clinics in Chest Medicine*, we have tried to bring together the accumulated knowledge of over 200 years of information related to COPD, aiming to provide the readers with a compendium of facts useful to clinicians, trainees, and health care providers as they face potential and actual patients with this disease.

During these 2 centuries and just as Laennec had predicted, we have rediscovered that COPD may actually begin not only in infancy, but much earlier. Indeed, COPD has an important genetic origin that modulates its response to the environment from the moment of conception and thereafter. While in uterus through the mother, after birth with its close surroundings, and throughout the period of growth, the human lung has an intimate interaction with the environment that will in the end determine whether the result is an optimally developed respiratory system or an impaired organ, likely to decline in function more rapidly if encountering injurious interactions with the environment. Although cigarette smoking captured our attention as the main culprit of COPD, we now know that this is true for high-income societies, but that several other factors, particularly biomass and pollution, cause the vast majority of cases in the less developed portion of the world. During this period, we have also learned that patients with COPD may develop and actually suffer from many extrapulmonary morbidities, and these profoundly impact the outcomes of the patients.

We can thus envision a sequence as depicted in **Fig. 1**, where our genetic makeup interacts with the various causes that are known to result in airflow limitation.[2] In this natural course, there is a "silent" period of little clinical expression that

Clin Chest Med 41 (2020) xv–xvii
https://doi.org/10.1016/j.ccm.2020.06.015
0272-5231/20/© 2020 Published by Elsevier Inc.

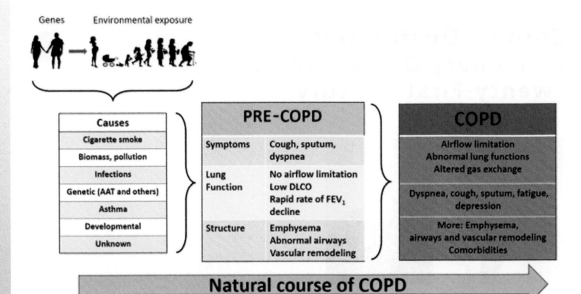

Fig. 1. COPD results from the interaction of the genetic makeup inherited from our parents and the interaction with causative agents present in the environment. It goes through a period without airflow limitation in many subjects, whereas in some it reaches a stage characterized by spirometrically defined airflow limitation. AAT, alpha-1-antitrypsin; DLCO, diffusing capacity of the lungs for carbon monoxide; FEV$_1$, forced expiratory volume in 1 second. (*Modified from* Celli BR, Wedzicha JA. Update on clinical aspects of chronic obstructive pulmonary disease. N Engl J Med 2019;381:1257-1266.)

can be detected by symptoms of cough and phlegm (just as Laennec had expressed) or identified, if not with a stethoscope, using computerized tomography, or certain pulmonary function tests, such as the diffusion capacity for carbon monoxide or rapid decline of spirometric lung function. Due to the delay in diagnosing the clinical disease, it is only now that we are beginning to explore this "pre-COPD" phase, which offers us the opportunity of primary and secondary prevention. In addition, during this period, we have identified one genetic cause of COPD, alpha-1-antitrypsin deficiency, the identification of which is mandatory, because we now know that replacement therapy improves the outcome of these patients.

More than 200 years, we have also learned about the deleterious consequences that exacerbations have on the natural course of COPD. Those episodes so well described by Laennec not only impact on our patient's quality of life but also worsen disease progression and increase risk of death. Prevention and treatment of those episodes remain at the center of treatment, and fortunately, over the last decades, many well-conducted clinical trials have proven that inhaled long-acting bronchodilators and appropriately dosed inhaled corticosteroids are effective in symptomatic patients with the disease.

Finally, for the most severely affected patients, we need not lose perspective of the advances that have shown the greatest documented impact on outcomes, including death. Pulmonary rehabilitation for functionally limited patients, oxygen therapy for hypoxemic individuals, and lung volume reduction approaches for patients with emphysema and severe hyperinflation have all shown improvement in dyspnea, health status, and functional capacity; importantly, they all decrease the risk of exacerbations and death.

If René Laennec could return, he would be very proud of the advances reviewed in this issue. He would view with some pleasure the fact that although COPD is currently the third leading cause of death worldwide, its overall impact has been decreasing over the last decade. It is our hope that with more emphasis on prevention, and better implementation of pharmacologic and nonpharmacologic therapies, we may be able to eradicate COPD's impact on society.

Bartolome R. Celli, MD
Pulmonary and Critical Care Division
Brigham and Women's Hospital
Harvard Medical School
75 Francis Street
Boston, MA 02460, USA

Gerard J. Criner, MD
Department of Thoracic Medicine and Surgery
Lewis Katz School of Medicine at Temple
University
712 Parkinson Pavilion
3401 North Broad Street
Philadelphia, PA 19140, USA

E-mail addresses:
bcelli@copdnet.org (B.R. Celli)
gerard.criner@tuhs.temple.edu (G.J. Criner)

REFERENCES

1. Laennec R. A treatise on the diseases of the chest. London: T. Underwood, and C. Underwood; 1821.
2. Celli BR, Wedzicha JA. Update on clinical aspects of chronic obstructive pulmonary disease. N Engl J Med 2019;381:1257–66.

Section I : COPD Pathogenesis and Risk Factors

Chronic Obstructive Pulmonary Disease Pathogenesis

Alvar Agusti, MD, PhD[a,b,c,d,*], Rosa Faner, PhD[c,d,1]

KEYWORDS

- Airway diseases • Chronic bronchitis • Chronic obstructive pulmonary disease • Emphysema
- Smoking

KEY POINTS

- Tobacco smoking is the main, but not the sole risk factor for COPD.
- COPD can start early in life. About 4% to 12% of individuals in the general population never achieve normal peak lung function in early adulthood and are at risk for developing COPD (and other concomitant diseases) later in life, and of dying prematurely.
- The pathogenesis of COPD involves a series of dynamic, cumulative, environment-host interactions that occur throughout life and determine lung development, repair, and aging, hence the vital trajectory of lung function.
- Prevention beyond smoking avoidance/cessation, prompt detection, and early intervention are likely to be important to reduce disease burden and to improve health status and the prognosis of patients.

INTRODUCTION

Chronic obstructive pulmonary disease (COPD) has been traditionally considered a self-inflicted disease induced by tobacco smoking and characterized by an accelerated decline of lung function with aging.[1] Tobacco smoking continues to be the main, environmental and preventable, risk factor of COPD, so every effort needs to be made to prevent smoking initiation and/or to favor early smoking cessation; however, this classical paradigm is changing rapidly[2] and goes well beyond smoking.[3] This new understanding of the pathogenesis of the disease can open novel windows for prevention and early intervention.[3]

THE TRADITIONAL UNDERSTANDING OF CHRONIC OBSTRUCTIVE PULMONARY DISEASE: A SELF-INFLICTED DISEASE CAUSED BY TOBACCO SMOKING (IN MALES)

In 1976, Fletcher and coworkers[4] published the classic book *The Natural History of Chronic Bronchitis and Emphysema*. It details the results of a study in a stratified, relatively small (n = 792), random sample of men (no females were included in the study) aged 30 to 59 working in West London, who were followed the next 8 years.[4] Results were summarized 1 year later.[1] **Fig. 1** here and in that review became, until recently,[2] the holy grail of the understanding of the pathogenesis of

[a] Respiratory Institute, Hospital Clinic, Villarroel 170, Barcelona 08036, Spain; [b] University of Barcelona, Barcelona, Spain; [c] Institut d'Investigacio August Pi I Sunyer (IDIBAPS), Barcelona, Spain; [d] Centro de Investigación Biomédica en Red (CIBER) Enfermedades Respiratorias, Instituto de Salud Carlos III, Spain
[1] Present address: CIBERES, C/Casanova 143, Cellex, P2A, Barcelona 08036, Spain.
* Corresponding author. Respiratory Institute, Hospital Clinic, Villarroel 170, Barcelona 08036, Spain.
E-mail address: aagusti@clinic.cat

Clin Chest Med 41 (2020) 307–314
https://doi.org/10.1016/j.ccm.2020.05.001

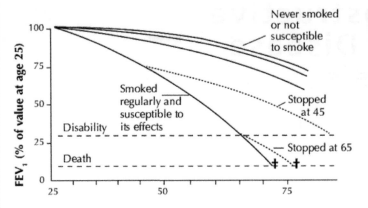

Fig. 1. The traditional COPD paradigm, as described by Fletcher and Peto in 1977. For further explanations, see text. (*From* Fletcher C, Peto R. The natural history of chronic airflow obstruction. Br Med J. 1977 1(6077):1645-1648; with permission.)

COPD. It stated that a proportion of so-called "susceptible smokers" developed chronic airflow obstruction (COPD) caused by an accelerated decline of lung function with age.[1] This understanding implied that tobacco smoking was the cause of COPD, and that COPD was an irremediable progressive disease that always leads to disability and early death. Yet, as discussed next, evidence over the past decade, or so, contradicts this interpretation.

SOME OBSERVATIONS DO NOT FIT THIS TRADITIONAL PATHOGENIC PARADIGM

The following recent epidemiologic and clinical observations do not fit this traditional paradigm and, overall, partially challenge its validity.

Chronic Obstructive Pulmonary Disease in Never Smokers

Between 20% and 40% of patients with COPD around the world are never smokers.[5] This clearly indicates that there must be other environmental and/or biologic factors than smoking that contribute to the pathogenesis of the disease. In this context, it is well established now that other environmental pollutants, such as those derived from biomass exposure and others, can also contribute to a significant proportion of COPD cases.[6]

Individual Susceptibility

As originally recognized by Fletcher and Peto,[1] there is an element of individual susceptibility to environmental exposures (smoking and others), likely related to the genetic and/or epigenetic background of the individual.[3] A large epidemiologic study (15,256 cases and 47,936 control subjects, with replication of top results [$P < 5 \times 10^{-6}$] in another 9498 cases and 9748 control subjects) identified 22 genetic loci associated with COPD (**Table 1**).[7] Yet, the individual effect size (odds ratio) of each of these 22 genes is small (see **Table 1**), clearly indicating the polygenic basis of COPD.[7]

More recent research also emphasizes the role of epigenetic changes,[8] thus contributing to a great level of genetic complexity and interaction with the environmental exposures discussed previously.

Chronic Obstructive Pulmonary Disease Is a Progressive Disease

The notion that COPD always is irremediable and progressive (at least in terms of lung function decline) is not sustained by evidence. In the ECLIPSE (Evaluation of COPD Longitudinally to Identify Predictive Surrogate Endpoints) study, investigators found that during 3-year follow-up forced expiratory volume in 1 second (FEV_1) declined substantially (>60 mL/y) in 31% of patients and modestly (60–30 mL/y) in 29%, but remained stable in 29% and even improved in 10%,[9] an observation also reported by Fletcher and colleagues.[4] Admittedly, the patients included in the ECLIPSE study were being treated according to their attending physician, so they do not represent the natural history of "untreated" COPD. Yet, these observations clearly argue against the nihilistic view that COPD is untreatable and always progressive. Furthermore, as discussed later, COPD is a complex disease with numerous and varied pulmonary and extrapulmonary manifestations, so the concept of disease progression goes beyond FEV_1 changes and requires careful consideration.[2]

Parallel FEV₁ Decline Trajectories

By putting together data gathered from the TORCH (Toward a Revolution in COPD Health)[10] and UPLIFT (Understanding Potential Long-Term Impacts on Function with Tiotropium)[11] studies, Decramer and Cooper[12] clearly illustrated that FEV_1 basically declined in parallel in patients with COPD with different degrees of airflow limitation severity (**Fig. 2**), thus questioning the validity of a single lung function trajectory as originally interpreted from the observations by Fletcher and Peto[1] in healthy British workers.

Table 1
Twenty two genetic loci significantly associated with COPD as identified by Hobbs et al[7]

rsID	Closest Gene	Risk Allele Frequency Mean		Odds Ratio	95% Confidence Interval	P Value
		Mean	Range			
rs1314164	HHIP	0.59	0.52–0.89	1.21	1.16–1.27	9.10×10^{-41}
rs17486278	CHRNA5	0.35	0.24–0.44	1.13	1.08–1.18	1.77×10^{-28}
rs7733088	HTR4	0.60	0.47–0.69	1.18	1 13–1.23	5.33×10^{-26}
rs9399401	ADGRG6	0.72	0.61–0.75	1.17	1.12–1.23	1.81×10^{-19}
rs1441358	THSD4	0.33	0.19–0.55	1.12	1.07–1.17	8.22×10^{-16}
rs6837671	FAM13A	0.41	0.36–0.58	1.07	1.02–1.11	7.48×10^{-15}
rs11727735	GSTCD	0.94	0.93–0.99	1.25	1.14–1.36	3.84×10^{-14}
rs754388	RIN3	0.82	0.80–0.86	1.11	1.05–1.17	4.96×10^{-14}
rs113897301	ADAM 19	0.17	0.05–0.19	1.13	1.07–1.19	1.58×10^{-13}
rs2047409*	TET2	0.62	0.22–0.65	1 14	1.09–1.19	2.46×10^{-13}
rs2955083	KLFSEC	0.88	0.85–0.89	1.17	1.09–1.25	4.16×10^{-13}
rs7186831*	CFDP1	0.43	0.23–0.47	1.12	1.07–1.17	1.12×10^{-11}
rs10429950*	TGFB2	0.73	0.22–0.77	1.10	1.04–1.15	1.66×10^{-10}
rs2070600*	AGER	0.95	0.85–0.99	1.21	1.10–1.32	5.94×10^{-10}
rs17707300	CCDC101	0.37	0.11–0.43	1.06	1.02–1.11	6.75×10^{-10}
rs2806356*	ARMC2	0.18	0.05–0.24	1.12	1.06–1.18	8.34×10^{-10}
rsl6825267*	PID1	0.93	0.87–0.94	1.13	1.04–1.22	1.68×10^{-9}
rs2076295	DSP	0.55	0.44–0.58	1.06	1.02–1.14	3.97×10^{-9}
rs647097*	MTCL1	0.27	0.26–0.40	1.09	1.04–1.11	6.14×10^{-9}
rs1529672	RA RH	0.83	0.68–0.86	1.05	0.99–1.11	2.47×10^{-8}
rs721917*	SFTPD	0.42	0.39–0.63	1.07	1.02–1.13	2.49×10^{-8}
rs12459249*	CYP2A6	0.66	0.62–0.70	1.08	1.03–1.13	3.42×10^{-8}

* Indicates genome-wide significant loci in overall meta-analysis only.
From Agusti A, Hogg JC. Update on the pathogenesis of Chronic Obstructive Pulmonary Disease. New Engl J Med 2019;381:1248-1256; with permission.

Females Also Suffer (Perhaps a Different Form of) Chronic Obstructive Pulmonary Disease

Because the seminal study by Fletcher and co-workers[4] did not include females, until recently COPD was considered a disease of "old men." This is certainly not the case because it is now widely recognized that females can suffer COPD too.[13] It is even possible that females and males have different forms of COPD as suggested by a higher proportion of females among an early onset severe COPD cohort studied in Boston[14] and the different systemic inflammatory response elicited by smoking in males and females.[15]

A NEW PATHOGENIC UNDERSTANDING OF CHRONIC OBSTRUCTIVE PULMONARY DISEASE: A BALANCED LUNG DEVELOPMENT AND AGING PROCESS DETERMINES LIFELONG LUNG FUNCTION TRAJECTORIES

As summarized graphically in **Fig. 3**, and discussed in detail next, we propose that COPD should be considered the end result of several dynamic, cumulative, and lifelong gene-environment interactions that modulate the intensity and interaction of two key biologic phenomena[3]: organ development, maintenance, and repair; and cumulative tissue injury and aging. The interaction of these two mechanisms determines the trajectory followed by lung function throughout life (**Figs. 4** and **5**), and by doing so, contributes to lung health or the occurrence of lung disease including, among others, COPD.

Normal Lung Function Trajectory

After birth, the normal lung continues to grow and develop during infancy and adolescence.[16] In healthy males, lung function achieves its peak value at around 20 to 25 years of age; this occurs about 5 years earlier in females.[17] Following this peak, there is a relatively brief plateau, after which lung function declines physiologically with age because of lung aging.[18] These three phases determine the normal lung function trajectory throughout life (see **Fig. 4**, normal trajectory). It is now well established, however, that these three phases (growth,

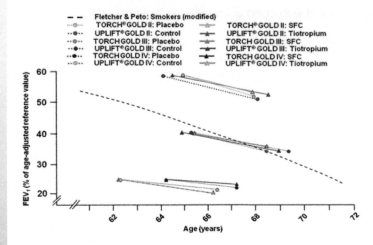

Fig. 2. FEV$_1$ decline determined in the different arms of the TORCH[10] and UPLIFT[11] studies, superimposed on the trajectory described by Fletcher and Peto in 1977 (dashed line). Note that, independently of the study and arm, the observed FEV$_1$ trajectories run in parallel in patients with different degrees of airflow limitation. Note too, the narrow age range studied. For further explanations, see text. (*From* Decramer M, Cooper CB. Treatment of COPD: the sooner the better? Thorax. 2010 65(9):837-841.)

maintenance, and aging) are altered by several gene and/or environmental factors,[19] leading to abnormal lung function trajectories (discussed later).[18]

Early Decline Trajectory

As originally described by Fletcher and Peto (see **Fig. 1**),[1] there are certainly individuals who suffer an accelerated loss of lung function in early adulthood starting from a normal peak lung function value, and they go on to develop airflow limitation (hence, COPD) in late adulthood (early decline trajectory in **Fig. 4**). Given that in a healthy individual lung function declines with age because of lung aging, this accelerated decline trajectory is interpreted as accelerated lung aging.[20] Indeed, there is evidence of many markers of accelerated lung

aging occurring in patients with COPD.[21] However, although often difficult to disentangle, it should also be considered that the repetitive injury caused by smoking can damage the lung parenchyma directly and contribute also to this rapid lung function decline, which may not be directly related to lung aging.[2]

Poor Lung Development Trajectories

By contrast, estimates from several large general population studies suggest that between 4% and 12% of individuals never reach a normal value of peak lung function in early adulthood.[18,22,23] This is caused by genetic (see **Table 1**) and/or environmental influences, including exposure to pollutants (eg, maternal smoking during pregnancy),

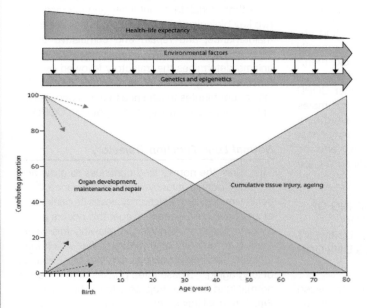

Fig. 3. The capacity of organ development, maintenance, and repair (*green triangle*) is maximal early in life and decreases with age. By contrast, cumulative tissue injury and aging (*red triangle*) increase progressively with age. *Dashed green* and *red arrows* indicate that the slope of these lines can vary (for better or worse) in different individuals, likely in relation to a dynamic and cumulative number of environment-host interactions (*vertical black arrows*) that occur over a lifetime. In essence, it is the balance between these two basic biologic phenomena during life that determines health and life expectancy (*top triangle*). Contributing proportion refers to the proportion of the processes represented by the *green* and *red triangles* contributing to health and life expectancy. (*From* Agusti A, Faner R. COPD beyond smoking: new paradigm, novel opportunities. Lancet Respir Med. 2018 6(5):324-326; with permission.)

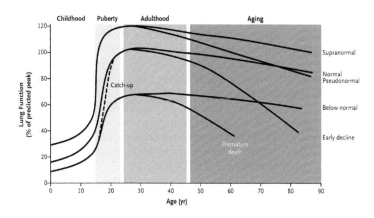

Fig. 4. Different lung function trajectories through life. For further explanations, see text. (*From* Agusti A, Hogg JC. Update on the pathogenesis of Chronic Obstructive Pulmonary Disease. New Engl J Med. 2019 381:1248-1256; with permission.)

prematurity, reduced intrauterine growth, and/or poor nutrition or repeated infections during infancy and adolescence.[19] Individuals with low peak lung function in early adulthood may live their life with a below normal lung function (small lungs)[24] or die prematurely (see **Fig. 4**).[23] The latter may occur because of unhealthy life exposures and/or, intriguingly, because of abnormal development of other organ systems.[23] **Fig. 5** shows that, indeed, these individuals have a higher prevalence and about a decade earlier incidence of other concomitant diseases, such as cardiovascular and/or endocrine ones associated abnormalities.[23] We interpret these observations as low lung function in early adulthood being a marker of poor development of other organ systems, such as the cardiovascular and metabolic systems.[23] After all, genes are the same in all our cells, and many environmental

influences (pollutants, infections, diet) also have the potential to reach many cells beyond the lungs. In this context, a low lung function in early life may be considered as the "canary in the coal mine," that is, a marker of poor development of other organs.[25]

Supranormal Trajectories

About 12% of individuals in the general population exhibit a supranormal trajectory.[22] This is higher than what is expected (around 5%) in any epidemiologic study in the general population.[17,26,27] It is unknown, but certainly possible, that if some of these supranormal individuals loose lung function over life starting from a high peak value (eg, by smoking), they may end up in their sixth or seventh decade of life with an apparently normal spirometry (pseudonormal trajectory in **Fig. 4**) but with

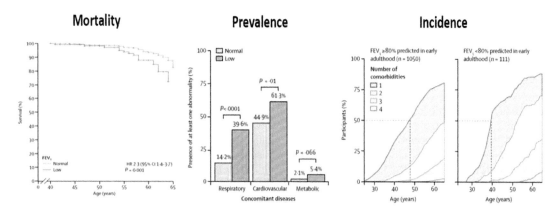

Fig. 5. All-cause mortality, prevalence (in early adulthood), and incidence (during follow-up) of concomitant diseases in participants in the Framingham Offspring Cohort stratified by their lung function determined in early adulthood (normal, FEV_1 >80% ref; low, FEV_1 <80% ref). For further explanations, see text. CI, confidence interval; HR, hazard ratio. (*From* Agustí A, Noell G, Brugada J, et al. Lung function in early adulthood and health in later life: a transgenerational cohort analysis. The Lancet Respiratory Medicine 2017;5(12):935-945; with permission.)

evidence of lung disease (eg, symptoms, exacerbations, and/or computed tomography [CT] emphysema).[2,28] This is extremely difficult to ascertain because lung function is rarely measured in early adulthood, but this hypothesis merits study because it may explain the observation of individuals with symptoms and/or clear evidence of lung damage (CT emphysema) but normal spirometry. This raises important issues about the diagnosis (and taxonomy) of COPD itself.[29,30]

Catch-up Trajectories

It is now known that about two-thirds of children born with low lung function are able to catch-up and regain a normal lung function trajectory, whereas a third cannot.[18] Why this is the case is unclear and likely dependent on their original causes for being born with low lung function.[18] For instance, if this was caused by some genetic deficiency, it is unlikely that this deficit is regained later in life. By contrast, if this was caused by some environmental reason (exposures, diet, infection), this may theoretically be overcome later in life.[18] In any case, understanding the potential mechanisms underlying catch-up in children is of great importance, not only to help these children to regain a normal lung function trajectory but, potentially, to promote lung regeneration and health in individuals with abnormal lung function in early or late adulthood.[2]

IMPLICATIONS

This new pathogenic understanding of COPD has numerous implications that clearly open new opportunities for its prevention and early therapy.

Mechanisms (Endotypes)

The consideration that tobacco smoking is not the only risk factor for COPD (albeit it clearly is an important, preventable, one) and that COPD is not always self-inflicted and that it can have its origins really early in life opens new avenues for research. The mechanisms of normal and abnormal lung development (endotypes[31]), and those that facilitate or limit catch-up, need to be better understood. Eventually, novel therapeutic targets (at the appropriate time points) need to be identified and tested.

It has long been recognized that COPD can affect the airways (bronchitis, bronchiolitis), the alveoli (emphysema), and the pulmonary vessels.[32] These pathologic abnormalities can result from abnormal development, poor tissue maintenance, chronic tissue injury, and/or defective repair.[33,34] For instance, using ex vivo micro-CT Hogg and coworkers have recently shown that the number of terminal bronchioles is significantly reduced in patients with COPD, particularly Global Initiative on Obstructive Lung Disease stage 3 to 4 individuals.[35,36] It is tempting to speculate that the repetitive nature of smoking-induced injury destroyed them but, given that these are cross-sectional analysis, it is equally possible that these "missing" airways have never been there because of abnormal lung development.[2]

Clinical Practice

It seems clear that COPD can no longer be considered a single disease[37] but rather a clinical syndrome[30,38] that, as any other clinical syndrome,[39] recognizes several causes (or risk factors) and presents clinically with several shared features (eg, airflow limitation). However, a better identification of the causes and presentations of the disease is essential to prevent and treat it adequately.[30,38] It is unlikely that patients with COPD who followed different lung function trajectories throughout life (see **Fig. 4**) really suffer the same disease, have the same prognosis, and/or require the same therapy.[2,18] Given that lung function is rarely measured early in life, lung function trajectories cannot be estimated from available clinical information in regular clinical practice. Yet, research should identify biomarkers associated with different lung function trajectories to explore the efficacy (and safety) of different therapeutic alternatives.

Randomized Clinical Trials

So far, all randomized clinical trials (RCTs) in COPD have selected participants based on their previous tobacco smoking exposure (typically more than 10 pack-years) and the presence of airflow limitation in late adulthood (typically in their sixth or seventh decade of age). Given that it is now known that neither smoking exposure nor age nor even airflow limitation are absolute requirements for the diagnosis of COPD, and that different lung function trajectories can lead to the disease (see **Fig. 4**), it is almost certain that all RCTs so far have included patients with different trajectories and mechanisms of disease (endotypes).[31] It is imperative to identify and validate disease trajectory associated biomarkers to go back to the results of these RCTs and try to stratify patients according to them. It is possible that, by doing so, the efficacy and safety of some already available drugs (eg, inhaled corticosteroids) can be better assessed.

Public Health

Given that the prevalence of low peak lung function in early adulthood ranges between 4% and 12%,[18,22,23] and that these individuals are at a higher risk of comorbid diseases and premature death,[23] their early identification, assessment, and, it is hoped, treatment, should be a public health priority. The question is how and when to do it. The answer to how is easy: spirometry (remember, the canary in the coal mine[25]). The second question is trickier. It is certainly clear that diagnosing COPD in the sixth or seventh decade of life, as is the case most often today, is too late.[2,18] It has been recently proposed that efforts should focus on the diagnosis of so-called early COPD, which has been defined operationally as COPD in individuals younger than 50 years of age.[40] But, is that early enough? We have proposed previously that, when an individual applies for a driver license (most often in their early twenties) may offer a window of opportunity to measure spirometry (a cheap, noninvasive, reproducible, and easy measurement).[18] Is that early enough? Certainly, it is earlier than 50 years of age, but we can do better. We can (and probably should) measure spirometry in schools. A child is perfectly capable of performing a correct spirometry by the age of 6 to 7 years. By that time, we would still be in a (so far, theoretic) position to stimulate catch-up in those children with low lung function (see **Fig. 4**). These are alternatives that need to be rigorously tested but, waiting until the old individual consultates because of invalidating symptoms is clearly too late. At most, current therapies can at that time improve symptoms but it is unlikely that they can reverse the damage already caused by the disease. We arrive far too late.

SUMMARY

The understanding of the pathogenesis of COPD has changed significantly in recent years. Although tobacco smoking continues to be a key environmental risk factor for the development of the disease in some smokers, it is now recognized that there are many other risk factors that can significantly affect lung development and lung aging, both of which are key pathogenic mechanisms of the disease (see **Fig. 3**).[3] Eventually, it is the dynamic and cumulative interaction of environment and host factors what eventually determines lung health or disease.[18] A final important, and often forgotten, element in this conceptual construct is the precise timing (ie, the age of the individual) when these environment-gene interactions occur. This point is nicely illustrated by the study of Torres-González and colleagues[41] who showed acute murine γherpesvirus 68 infection in aged mice (≥18 months) resulted in severe pneumonitis and fibrosis, whereas the response to the same virus was much attenuated (and eventually cleared) when compared with young animals (2–3 months old).

COPD is a complex and heterogeneous condition caused by a variety of environmental and host factors, whose nature and precise timing eventually determine the emergence of the disease. Understanding these temporal relationships is essential to preventing and treating this disease much more effectively.

DISCLOSURE

Supported, in part, by FIS (PI17/00369, PI18/01008)CIBERES and SEPAR. RF is a recipient of a Miguel Servet Research Contract supported by FEDER funds (CP16/00039).

REFERENCES

1. Fletcher C, Peto R. The natural history of chronic airflow obstruction. Br Med J 1977;1(6077):1645–8.
2. Agusti A, Hogg JC. Update on the pathogenesis of chronic obstructive pulmonary disease. N Engl J Med 2019;381:1248–56.
3. Agusti A, Faner R. COPD beyond smoking: new paradigm, novel opportunities. Lancet Respir Med 2018;6(5):324–6.
4. Fletcher C, Peto R, Tinker C, et al. The natural history of chronic bronchitis and emphysema. New York: Oxford University Press; 1976.
5. Salvi SS, Barnes PJ. Chronic obstructive pulmonary disease in non-smokers. Lancet 2009;374(9691):733–43.
6. Salvi S, Barnes PJ. Is exposure to biomass smoke the biggest risk factor for COPD globally? Chest 2010;138(1):3–6.
7. Hobbs BD, de Jong K, Lamontagne M, et al. Genetic loci associated with chronic obstructive pulmonary disease overlap with loci for lung function and pulmonary fibrosis. Nat Genet 2017;49(3):426–32.
8. Morrow JD, Glass K, Cho MH, et al. Human lung DNA methylation quantitative trait loci colocalize with chronic obstructive pulmonary disease genome-wide association loci. Am J Respir Crit Care Med 2018;197(10):1275–84.
9. Vestbo J, Edwards LD, Scanlon PD, et al. Changes in forced expiratory volume in 1 second over time in COPD. N Engl J Med 2011;365(13):1184–92.

10. Jenkins CR, Jones PW, Calverley PM, et al. Efficacy of salmeterol/fluticasone propionate by GOLD stage of chronic obstructive pulmonary disease: analysis from the randomised, placebo-controlled TORCH study. Respir Res 2009;10(1):59.

11. Decramer M, Celli B, Kesten S, et al. Effect of tiotropium on outcomes in patients with moderate chronic obstructive pulmonary disease (UPLIFT): a prespecified subgroup analysis of a randomised controlled trial. Lancet 2009;374(9696):1171–8.

12. Decramer M, Cooper CB. Treatment of COPD: the sooner the better? Thorax 2010;65(9):837–41.

13. Anto JM, Vermeire P, Vestbo J, et al. Epidemiology of chronic obstructive pulmonary disease. Eur Respir J 2001;17(5):982–94.

14. Silverman EK, Chapman HA, Drazen JM, et al. Genetic epidemiology of severe, early-onset chronic obstructive pulmonary disease. Risk to relatives for airflow obstruction and chronic bronchitis. Am J Respir Crit Care Med 1998;157(6 Pt 1):1770–8.

15. Faner R, Gonzalez N, Cruz T, et al. Systemic inflammatory response to smoking in chronic obstructive pulmonary disease: evidence of a gender effect. PLoS One 2014;9(5):e97491.

16. Jobe AH, Whitsset JA, Abman SH. Fetal & neonatal lung development. Clinical correlates and technologies for the future. New York: Cambridge University Press; 2016.

17. Kohansal R, Martinez-Camblor P, Agusti A, et al. The natural history of chronic airflow obstruction revisited: an analysis of the Framingham offspring cohort. Am J Respir Crit Care Med 2009;180:3–10.

18. Agusti A, Faner R. Lung function trajectories in health and disease. Lancet Respir Med 2019;4:358–64.

19. Martinez FD. Early-life origins of chronic obstructive pulmonary disease. N Engl J Med 2016;375(9):871–8.

20. Ito K, Barnes PJ. COPD as a disease of accelerated lung aging. Chest 2009;135(1):173–80.

21. Meiners S, Eickelberg O, Konigshoff M. Hallmarks of the ageing lung. Eur Respir J 2015;45(3):807–27.

22. Bui DS, Lodge CJ, Burgess JA, et al. Childhood predictors of lung function trajectories and future COPD risk: a prospective cohort study from the first to the sixth decade of life. Lancet Respir Med 2018;6(7):535–44.

23. Agusti A, Noell G, Brugada J, et al. Lung function in early adulthood and health in later life: a transgenerational cohort analysis. Lancet Respir Med 2017;5(12):935–45.

24. Lange P, Celli B, Agusti A, et al. Lung-function trajectories leading to chronic obstructive pulmonary disease. N Engl J Med 2015;373(2):111–22.

25. Bush A. Lung development and aging. Ann Am Thorac Soc 2016;13(Supplement_5):S438–46.

26. Quanjer PH, Stanojevic S, Cole TJ, et al. Multi-ethnic reference values for spirometry for the 3-95-yr age range: the global lung function 2012 equations. European Respiratory Journal 2012;40(6):1324–43.

27. Breyer-Kohansal R, Hartl S, Burghuber OC, et al. The LEAD (lung, heart, social, body) study: objectives, methodology, and external validity of the population-based cohort study. J Epidemiol 2019;29(8):315–24.

28. Woodruff PG, Barr RG, Bleecker E, et al. Clinical significance of symptoms in smokers with preserved pulmonary function. N Engl J Med 2016;374(19):1811–21.

29. Celli BR, Agustí A. COPD: time to improve its taxonomy? ERJ Open Res 2018;4(1) [pii: 00132-02017].

30. Barnes PJ, Vestbo J, Calverley PM. The pressing need to redefine "COPD". Chronic Obstr Pulm Dis 2019;6(5):380–3.

31. Woodruff PG, Agusti A, Roche N, et al. Current concepts in targeting chronic obstructive pulmonary disease pharmacotherapy: making progress towards personalised management. Lancet 2015;385(9979):1789–98.

32. Hogg JC, Timens W. The pathology of chronic obstructive pulmonary disease. Annu Rev Pathol 2009;4:435–59.

33. Barbera JA, Peinado VI. Disruption of the lung structure maintenance programme: a comprehensive view of emphysema development. Eur Respir J 2011;37(4):752–4.

34. Tuder RM, Yoshida T, Fijalkowka I, et al. Role of lung maintenance program in the heterogeneity of lung destruction in emphysema. Proc Am Thorac Soc 2006;3(8):673–9.

35. McDonough JE, Yuan R, Suzuki M, et al. Small-airway obstruction and emphysema in chronic obstructive pulmonary disease. N Engl J Med 2011;365(17):1567–75.

36. Tanabe N, Vasilescu DM, McDonough JE, et al. Micro-computed tomography comparison of preterminal bronchioles in centrilobular and panlobular emphysema. Am J Respir Crit Care Med 2017;195(5):630–8.

37. Vogelmeier CF, Criner GJ, Martinez FJ, et al. Global strategy for the diagnosis, management, and prevention of chronic obstructive lung disease 2017 report: GOLD executive summary. Am J Respir Crit Care Med 2017;195(5):557–82.

38. Celli B, Wedzicha AJ. Update on clinical aspects of chronic obstructive pulmonary disease. N Engl J Med 2019;381:1257–66.

39. Scadding JG. Health and disease: what can medicine do for philosophy? J Med Ethics 1988;14(3):118–24.

40. Martinez FJ, Han MK, Allinson JP, et al. At the root: defining and halting progression of early chronic obstructive pulmonary disease. Am J Respir Crit Care Med 2018;197(12):1540–51.

41. Torres-González E, Bueno M, Tanaka A, et al. Role of endoplasmic reticulum stress in age-related susceptibility to lung fibrosis. Am J Respir Cell Mol Biol 2012;46(6):748 56.

Epidemiology of Chronic Obstructive Pulmonary Disease

Lisa Ruvuna, MD, Akshay Sood, MD, MPH*

KEYWORDS

- Global burden • Racial/ethnic disparities • Rural/urban disparities • Occupational COPD
- Air pollution

KEY POINTS

- Household air pollution from solid fuel combustion affects almost 3 billion people worldwide and is a major risk factor for COPD.
- An estimated 25% to 45% of patients with COPD worldwide have never smoked.
- Fourteen percent of the overall COPD burden can be attributed to occupational exposures.
- Rural populations show a greater prevalence and mortality from COPD than urban residents.
- African American never-smokers have a disproportionately high prevalence and Hispanic people have a low prevalence of COPD.

 Video content accompanies this article at http://www.chestmed.theclinics.com.

INTRODUCTION

Chronic obstructive pulmonary disease (COPD) is a slowly progressing chronic respiratory disorder. It is characterized by an obstructive ventilatory pattern, which is often partially reversible, commonly related to tobacco smoking, and can lead to chronic respiratory failure. COPD occurs as the clinical consequence of an interaction between multiple occupational and environmental factors on the one hand and the existence of a not yet properly understood genetic predisposition on the other. In developed nations, the most important cause of COPD is cigarette smoking, with a progressive increase in the number of women as the habit of smoking has taken hold in that sex. However, an estimated 25% to 45% of patients with COPD have never smoked; the burden of nonsmoking COPD is therefore much higher than was previously thought.[1] COPD may result from rapid lung function decline or inadequate growth and development of the lung.[2] This disorder is still underdiagnosed by treating providers, and is sometimes diagnosed too late.

SPIROMETRIC DEFINITION OF CHRONIC OBSTRUCTIVE PULMONARY DISEASE

Two widely accepted definitions of COPD exist, based on the presence of spirometric airflow limitation. The existence of 2 separate definitions has been a barrier to interpreting epidemiologic studies. The GOLD (Global Initiative for Chronic Obstructive Lung Disease) definition uses a fixed ratio of the postbronchodilator forced expiratory volume in 1 second (FEV_1)/forced vital capacity (FVC) of less than 0.70 to define obstruction,[3] a position endorsed by the American Thoracic Society (ATS) and European Respiratory Society (ERS).[4] Another document by the ATS and ERS that deals

Department of Internal Medicine, University of New Mexico School of Medicine, 1 University of New Mexico, MSC 10 5550, Albuquerque, NM 87131, USA
* Corresponding author.
E-mail address: asood@salud.unm.edu

Clin Chest Med 41 (2020) 315–327
https://doi.org/10.1016/j.ccm.2020.05.002
0272-5231/20/

with interpretative strategies of spirometry advocates using the lower limit of normal (LLN) for the FEV$_1$/FVC ratio to define obstruction.[5] An Analysis of the Third National Health and Nutrition Examination Survey (NHANES III) from 2007 to 2010, reporting both definitions, clearly showed that the prevalence of COPD changed from 10.2% with the postbronchodilator LLN criteria to 20.9% with the prebronchodilator fixed ratio criteria.[6] Studies have shown that the fixed ratio criteria overdiagnose the elderly and underdiagnose younger populations.[7,8] Although the scientific community debates which criteria accurately represent COPD, it is clear that patients who are obstructed using the fixed ratio criteria but normal using the LLN criteria are not normal. In the NHANES III data, subjects classified as normal using LLN criteria but abnormal using GOLD criteria had a higher risk of mortality than those with normal lung function using both criteria.[9]

GLOBAL EPIDEMIOLOGY OF CHRONIC OBSTRUCTIVE PULMONARY DISEASE
Prevalence

Comparisons of COPD prevalence and mortality between countries and over time are important, because the disease is largely preventable.[10] Studying global prevalence of COPD was previously difficult because of the lack of data representative of the world population and lack of consensus on case definitions. The initiation of multinational studies on COPD have improved the understanding of its global burden and shown variable disease prevalence among countries. An example of these studies is the Global Burden of Disease (GBD) study,[10] which used a central database of registries, national surveys, and census data, among other sources, from more than 100 countries, stratified by sociodemographic index (SDI), a composite measure of income, education, and fertility. Using the fixed ratio diagnostic criteria, COPD affected an estimated 299 million people in 2015, which was an increase from 174 million or 44% since 1990.[10]

In a 2015 systematic search of population-based studies across 52 countries, the highest COPD prevalence was estimated in the Americas (15% in 2010), and the lowest in Southeast Asia (10%). The study estimated a global prevalence of 12%, corresponding with 384 million cases in 2010,[11] a number substantially higher than that estimated by the GBD study. The percentage increase in COPD cases between 1990 and 2010 was the highest in the eastern Mediterranean region (119%), followed by the African region (102%), whereas the European region recorded

the lowest increase (23%).[11] The COPD guidelines used across selected studies varied, but 92% of all retained studies used the fixed ratio diagnostic criteria.

Mortality

In 2015, more than 3 million people died of COPD worldwide, an increase of 12% compared with 1990.[10] Disability-adjusted life years (DALYs), a summary measure of fatal and nonfatal disease outcomes, is defined as the total number of years lived with the disease plus the total number of years lost to the disease. In 2015, COPD represented about 64 million DALYs, ranking eighth among causes of global disease burden worldwide.[10] Age-standardized DALY rates caused by COPD were highest (>2000 per 100,000 people) in Papua New Guinea, India, Lesotho, and Nepal (Fig. 1). These rates were higher in countries between the low to middle range of the SDI, before reducing sharply from the middle to high range of the SDI. Other investigators have also reported that as much as 90% of COPD deaths worldwide occur in low-income and middle-income countries.[11–13]

Causes of Variation in Global Trends

The variations in trends between different world regions and countries are largely explained by the variations in smoking, secondhand smoke, and outdoor and household air pollution, including ozone, and occupational exposures. Together, these risks explain 73% of DALYs caused by COPD.[10] Another important reason for global differences is the varying rates of COPD underdiagnosis[14] in many jurisdictions.[15]

RISK FACTORS FOR CHRONIC OBSTRUCTIVE PULMONARY DISEASE
Tobacco Smoke Exposure

Cigarette smoking is the most common risk factor for the development of COPD in the United States and high-income countries. However, it is the second most common risk factor worldwide after air pollution. Worldwide, more than 1 billion people smoked tobacco in 2015, but the rates of tobacco use are declining in most countries, except for the eastern Mediterranean and African regions.[16] By 2015, the age-standardized global prevalence of daily smoking decreased to 15%, an overall 29% decrease since 1990.[17] However, in 2015, 1 in every 4 men and 1 in every 20 women in the world continued to smoke daily.[17] In 2017, active smoking contributed to 1.23 million COPD-related

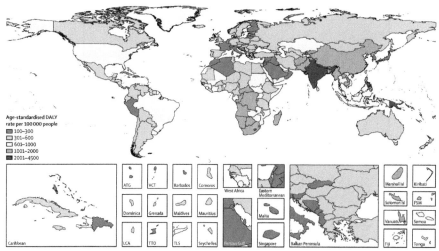

Fig. 1. Age-standardized DALY rate per 100,000 people caused by COPD by country, both sexes, 2015. ATG, Antigua and Barbuda; FSM, Federated States of Micronesia; Isl, islands; LCA, Saint Lucia; TLS, Timor-Leste; TTO, Trinidad and Tobago; VCT, Saint Vincent and the Grenadines. (*Reprinted* with permission from Elsevier; GBD 2015 Chronic Respiratory Disease Collaborators. Global, regional, and national deaths, prevalence, disability-adjusted life years, and years lived with disability for chronic obstructive pulmonary disease and asthma, 1990–2015: a systematic analysis for the Global Burden of Disease Study 2015. Lancet Respir Med 2017; 5(9):691-706.)

deaths and 28.28 million COPD-related DALYs (**Table 1**).[18]

To significantly and permanently bend the tobacco epidemic's trajectory, a renewed and sustained focus is needed on comprehensive tobacco control policies and laws worldwide and in the United States.[17] In 2003, the World Health Organization (WHO) adopted the Framework Convention on Tobacco Control to call on nations for stricter control of tobacco use.[19] In addition, the WHO has drafted the 25 × 25 noncommunicable disease (NCD) targets, which include decreasing tobacco use by 30% between 2010 and 2025.[19] Further reduction in cigarette smoking will help decrease the prevalence, morbidity, and mortality of COPD worldwide and in the United States.

Secondhand Smoke Exposure

The sidestream smoke from the burning of cigarettes is called secondhand smoke or environmental tobacco smoke. In a 2011 analysis, exposure to secondhand smoke was estimated to globally account for nearly 600,000 all-cause deaths and nearly 11 million DALYs annually.[20] During 2011 to 2012, about 58 million nonsmokers in the United States, including 47% of African American nonsmokers, were exposed to secondhand smoke.[21] During the same time frame, 2 out of every 5 children of ages 3 to 11 years, including 7 out of every 10 African American children, were exposed to secondhand smoke regularly.[21]

Secondhand smoke exposure, particularly during childhood, is an important risk factor for COPD worldwide, including the United States.[22] A cross-sectional population-based study from the United States involving 2113 adults between the ages of 55 and 75 years reported that the highest quartile of lifetime workplace exposure to secondhand smoke was associated with 36% greater odds of contracting COPD.[23] The population-attributable fraction (PAF) for COPD was 11% for the highest quartile of home-based secondhand smoke exposure and 7% for work-based exposure.[23] The respiratory health effects of secondhand smoke exposure provide a compelling rationale for legislation that mandates 100% smoke-free public places.[24]

Ambient (Outdoor) Air Pollution

Industries, households, cars, and trucks emit complex mixtures of ambient air pollutants, many of which are harmful to health. Of all ambient air pollutants, fine particulate matter less than 2.5 μm in aerodynamic diameter (PM2.5) has the greatest effect on respiratory health. Although, in many Western countries, levels of ambient air pollution have been improving with the setting of upper limits and better urban planning, air pollution in developing countries, and particularly those with rapid industrialization, has become a major global problem.

Table 1
Global all-age attributable deaths and disability-adjusted life years, and percentage change of age-standardized death rates and disability-adjusted life year rates of chronic obstructive pulmonary disease caused by environment exposure between 2007 and 2017

Exposure Risk	2007 Deaths (Millions)	2017 Deaths (Millions)	Change in Age-Standardized Death Rate During 2007–2017 (%)	2007 DALYs (Millions)	2017 DALYs (Millions)	Change in Age-Standardized DALYs Rate During 2007–2017 (%)
Active smoking	1.13	1.23	−19.1	26.10	28.20	−18.4
Ambient particulate matter pollution	0.519	0.633	−10.5	12 80	15.70	−6.0
Occupational particulate matter, gases, and fumes	0.425	0.481	−16.1	10.40	11.90	−12.7
Ambient ozone pollution	0.392	0.472	−11.6	6.33	7.37	−12.2
Household air pollution from solid fuels	0.421	0.362	−36.3	10.800	9.37	−33.5
Secondhand smoke	0.244	0.266	−20.0	6.23	6.91	−15.3
Lead exposure	0.009	0.011	−3.3	0.286	0.327	−11.0

From Huang X, Mu X, Deng L, et al. The etiologic origins for chronic obstructive pulmonary disease. Int J Chron Obstruct Pulmon Dis. 2019; 14: 1139–1158. Published online 2019 May 27. With permission.

Ambient air PM2.5 was the fifth-ranking mortality risk factor in 2015.[25] Exposure to PM2.5 caused 4.2 million deaths and 103.1 million DALYs in 2015, representing 8% of total global deaths and 4% of global DALYs.[25] Most deaths were in low-income and middle-income countries, particularly in east and south Asia.[25] Deaths worldwide attributable to ambient PM2.5 increased from 3.5 million in 1990 to 4.2 million in 2015.[25] In the contiguous United States, PM2.5 pollution in excess of the lowest observed concentration (2.8 $\mu g/m^3$) was responsible for an estimated 30,000 excess deaths during the time frame 1999 to 2015.[26] The life expectancy loss caused by PM2.5 was largest around Los Angeles and in some southern states, such as Arkansas, Oklahoma, and Alabama.

Exposure to ambient air pollutants is associated with rapid decline in lung function in healthy populations[27,28] as well as a greater level of emphysema assessed quantitatively using computed tomography (CT) imaging,[28] greater risk of acute exacerbations of COPD,[29] and greater risk of death from chronic lower respiratory diseases.[30] The pathologic effects in the lung are mediated via inflammatory pathways and involve oxidative stress similar to cigarette smoking. Reducing exposure to ambient air pollution has important health benefits but also reduces greenhouse gas emissions that contribute to climate change.

Household Air Pollution

Almost 3 billion people worldwide use solid fuel (eg, wood, charcoal, crop residues, animal dung) for cooking, with many more using solid fuels for heating homes.[31] These so-called biomass fuels contribute to household air pollution. With inefficient combustion of these solid fuels, a complex mixture of carbon-based particles, inorganic particles, and irritant gases is generated indoors, which shares some characteristics with tobacco smoke.

The greatest proportions of the populations exposed to household air pollution are in countries of sub-Saharan Africa, India, China, and Central America.[31] Although the exposure burden is highest in low-income countries, a significant number of households in high-income countries, including the United States, rely on solid fuel for heating homes.[32] According to the GBD study, an estimated 2 million deaths and 60 million DALYs were attributable to household air pollution worldwide in 2017, almost all in low-income and middle-income countries, the published WHO estimates are even higher.[33]

Observational studies show strong associations between household air pollution exposures and COPD, among other illnesses.[34] The Global Alliance for Clean Cookstoves initiative hosted by the United Nations Foundation to enable the distribution of clean stoves and the initiatives of several governments to accelerate the progression away from biomass to clean fuels may help decrease the prevalence, morbidity, and mortality of COPD from household air pollution exposure.

Occupational Exposures

A 2019 ATS statement[35] concluded that pooled estimates of the PAF are 14% for the occupational contribution to the burden of COPD and 13% for chronic bronchitis. Moreover, a higher occupational PAF for COPD among never smokers (31%) suggests that occupational exposures contribute more substantially to the burden of COPD in nonsmokers. This finding means that, as the prevalence of cigarette smoking in the general population decreases, other COPD-related risk factors may become more prominent. Cigarette smoking and occupation act as additive risks for COPD,[35] which is plausible given that each of these exposures subsumes a heterogeneous mix of toxic materials.

Occupational exposures to vapors, gas, dust, or fumes (VGDF) are associated with COPD.[36–39] Causal associations with coal dust, silica, construction dust, cotton dust, asbestos, and grain dust are well documented in the literature.[40–42] The Faces of Black Lung series by the National Institute of Occupational Safety and Health (NIOSH) provides useful information on the impact of coal mine dust and other work-related exposures on patients with COPD Video 1: Available at: https://youtu.be/H2U9Onrxepg and Video 2: Available at: https://youtu.be/X-agtyN4py4. However, there are multiple other at-risk occupations that are not well studied. For example, a recent study indicated that the highest COPD prevalence in industries or occupations was noted among workers in the information industry (including publishing, telecommunications, broadcasting, and data processing workers) and office and administrative support occupations (including secretaries, administrative and dental assistants, and clerks).[43] Often overlooked, workers in these industries are exposed to organic and inorganic dusts, isocyanates, irritant gases, paper dust, fumes from photocopiers, chemicals, oil-based ink, paints, glues, toxic metals, and solvents, all of which are known respiratory irritants associated with COPD.[43]

Prevention of occupational COPD relies on worker education; governmental regulation for appropriately protective work setting and effective enforcement of the same[44]; continued surveillance; early identification of COPD; and reduction or elimination of COPD-associated risk factors, such as VGDF, chemicals, and exposure to indoor and outdoor air pollutants.[43]

RURAL-URBAN DISPARITIES

Heath disparities, as defined by significant differences in heath between populations, are more common among respiratory diseases than for those for other organ systems, because of the environmental influence on breathing and the variation of the environment among different segments of the population.[45] Rural-urban disparities in COPD are a new focus of research. In 2010, 65% of US counties were classified as rural, which encompassed 17% of the total population.[46] Despite their smaller population, rural residents are prone to worse health outcomes than urban residents, including greater prevalence, hospitalization, and death rates.[47]

Prevalence

Information on rural-urban disparities in the prevalence of self-diagnosed COPD comes from 3 national surveys in the United States: the Behavioral Risk Factor Surveillance System (BRFSS), the National Health Interview Survey (NHIS), and NHANES, and the results are remarkably similar.

BRFSS uses the random digit dialing system to collect self-reported population-based data on exposures and diseases. A 2015 analysis of the BRFSS data identified an age-adjusted national prevalence of 6% of self-reported COPD.[47] The prevalence in noncore rural areas (8%) was much higher than in large metropolitan centers (5%). Similarly, a review of the NHIS data from 2012 to 2015 on self-reported COPD reported an estimated overall prevalence of 8%.[48] The prevalence of 16% in rural poor regions was more than twice that in the urban nonpoor region (6%).[48] Even when adjusted for confounders such as smoking, sex, age, race, wealth, and education, rural residence was associated with 23% greater odds for COPD than urban residence.[48] Raju and colleagues[49] reviewed the NHANES data from 2007 to 2012 and showed that rural residence was associated with 106% greater odds for COPD than urban residence. Despite the variation in the absolute prevalence rates reported, these surveys consistently show that rural populations are at high risk for COPD.

Mortality

Based on data from the National Vital Statistics, chronic lower respiratory disease, consisting primarily of COPD, was the third leading cause of death in the United States in 2015 and the fourth leading cause of death from 2016 through 2018.[50] The year-on-year nationwide COPD mortality decreased by about 2% in 2018, to 40 per 100,000.[50] The year-on-year nationwide mortality increased in 2017 but decreased in 2016. Despite these sinusoidal fluctuations, the overall mortality trend for COPD within the United States has decreased since 2002.[50]

Causes of Rural-Urban Disparity

The basis for rural-urban disparity in COPD is likely multifactorial. Rural populations may have higher COPD risk because these populations have a greater proportion with a history of smoking,[51] and more secondhand smoke exposure but less access to smoking cessation programs. Occupational exposures to VGDF is a risk factor for COPD, and rural residents are more likely than urban residents to work in dusty jobs such as crop farming and coal mining.[52,53] Environmental exposures to wood smoke[32] and coal smoke[48] also place rural residents at risk for COPD. The 2015 cross-sectional analysis of the BRFSS data showed that rural residents had the highest Medicare hospitalizations and death rates from COPD.[47]

The WHO defines social determinants of health as "the conditions in which people are born, grow, live, work, and age. These circumstances are shaped by the distribution of money, power, and resources at global, national and local levels."[54] Relevant social determinants of health for rural residents include low socioeconomic status (SES), inadequate access to health care, lack of healthy lifestyles,[54] and low levels of education and income. Low SES is a risk factor for COPD in the United States and other parts of the world.[48] Inadequate access to health care for rural residents is related to the lower rates of those insured, unavailability of clinical expertise, long travel distance, and unavailability of transportation. Despite higher rates of COPD-related hospitalizations,[55] rural residents are less likely to receive and complete outpatient pulmonary rehabilitation.[56] As the disease progresses, patients require specialist management from a pulmonologist. Only about 30% of rural residents have access to pulmonologist services within a 16-km (10-mile) radius, compared with more than 90% of urban residents.[57] Because of the shortage of pulmonologists, COPD management in rural areas is provided by primary care providers (PCPs), often without access to quality spirometry. COPD care by PCPs may not be consistent and may differ from guideline practices.[58]

RACIAL/ETHNIC DISPARITIES

Racial/ethnic heath disparities in COPD are being increasingly recognized.[45] The US Office Management and Budget divides race into a minimum of 5 categories, based on self-identification: white, black or African American, American Indian or Alaska Native, Asian, and Native Hawaiian or other Pacific Islander, and similarly divides ethnicity into 2 categories, Hispanic and non-Hispanic.

Prevalence

The estimated age-adjusted prevalence of self-reported COPD in 2017 in the United States, based on the BRFSS data, varied by race/ethnicity: American Indian/Alaska Native 11.9%, white 6.7%, black 6.6%, Hispanic 3.6%, Asian 1.7%, and Native Hawaiian/Pacific Islander 3.3%.[59] By using the definition of self-reported physician diagnosis of COPD, BRFSS data may underestimate true disease prevalence.[8] This underestimation may occur because of recall and social desirability biases, differing likelihoods of COPD diagnosis by physicians in states with high smoking rates and rurality, and exclusion of institutionalized adults who live in long-term care facilities or prisons.[59] Using postbronchodilator spirometry as the gold standard, a study found that as much as 81% of spirometrically defined COPD cases were underdiagnosed, with greater probability of underdiagnosis associated with male sex, younger age, never and current smoking, lower education, no previous spirometry, and less severe airflow limitation.[8]

Racial/ethnic disparities in COPD may be confounded by the presence of similar disparities in smoking behavior, which, despite recent decline, remains the biggest risk factor for the development of COPD in the United States. Thus, American Indian/Alaska Native populations are the racial/ethnic category with the highest prevalence of self-reported current cigarette smoking at 32%, whereas Hispanic and Asian populations have the lowest rates of 11% and 9%, and white people and African Americans have intermediate rates of 17% and 17% respectively.[60] By limiting comparisons to never-smokers, the confounding effect of smoking can be excluded. Using data from the self-reported never-smokers, the comparison of prevalence of self-reported COPD among racial/ethnic groups reveals an interesting trend. American Indians/

Alaska Natives and African Americans have the highest prevalence rates of COPD at 5.7% and 4.1% respectively, Hispanic and white people have intermediate prevalence rates at 2.3% and 2.7% respectively, and the lowest prevalence is noted among Asian people and Native Hawaiian/Pacific Islanders at 1.2% and 0.9% respectively.[59] When examining the population of employed never-smokers from 2013 to 2017, the prevalence of self-reported physician diagnosis of COPD was lower among Hispanic people at 1.7% compared with non-Hispanic white people at 2.5% and non-Hispanic African Americans at 2.6%, with greater differences noted among women than among men.[60]

Racial/ethnic disparities are confirmed with studies using objective COPD outcomes rather than self-report. Multiple studies, using spirometric end points, indicate that Hispanic people have a lower prevalence of self-reported COPD than non-Hispanic white people. In a national study using the NHANES III data, an obstructive pattern was less common in Mexican Americans (8%) than non-Hispanic white people (15%).[61] Several studies, many from New Mexico, have shown reduced prevalence of COPD, higher baseline lung function, and lower decline in lung function in Hispanic groups, compared with non-Hispanic white people.[62–67]

Although national studies report high prevalence rates of COPD in American Indians, there are remarkable differences among American Indian groups in different parts of the country. For instance, some investigators have shown a protective effect of an American Indian ancestry component in racially admixed populations in New Mexico and Costa Rica[67,68] on the spirometric prevalence of COPD and lung function decline.

In addition to the higher prevalence of COPD in African American than white never-smokers in the Wheaton and colleagues[59] study, several reports have shown that African Americans develop COPD with less intense cumulative smoking and at a younger age, possibly because of differences in nicotine metabolism.[69–71] Among patients with severe COPD, African Americans were disproportionately represented among those with early-onset disease (occurring before the age of 55 years) compared with those with late-onset disease.[72] African genetic ancestry has been associated with reduced FEV_1 and faster decline in lung function.[73]

Mortality

The 2016 data from the National Vital Statistics System showed the following age-adjusted death rates per 100,000 standard US population for chronic lower respiratory disease (mostly COPD) by race: white 46, American Indian/Alaska Native 41, black 30, Hispanic 17, and Asian 12, with overall estimated death rate of 41.[74] Although mortality is lower among African Americans than among white people, some reports indicate that COPD mortalities may be increasing faster among African Americans than among white Americans.[75] Although national studies report high mortalities of COPD in American Indians, there are remarkable differences among American Indian groups in different parts of the country. For instance, county-level mortalities from COPD in American Indian communities of New Mexico are generally low.[76]

Although many studies show that Hispanic people have disproportionately low COPD mortalities, 1 study suggested that the risk of death was similar to that of white people and African Americans.[65] Kinney and colleagues[63] showed that the protective effect of Hispanic ethnicity on COPD mortality was not explained away by their lower cumulative exposure to tobacco smoke. In 2013, the age-adjusted death rates (per 100,000 people) from COPD among US Hispanic people were highest in Cubans[28] and Puerto Ricans[27] and lowest in Mexican Americans,[18] showing significant variability within Hispanic ethnic subgroups.[77]

Causes for Racial/Ethnic Disparities

Health disparities in racial/ethnic groups are largely affected by social determinants of health indices.[78] These indices include low SES, lack of health care access, lack of insurance, health literacy, cultural beliefs, social and family situations, governmental structure or laws that do not protect vulnerable individuals, individual preferences, availability of quality health care providers, and racial and ethnic discrimination. Racial/ethnic minority groups are more likely to live in cities with poorer air quality and, therefore, experience a disparately larger impact on chronic lung disease. Household air pollution from smoky cooking or heating fires is more common in racial/ethnic minority households, particularly among American Indian communities.

Possible causes for the disproportionately high prevalence of COPD in African American never-smokers[59] include increased likelihood of exposure to secondhand smoke (especially caused by living conditions and poverty), smaller/lower lung function that increases the likelihood of development of COPD with very little irritant exposure, and higher contribution of occupational exposures.[79] In addition, African Americans report worse dyspnea and health-related quality of life

than white people, after adjustment for lung function. One possible explanation may be their use of fewer respiratory medications, lower use of medical care, and poorer access to care.[80,81] Another possible explanation is that African Americans are twice as likely than non-Hispanic white people to report a history of asthma.[82] Patients with COPD with concomitant asthma experience poor quality of life and greater dyspnea. The presence of comorbidities such as gastroesophageal reflux has a greater negative impact on dyspnea on African Americans than on non-Hispanic white people, which may also help explain their greater report of dyspnea.[83]

The so-called Hispanic paradox refers to the fact that, despite their lower social determinants of health indices, Hispanic people have a lower all-cause mortality than non-Hispanic white people.[84] Although some investigators have attributed the paradox to the lower cumulative exposure to tobacco smoke,[63] others show a protective effect of an American Indian ancestry component in racially admixed Hispanic populations of New Mexico and Costa Rica.[67,68] Furthermore, disparities in COPD prevalence across US Hispanic subgroups are seen, and may be partly explained by differences in racial ancestry. For example, Puerto Ricans have a greater proportion of African ancestry but a lower proportion of Native American ancestry than New Mexican Hispanic people.[67] Studies have also identified unique genetic loci that may play a role in COPD pathogenesis in Hispanic populations.[85] Despite the lower prevalence and mortality of COPD, Hispanic smokers report greater dyspnea than non-Hispanic white smokers, which is consistent with their lower health-related quality of life[86] and is not explained by differences in either lung function or CT measure of lung structure.[87] It is possible that social determinants of health may explain the difference in dyspnea and health-related quality of life among Hispanic people.[86]

USEFUL INTERVENTIONS TO ADDRESS CHRONIC OBSTRUCTIVE PULMONARY DISEASE DISPARITIES

The COPD National Action Plan is one effort to address health disparities related to COPD.[88] Drafted in May 2017 by the National Institutes of Health (NIH) and the Centers for Disease Control and Prevention (CDC), the plan provides a coordinated, unified, national approach to tackling COPD. It identifies goals targeted at improvement of COPD within vulnerable populations, which include improvement of patient education, provider education to improve and standardize management, enhancement of research to identify

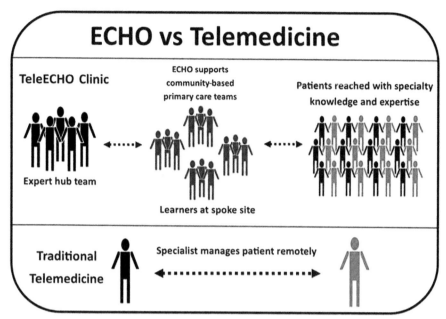

Fig. 2. ECHO versus telemedicine data from ECHO Institute at the University of New Mexico's Health Science Center. (*From* NH Citizen's Health Initiative. Project ECHO. Available at: https://www.citizenshealthinitiative.org/project-echo. With permission.)

other key areas for improvement, and use of this research to effect change and further drive policy.

Another useful approach is to provide structured longitudinal telementoring to PCPs serving vulnerable populations, using the Extension for Community Health Outcomes (ECHO) model to create a virtual community of practice.[89–91] The approach of moving knowledge instead of moving patients has been effective in managing other chronic diseases in medically underserved areas by reducing variation in processes of care and sharing best practices.[92] Distinct from telemedicine, this telementoring model, as shown in **Fig. 2**, is based on the principle of case-based learning. Over time with iterative practice and feedback, PCPs who share cases from their practice with specialists begin to comanage these patients with the specialists. This model, developed at the University of New Mexico, is currently being used at 2 ECHO hub sites in New Mexico and West Virginia. The presence of limited data regarding the effectiveness of the virtual community of practice approach in rural patients with COPD necessitates building more evidence basis.

SUMMARY

Approximately 300 million people have COPD worldwide, most in low-income and middle-income countries.[11] The 2008 to 2013 WHO action plan on NCDs lists chronic respiratory diseases as

1 of its 4 priorities for research.[93] Additional research is needed to understand the reasons for global, rural-urban, and racial/ethnic disparities in COPD. Given that a large proportion of individuals with COPD have never smoked, the role of ambient and householder pollution and occupational and other environmental exposures needs to be better understood.[31] Research priorities should also focus on studies to evaluate different approaches to health care delivery (eg, spirometry for diagnosis and treatment, and integrated health care strategies during transitions in care) and telementoring.[94] As with any other public health problem, increased political commitment and funding remains crucial, particularly in low-income and middle-income country settings. Governments and policymakers must consider strengthening regulations to address occupational and environmental risk factors, regulate tobacco use, improve public awareness, and educate physicians.

DISCLOSURE

The authors have no commercial or financial conflicts of interest and no funding sources to disclose.

REFERENCES

1. Salvi SS, Barnes PJ. Chronic obstructive pulmonary disease in non-smokers. Lancet 2009;374:733–43.

2. Lange P, Celli B, Agusti A. Lung-function trajectories and chronic obstructive pulmonary disease. N Engl J Med 2015;373:1575.

3. Pauwels RA, Buist AS, Calverley PM, et al. Global strategy for the diagnosis, management, and prevention of chronic obstructive pulmonary disease. NHLBI/WHO Global Initiative for Chronic Obstructive Lung Disease (GOLD) workshop summary. Am J Respir Crit Care Med 2001;163:1256–76.

4. Celli BR, MacNee W. Standards for the diagnosis and treatment of patients with COPD: a summary of the ATS/ERS position paper. Eur Respir J 2004; 23:932–46.

5. Pellegrino R, Viegi G, Brusasco V, et al. Interpretative strategies for lung function tests. Eur Respir J 2005;26:948–68.

6. Tilert T, Dillon C, Paulose-Ram R, et al. Estimating the U.S. prevalence of chronic obstructive pulmonary disease using pre- and post-bronchodilator spirometry: the National Health and Nutrition Examination Survey (NHANES) 2007-2010. Respir Res 2013;14:103.

7. Diab N, Gershon AS, Sin DD, et al. Underdiagnosis and overdiagnosis of chronic obstructive pulmonary disease. Am J Respir Crit Care Med 2018;198:1130–9.

8. Lamprecht B, Soriano JB, Studnicka M, et al, Bold Collaborative Research Group tEPISTtPT, the PSG. Determinants of underdiagnosis of COPD in national and international surveys. Chest 2015;148: 971–85.

9. Mannino DM, Diaz-Guzman E. Interpreting lung function data using 80% predicted and fixed thresholds identifies patients at increased risk of mortality. Chest 2012;141:73–80.

10. G. B. D. Chronic Respiratory Disease Collaborators. Global, regional, and national deaths, prevalence, disability-adjusted life years, and years lived with disability for chronic obstructive pulmonary disease and asthma, 1990-2015: a systematic analysis for the Global Burden of Disease Study 2015. Lancet Respir Med 2017;5:691–706.

11. Adeloye D, Chua S, Lee C, et al. Global and regional estimates of COPD prevalence: systematic review and meta-analysis. J Glob Health 2015;5:020415.

12. Barnes PJ. Chronic obstructive pulmonary disease: a growing but neglected global epidemic. Plos Med 2007;4:e112.

13. Alwan A. Global status report on non-communicable diseases. Geneva (Switzerland): World Health Organization; 2010.

14. Ehteshami-Afshar S, FitzGerald JM, Doyle-Waters MM, et al. The global economic burden of asthma and chronic obstructive pulmonary disease. Int J Tuberc Lung Dis 2016;20:11–23.

15. Soriano JB, Zielinski J, Price D. Screening for and early detection of chronic obstructive pulmonary disease. Lancet 2009;374:721–32.

16. World Health Organization. Global Health Observatory data. Prevalence of tobacco smoking. 2015. Available at: https://www.who.int/gho/tobacco/use/en/. Accessed May 7, 2020.

17. Collaborators GBDT. Smoking prevalence and attributable disease burden in 195 countries and territories, 1990-2015: a systematic analysis from the Global Burden of Disease Study 2015. Lancet 2017;389:1885–906.

18. Huang X, Mu X, Deng L, et al. The etiologic origins for chronic obstructive pulmonary disease. Int J Chron Obstruct Pulmon Dis 2019;14:1139–58.

19. World Health Organization. Noncommunicable diseases and mental health. NCD global Monitoring Framework. Available at: https://www.who.int/nmh/global_monitoring_framework/en/. Accessed May 7, 2020.

20. Oberg M, Jaakkola MS, Woodward A, et al. Worldwide burden of disease from exposure to secondhand smoke: a retrospective analysis of data from 192 countries. Lancet 2011;377:139–46.

21. Homa DM, Neff LJ, King BA, et al, Centers for Disease Control and Prevention. Vital signs: disparities in nonsmokers' exposure to secondhand smoke–United States, 1999-2012. MMWR Morb Mortal Wkly Rep 2015;64:103–8.

22. Diver WR, Jacobs EJ, Gapstur SM. Secondhand smoke exposure in childhood and adulthood in relation to adult mortality among never smokers. Am J Prev Med 2018;55:345–52.

23. Eisner MD, Balmes J, Katz PP, et al. Lifetime environmental tobacco smoke exposure and the risk of chronic obstructive pulmonary disease. Environ Health 2005;4:7.

24. Eisner MD. Secondhand smoke and obstructive lung disease: a causal effect? Am J Respir Crit Care Med 2009;179:973–4.

25. Cohen AJ, Brauer M, Burnett R, et al. Estimates and 25-year trends of the global burden of disease attributable to ambient air pollution: an analysis of data from the Global Burden of Diseases Study 2015. Lancet 2017;389:1907–18.

26. Bennett JE, Tamura-Wicks H, Parks RM, et al. Particulate matter air pollution and national and county life expectancy loss in the USA: a spatiotemporal analysis. PLoS Med 2019;16:e1002856.

27. Rice MB, Ljungman PL, Wilker EH, et al. Long-term exposure to traffic emissions and fine particulate matter and lung function decline in the Framingham heart study. Am J Respir Crit Care Med 2015;191: 656–64.

28. Wang M, Aaron CP, Madrigano J, et al. Association between long-term exposure to ambient air pollution and change in quantitatively assessed emphysema and lung function. JAMA 2019;322:546–56.

29. Li J, Sun S, Tang R, et al. Major air pollutants and risk of COPD exacerbations: a systematic review and

meta-analysis. Int J Chron Obstruct Pulmon Dis 2016;11:3079–91.

30. Hao Y, Balluz L, Strosnider H, et al. Ozone, fine particulate matter, and chronic lower respiratory disease mortality in the United States. Am J Respir Crit Care Med 2015;192:337–41.

31. Sood A, Assad NA, Barnes PJ, et al. ERS/ATS workshop report on respiratory health effects of household air pollution. Eur Respir J 2018;51:1700698.

32. Sood A, Petersen H, Blanchette CM, et al. Wood smoke exposure and gene promoter methylation are associated with increased risk for COPD in smokers. Am J Respir Crit Care Med 2010;182: 1098–104.

33. Collaborators GBDRF. Global, regional, and national comparative risk assessment of 84 behavioural, environmental and occupational, and metabolic risks or clusters of risks for 195 countries and territories, 1990-2017: a systematic analysis for the Global Burden of Disease Study 2017. Lancet 2018;392:1923–94.

34. Gordon SB, Bruce NG, Grigg J, et al. Respiratory risks from household air pollution in low and middle income countries. Lancet Respir Med 2014;2: 823–60.

35. Blanc PD, Annesi-Maesano I, Balmes JR, et al. The occupational burden of Nonmalignant respiratory diseases. An official American Thoracic Society and European Respiratory Society Statement. Am J Respir Crit Care Med 2019;199:1312–34.

36. Bang KM, Syamlal G, Mazurek JM. Prevalence of chronic obstructive pulmonary disease in the U.S. working population: an analysis of data from the 1997-2004 National Health Interview Survey. COPD 2009;6:380–7.

37. Bang KM, Syamlal G, Mazurek JM, et al. Chronic obstructive pulmonary disease prevalence among nonsmokers by occupation in the United States. J Occup Environ Med 2013;55:1021–6.

38. De Matteis S, Consonni D, Bertazzi PA. Exposure to occupational carcinogens and lung cancer risk. Evolution of epidemiological estimates of attributable fraction. Acta Biomed 2008;79(Suppl 1):34–42.

39. Blanc PD, Eisner MD, Balmes JR, et al. Exposure to vapors, gas, dust, or fumes: assessment by a single survey item compared to a detailed exposure battery and a job exposure matrix. Am J Ind Med 2005;48:110–7.

40. Bang KM. Chronic obstructive pulmonary disease in nonsmokers by occupation and exposure: a brief review. Curr Opin Pulm Med 2015;21:149–54.

41. Bergdahl IA, Toren K, Eriksson K, et al. Increased mortality in COPD among construction workers exposed to inorganic dust. Eur Respir J 2004;23: 402–6.

42. Toren K, Jarvholm B. Effect of occupational exposure to vapors, gases, dusts, and fumes on COPD mortality risk among Swedish construction workers: a longitudinal cohort study. Chest 2014;145:992–7.

43. Syamlal G, Doney B, Mazurek JM. Chronic obstructive pulmonary disease prevalence among adults who have never smoked, by industry and occupation - United States, 2013-2017. MMWR Morb Mortal Wkly Rep 2019;68:303–7.

44. Blanc PD, Toren K. COPD and occupation: resetting the agenda. Occup Environ Med 2016;73:357–8.

45. Schraufnagel DE, Blasi F, Kraft M, et al. An official American Thoracic Society/European Respiratory Society policy statement: disparities in respiratory health. Am J Respir Crit Care Med 2013;188:865–71.

46. Meit M, Knudson A, Gilbert T, et al. S. The 2014 Update of the Rural-Urban Chartbook. Bethesda (MD): The Rural Health Reform Policy Research Center; 2014.

47. Croft JB, Wheaton AG, Liu Y, et al. Urban-rural county and state differences in chronic obstructive pulmonary disease - United States, 2015. MMWR Morb Mortal Wkly Rep 2018;67:205–11.

48. Raju S, Keet CA, Paulin LM, et al. Rural residence and poverty are independent risk factors for chronic obstructive pulmonary disease in the United States. Am J Respir Crit Care Med 2019;199:961–9.

49. Raju S, Brigham EP, Paulin LM, et al. The burden of rural chronic obstructive pulmonary disease: analyses from the national health and nutrition examination survey. Am J Respir Crit Care Med 2020;201: 488–91.

50. National Center for Health Statistics. Chronic Obstructive Pulmonary Disease (COPD) includes: chronic bronchitis and emphysema. 2017. Available at: https://www.cdc.gov/nchs/fastats/copd.htm. Accessed May 6, 2020.

51. Matthews KA, Croft JB, Liu Y, et al. Health-related behaviors by urban-rural county classification - United States, 2013. MMWR Surveill Summ 2017; 66:1–8.

52. Eduard W, Pearce N, Douwes J. Chronic bronchitis, COPD, and lung function in farmers: the role of biological agents. Chest 2009;136:716–25.

53. Sood A, Shore X, Myers O, et al. Among all miners, coal miners demonstrate a disproportionately high prevalence of obstructive spirometric abnormality and chronic bronchitis. J Occup Environ Med 2019;61:328–34.

54. World Health Organization. Social determinants of health. Available at: https://www.who.int/social_determinants/sdh_definition/en/. Accessed April 19, 2020.

55. Burkes RM, Gassett AJ, Ceppe AS, et al. Rural residence and COPD exacerbations: analysis of the SPIROMICS cohort. Ann Am Thorac Soc 2018; 15(7):808–16.

56. Fan VS, Giardino ND, Blough DK, et al. Costs of pulmonary rehabilitation and predictors of adherence in

the national emphysema treatment Trial. COPD 2008;5:105–16.

57. Croft JB, Lu H, Zhang X, et al. Geographic accessibility of pulmonologists for adults with COPD: United States, 2013. Chest 2016;150:544–53.

58. Han MK, Martinez CH, Au DH, et al. Meeting the challenge of COPD care delivery in the USA: a multiprovider perspective. Lancet Respir Med 2016;4: 473–526.

59. Wheaton AG, Liu Y, Croft JB, et al. Chronic obstructive pulmonary disease and smoking status - United States, 2017. MMWR Morb Mortal Wkly Rep 2019; 68:533–8.

60. Jamal A, Phillips E, Gentzke AS, et al. Current cigarette smoking among adults - United States, 2016. MMWR Morb Mortal Wkly Rep 2018;67:53–9.

61. Vaz Fragoso CA, McAvay G, Gill TM, et al. Ethnic differences in respiratory impairment. Thorax 2014;69: 55–62.

62. Sood A, Stidley CA, Picchi MA, et al. Difference in airflow obstruction between Hispanic and non-Hispanic White female smokers. COPD 2008;5: 274–81.

63. Kinney GL, Thomas DS, Cicutto L, et al. The protective effect of hispanic ethnicity on chronic obstructive pulmonary disease mortality is mitigated by smoking behavior. J Pulm Respir Med 2014;4:220.

64. Samet JM, Wiggins CL, Key CR, et al. Mortality from lung cancer and chronic obstructive pulmonary disease in New Mexico, 1958-82. Am J Public Health 1988;78:1182–6.

65. Diaz AA, Come CE, Mannino DM, et al. Obstructive lung disease in Mexican Americans and non-hispanic whites: an analysis of diagnosis and survival in the national health and Nutritional examination survey III follow-up study. Chest 2014;145: 282–9.

66. Kurth L, Doney B, Halldin C. Prevalence of airflow obstruction among ever-employed US adults aged 18-79 years by longest held occupation group: national Health and Nutrition Examination Survey 2007-2008. Occup Environ Med 2016;73: 482–6.

67. Bruse S, Sood A, Petersen H, et al. New Mexican Hispanic smokers have lower odds of chronic obstructive pulmonary disease and less decline in lung function than non-Hispanic whites. Am J Respir Crit Care Med 2011;184:1254–60.

68. Chen W, Brehm JM, Boutaoui N, et al. Native American ancestry, lung function, and COPD in Costa Ricans. Chest 2014;145:704–10.

69. Kamil F, Pinzon I, Foreman MG. Sex and race factors in early-onset COPD. Curr Opin Pulm Med 2013;19: 140–4.

70. Chatila WM, Wynkoop WA, Vance G, et al. Smoking patterns in African Americans and whites with advanced COPD. Chest 2004;125:15–21.

71. Mehari A, Gillum RF. Chronic obstructive pulmonary disease in African- and European-American women: morbidity, mortality and healthcare utilization in the USA. Expert Rev Respir Med 2015;9:161–70.

72. Foreman MG, Zhang L, Murphy J, et al. Early-onset chronic obstructive pulmonary disease is associated with female sex, maternal factors, and African American race in the COPDGene Study. Am J Respir Crit Care Med 2011;184:414–20.

73. Aldrich MC, Kumar R, Colangelo LA, et al. Genetic ancestry-smoking interactions and lung function in African Americans: a cohort study. PLoS One 2012;7:e39541.

74. Kochanek KD, Murphy SL, Xu JQ, et al. Mortality in the United States, 2016. Hyattsville (MD): National Center for Health Statistics; 2017.

75. Dransfield MT, Bailey WC. COPD: racial disparities in susceptibility, treatment, and outcomes. Clin Chest Med 2006;27:463–71, vii.

76. Dwyer-Lindgren L, Bertozzi-Villa A, Stubbs RW, et al. Trends and patterns of differences in chronic respiratory disease mortality among US Counties, 1980-2014. JAMA 2017;318:1136–49.

77. Dominguez K, Penman-Aguilar A, Chang MH, et al, Centers for Disease Control and Prevention. Vital signs: leading causes of death, prevalence of diseases and risk factors, and use of health services among Hispanics in the United States - 2009-2013. MMWR Morb Mortal Wkly Rep 2015;64:469–78.

78. Singh GK, Daus GP, Allender M, et al. Social determinants of health in the United States: addressing major health inequality trends for the Nation, 1935-2016. Int J MCH AIDS 2017;6:139–64.

79. Ejike CO, Dransfield MT, Hansel NN, et al. Chronic obstructive pulmonary disease in America's black population. Am J Respir Crit Care Med 2019;200:423–30.

80. Rice KL, Leimer I, Kesten S, et al. Responses to tiotropium in African-American and Caucasian patients with chronic obstructive pulmonary disease. Transl Res 2008;152:88–94.

81. Shaya FT, Maneval MS, Gbarayor CM, et al. Burden of COPD, asthma, and concomitant COPD and asthma among adults: racial disparities in a medicaid population. Chest 2009;136:405–11.

82. Hardin M, Silverman EK, Barr RG, et al. The clinical features of the overlap between COPD and asthma. Respir Res 2011;12:127.

83. Putcha N, Han MK, Martinez CH, et al. Comorbidities of COPD have a major impact on clinical outcomes, particularly in African Americans. Chronic Obstr Pulm Dis 2014;1:105–14.

84. Ruiz JM, Steffen P, Smith TB. Hispanic mortality paradox: a systematic review and meta-analysis of the longitudinal literature. Am J Public Health 2013; 103:e52–60.

85. Chen W, Brehm JM, Manichaikul A, et al. A genome-wide association study of chronic obstructive

pulmonary disease in Hispanics. Ann Am Thorac Soc 2015;12:340–8.

86. Diaz AA, Petersen H, Meek P, et al. Differences in health-related quality of life between new Mexican hispanic and non-hispanic white smokers. Chest 2016;150(4):869–76.

87. Diaz AA, Rahaghi FN, Doyle TJ, et al. Differences in respiratory symptoms and lung structure between hispanic and non-hispanic white smokers: a comparative study. Chronic Obstr Pulm Dis 2017;4:297–304.

88. Moore P, Atkins GT, Cramb S, et al. COPD and rural health: a dialogue on the national action plan. J Rural Health 2019;35:424–8.

89. Wenger E. How we learn. Communities of practice. The social fabric of a learning organization. Healthc Forum J 1996;39:20–6.

90. Wenger E. Communities of practice: learning, meaning, and identity. New York: Cambridge University Press; 1998.

91. Parboosingh JT. Physician communities of practice: where learning and practice are inseparable. J Contin Educ Health Prof 2002;22:230–6.

92. Arora S, Thornton K, Murata G, et al. Outcomes of treatment for hepatitis C virus infection by primary care providers. N Engl J Med 2011;364: 2199–207.

93. Bousquet J, Kiley J, Bateman ED, et al. Prioritised research agenda for prevention and control of chronic respiratory diseases. Eur Respir J 2010;36: 995–1001.

94. Krishnan JA, Lindenauer PK, Au DH, et al, COPD Outcomes-based Network for Clinical Effectiveness and Research Translation. Stakeholder priorities for comparative effectiveness research in chronic obstructive pulmonary disease: a workshop report. Am J Respir Crit Care Med 2013; 187:320–6.

Host, Gender, and Early-Life Factors as Risks for Chronic Obstructive Pulmonary Disease

MeiLan K. Han, MD, MS[a], Fernando J. Martinez, MD, MS[b],*

KEYWORDS

- COPD • Gender • Genetics • Tobacco • Exposures

KEY POINTS

- Genetic susceptibility may account for as much as 30% of variation in risk for developing chronic obstructive pulmonary disease (COPD), although the attributable risk contribution from most individual genes to the development of COPD is likely small.
- Female gender may be associated with increased disease susceptibility, both from tobacco smoke but also non–tobacco-related COPD. It is important to remember that environmental and social factors all have the potential to impact disease presentation and progression.
- It has been estimated that exposures to vapors, gas, dust, or fumes contribute to the population burden of COPD by approximately 15%. Recent evidence also suggests outdoor air pollution may also contribute to COPD development.
- As many as half of individuals with COPD do not experience accelerated lung decline in adulthood, but rather have low attained peak lung function in early adulthood and normal age-related lung function decline through adulthood. This is likely related to early-life factors including preterm birth, maternal smoking, and respiratory infections in childhood.

INTRODUCTION

Although smoking results in lung pathology in many, still not all smokers develop COPD. Further, roughly a quarter of patients with chronic obstructive pulmonary disease (COPD) have never smoked. Hence, an understanding of both host and environmental factors beyond smoking that contribute to disease development remain critical to disease prevention and ultimately cure. In this article, we summarize host factors, including genetics and gender, as well as early-life events that contribute to the development of COPD.

HOST FACTORS
Genetics

Supporting a role for genetics in COPD susceptibility, family studies, as well as analyses of unrelated individuals suggests a heritable component to the disease, accounting for perhaps 30% of variation in risk.[1] Alpha-1 antitrypsin deficiency is the most well-described genetic association with COPD, caused by a single mutation in the alpha-1-antitrypsin gene (SERPINA1). It has been estimated that A1AT disease accounts for roughly 1% of COPD.[2] Several different gene mutations in this gene have been described, resulting in

[a] Division of Pulmonary and Critical Care Medicine, University of Michigan School of Medicine, 3916 Taubman Center, 1500 East Medical Center Drive, Ann Arbor, MI 48109, USA; [b] Division of Pulmonary and Critical Care Medicine, Internal Medicine, Weill Cornell Medicine, New York, NY, USA
* Corresponding author. 1330 First Avenue, Apartment 419, New York, NY 10021.
E-mail address: fjm2003@med.cornell.edu

Clin Chest Med 41 (2020) 329–337
https://doi.org/10.1016/j.ccm.2020.06.009
0272-5231/20/© 2020 Published by Elsevier Inc.

impaired production of the protein alpha-1 antitrypsin, which inactivates neutrophil elastase, which if left unchecked results in emphysematous destruction of the lung. Even individuals with MZ likely have lower lung function.[3]

Outside of A1AT deficiency, 2 well-described genes associated with lung function and COPD susceptibility include Hedgehog-Interacting Protein (HHIP)[4] and Family with frequency similarity 13 member A (FAM13 A).[5] The CHRNA3/CHRNA5/IREB2 region on chromosome 15q25 has also been associated with COPD susceptibility,[6] although some evidence supports the existence of 2 COPD genome-wide association study (GWAS) loci in that region, one related to nicotine addiction (the nicotinic acetylcholine receptor genes, such as CHRNA3 and CHRNA5) and one unrelated to nicotine addiction (related to IREB2).[7] Several GWAS loci have also been associated with emphysema on computed tomography (CT) imaging. These include the aforementioned CHRNA3 in addition to MMP12 and the AGER region that encodes the sRAGE protein biomarker that has also been strongly associated with emphysema.[8]

As the attributable risk contribution from individual genes to COPD development is relatively small, attempts have been made to combine data from multiple genes to create genetic risk scores. A recent analysis used data from the MESA Lung and SPIROMICS cohorts used 83 single nucleotide polymorphisms (SNPs) to create a genetic risk score that was associated with lower lung function and increased COPD risk, as well as lower lung density, smaller airway lumens, and fewer small airways without effect modification by smoking.[9] The COPD gene study has convincingly associated 20 genetic loci with COPD affection status; additional loci demonstrating associations with various COPD-related phenotypes.[10] Using data from 8 cohorts, a meta-analysis found 2 SNPs (rs112458284 and rs6860095) not previously described in genome-wide studies that were associated with Global Initiative for Chronic Obstructive Lung Disease spirometric stage III–IV COPD at genome-wide significance levels. One was believed to be related to SERPINA1 Z allele. Data from the UK Biobank was used to create a genetic risk score for COPD susceptibility with an odds ratio of 1.24 per 1 SD of the risk score ($\sim$6 alleles).[11] This analysis identified enrichment for genes involved in development, elastic fibers, and epigenetic regulation pathways. A recent investigative group completed a GWAS of 35,735 cases and 222,076 controls from the UK Biobank and studies from the International COPD Genetics Consortium; 82 loci associated with COPD or lung function measures. Forty-seven were previously known, whereas 13 of 35 new loci related principally to lung function.[12] COPD genetic risk loci were associated with quantitative imaging measures and comorbidities supporting COPD genetic susceptibility and heterogeneity.[12] Furthermore, gene-enrichment analysis confirmed the importance of developmental pathways suggesting that a substantial portion of COPD risk may relate to early life.[12] Interestingly, a combinatorial approach has suggested that incorporating a number of COPD risk alleles may improve the ability to define risk of lung function abnormality.[13] Integrated genomics has also been suggested to define potential biologically relevant biomarkers.[14] These approaches may yield insights to potentially druggable targets.[11] At this point, however, genetic testing beyond A1AT remains primarily suited for research as opposed to clinical purposes.

Gender

Female gender also appears to modify risk for disease.[15] When examining gender, however, we must think beyond simply the X chromosome and must also consider environmental or social factors that are unique to female gender. Smoking is arguably the biggest risk factor for the development of COPD. Although historically tobacco use was more common among men, women have been rapidly catching up.[16] In the United States, smoking among men peaked in the 1970s followed by women in the 1980s.[16] Global trends are similar.[17] Currently the prevalence of smoking among women varies dramatically by country, ethnicity, and socioeconomic status.[18] However, the absolute number of women who smoke is greater in developing countries, whereas the percentage of smokers who are women is higher in developed countries.[19] Moving forward, unfortunately global estimates suggest the proportion of female smokers will rise from approximately 12% in the first decade of this century to 20% by 2025.[20] Again this increase will be seen more predominantly in developing countries.[21–23] However, because of lag time between exposure and disease development, the historic trends toward increasing tobacco smoking by women are likely to be reflected in a high COPD burden among women for some time to come.[19]

Smoking habits themselves, the reasons why individuals choose to begin smoking and continue to smoke, differ between genders. The perception of tobacco representing female empowerment (widely promoted via advertising from tobacco companies) and body weight control are 2 reasons for smoking that may influence women more than men.[16,17,20] Further, some evidence suggests that it is more difficult for women to stop smoking[24]; and in fact, the US Surgeon General concluded that across all treatments for smoking cessation, women have more difficulty giving up smoking than men, both at short-term and long-term follow-up.[25]

Although not fully understood, several studies also suggest that women may be more susceptible to developing COPD or experience more rapid lung function decline than men with similar tobacco exposures.[26–34] A meta-analysis examining longitudinal loss of lung function concluded that female current smokers had significantly faster annual decline in forced expiratory volume in 1 second (FEV_1)% predicted than their male counterparts.[35] One of the largest single studies to examine this question comes from an analysis of nearly 250,000 individuals from the UK Biobank. In this study, the association between airflow obstruction and smoking status was stronger in women (odds ratio [OR] for ex-smokers 1.44; OR current smokers 3.45) than men (OR ex-smokers 1.25; OR current smokers 3.06), $P<.001$ for the interaction (**Fig. 1**).[36] Interestingly, the increase in risk at lower doses was also steeper among women. These data suggest it is even more important that women who do smoke quit, which is underscored by data from the Lung Health Study showing that pulmonary function improved more with smoking cessation in women than in men (ΔFEV_1, 3.7% vs 1.6%; $P<.001$).[37]

If women are more susceptible, the reason is not fully understood. A study of early-onset COPD families found a very high prevalence (71.4%) of affected women in particular.[38] In this study,

female first-degree relatives of probands who were also current or ex-smokers showed significantly greater bronchodilator responsiveness and reduced FEV_1 than their male first-degree relatives. As these differences were seen only among current and ex-smokers, the data suggest a genetic predisposition for smoking-related lung damage that is gender specific. Some have speculated that women may underreport tobacco consumption. However, a meta-analysis of 26 studies found that self-reported smoking data are generally accurate.[39] Another possible explanation for gender differences in tobacco susceptibility is that it is a dose-dependent effect with the lungs of women being smaller; hence, each cigarette represents a proportionately greater exposure for women than men. Social factors including secondhand smoke exposure and differences in cigarette brand preferences have also been hypothesized to play a role. Some have suggested that cigarette metabolites in the lungs of women,[40] sex-related differences in cigarette smoke metabolism,[34] and differences in smoking pattern, with women preferentially engaging the ribcage whereas men engage the abdominal compartment.[41]

Although tobacco smoke exposure remains an important risk factor for developing COPD in both genders, worldwide smoke generated from biomass fuel remains a major risk factor for the development of COPD in women in particular because of greater exposure due to cooking and domestic responsibilities.[18,42–44] Globally, roughly 50% of total households and 90% of rural households rely on biomass fuels as their primary source of domestic energy.[18] As an example of the potential damage, fewer than 1% of women in India

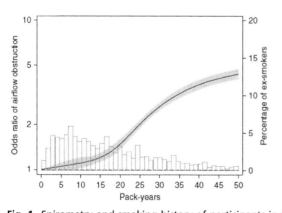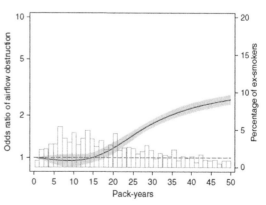

Fig. 1. Spirometry and smoking history of participants in the UK Biobank have similarly shown that women have higher risk of airflow obstruction when compared with men with comparable smoke exposure. Association of airflow obstruction and pack-years among women (*left*) and men (*right*) ex-smokers. Shaded area represents 95% confidence interval. Bars show the distribution of smoking characteristic (pack-years) among ex-smokers. (*Reprinted* with permission of the American Thoracic Society. Copyright © 2020 American Thoracic Society. All rights reserved. *From* Amaral AFS, Strachan DP, Burney PGJ, Jarvis DL. Female Smokers Are at Greater Risk of Airflow Obstruction Than Male Smokers. UK Biobank. Am J Respir Crit Care Med. 2017;195(9):1226-1235. The American Journal of Respiratory and Critical Care Medicine is an official journal of the American Thoracic Society.)

smoke, yet the prevalence of COPD in women is estimated between 1.2% and 19% in women.[45] Yet in certain parts of India, nonsmoker women with COPD constituted 65% of all female patients who meet spirometric criteria for COPD.[46] Women exposed to biomass fuel during the age period 5 to 9 years old have higher odds of developing COPD than those exposed at 20 years (OR 2.9 vs 1.3). The problem, however, is not isolated to developing countries. In the CanCOLD (Canadian Cohort Obstructive Lund Disease) study, a population-based study performed in Canada, exposure to passive smoke and biomass fuel for heating were independent risk factors for COPD in women.[47] Although we may not think that air pollution is a significant risk factor for lung impairment among developed countries, more than 11 million US homes are heated with a wood stove.[48] The World Health Organization (WHO) estimates that in North America, exposure to outdoor PM2.5 pollution from residential heating with solid fuels resulted in 9200 deaths in 2010, an increase from 7500 in 1990. Interestingly, women exposed to biomass fuel smoke may have an airway-predominant as opposed to emphysema-predominant phenotype.[49] A recent cohort study in rural India noted that nonsmoking-related COPD (NS-COPD) was seen in younger subjects with equal male-female predominance; NS-COPD was defined by a predominantly small-airway disease phenotype and slower rate of decline in lung function.[50]

ENVIRONMENTAL AND OCCUPATIONAL EXPOSURES

The role of environmental exposure in COPD causation is often underrecognised,[51] with the evidence of mechanistic causation poorly understood.[52] It has been estimated that exposures to vapors, gas, dust, or fumes contribute to the population burden of COPD by approximately 15%, whereas the attributable fraction of COPD due to cigarette smoking has been estimated to be between 80% and 90%.[53] Using survey data regarding exposures to vapors, gas, dust, or fumes, one study reported the risk for COPD development among exposed individuals was 2.5 (95% confidence interval [CI], 1.9–3.4).[53] Although certain occupations, such as coal mining, have been well studied, other cottage industries, such as brick making, fish smoking, tobacco curing, and leather working also pose potential respiratory health threats. Of particular concern are the significant number of women worldwide who are employed by or run cottage industries.[54]

Although the relationship between outdoor air pollution and exacerbations of respiratory disease has been reported, evidence now suggests outdoor air pollution may also contribute to COPD development.[55] A UK study of postmen documented the prevalence of COPD to be higher among those working in more polluted areas, independent of personal smoking history.[56] Data from other population studies of individuals living near roads with heavy motor vehicle traffic support these findings, in particular a large Danish study demonstrating a small but positive association between long-term exposure to traffic-related air pollution and incident COPD.[57] Similarly, a recent population-based study in Pisa, Italy, suggested a strong association of COPD incidence with PM10 exposure (OR 2.96; 95% CI 1.50–7.15).[58] Importantly, SPIROMICS investigator recently demonstrated that long-term historical ozone exposure was associated with reduced lung function, greater CT-defined emphysema, worse respiratory symptoms and quality of life, and higher odds of any and severe exacerbations.[59]

EARLY-LIFE FACTORS

Recent data suggest that although accelerated lung function decline in adulthood is part of the COPD picture, in roughly one-half of individuals, low attained peak lung function in early adulthood contributes to the development of COPD despite normal age-related lung function decline in adulthood (**Fig. 2**).[60] Hence, early-life risk factors, such as maternal smoking, maternal exposure to air pollution, preterm birth, low birth weight, and childhood respiratory infections, which have all been reported to impair respiratory health later in life, have the potential to increase risk for COPD.[61–63] In fact, a recent cohort study suggests that as much as 75% of adult COPD burden was associated with modifiable early-life exposures.[64]

Because the lungs are still developing during the latter half of pregnancy, intrauterine exposures and premature birth have the potential to negatively impact lung development.[65] Unfortunately, even in developed countries, such as the United States, roughly 20% of women report cigarette smoking during the 3 months before pregnancy and roughly 10% report cigarette smoking during the last 3 months of pregnancy.[66] Data suggest smoking during pregnancy is associated with lower lung function among offspring in childhood.[67] Further, maternal exposure to even low or moderate levels of environmental air pollution during pregnancy and in the subsequent first 2 years of life have also been associated with lower lung function in childhood.[68] Linking these

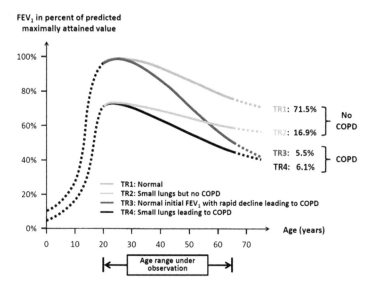

FEV₁ in percent of predicted
maximally attained value

Fig. 2. Distribution of the 2864 participants of Framingham Offspring Cohort and Copenhagen City Heart Study divided into 4 trajectories T1 to T4 defined according to baseline level of FEV_1 (below or above 80% of predicted value) and presence or absence of GOLD grade greater than 2 COPD at the final examination. The solid lines represent the schematic natural history of FEV_1 for the age range of this study, whereas the broken lines represent hypothetical trajectories. (*From* Lange P, Celli B, Agusti A, et al. Lung-Function Trajectories Leading to Chronic Obstructive Pulmonary Disease. *N Engl J Med.* 2015;373(2):111-122; with permission.)

abnormalities to COPD in adulthood has been somewhat more challenging. However, a systematic review of early-life insults and their association with subsequent COPD using a combination of cohort and case control studies identified tobacco exposure in utero and early life as some of the early-life risk factors most clearly linked to subsequent development of COPD.[62]

The impact of prematurity on lung function is well documented and inversely correlates with gestational age. The remarkable improvements in survival of premature infants we have witnessed in the past few decades could further increase the number of individuals in adulthood with lung impairment related to prematurity. Unfortunately, WHO also estimates that the number of preterm births are rising every year. The nature of injury in this patient population likely relates to the use of artificial ventilation and oxygen supplementation in the first few months of life and in some cases neonatal infection. Although the nature of injury can manifest in a variety of pathophysiologic abnormalities, development of bronchopulmonary dysplasia, the chronic lung disease of prematurity, is probably the most well described. Follow-up lung function and CT-imaging studies demonstrate that survivors of premature birth with chronic lung disease inherit a form of chronic lung disease characterized by airflow obstruction, although it still unclear to what degree such structural abnormalities persist in the long term and to what extent this type of lung injury contributes to what we see among adults who are currently diagnosed with COPD.[69,70]

A discussion of childhood risk factors for poor respiratory health would not be complete without a discussion of the potential impact of low socioeconomic status. WHO estimates that at least 250 million children younger than 5 years are at risk for suboptimal development in low-income to middle-income countries due to poverty.[71] Some studies suggest that early-life exposures may account for as many as 75% of COPD cases in adulthood.[72] Elegant work from the Medical Research Council National Survey of Health and Development confirmed a relationship between early-life exposures (infant lower respiratory tract infections, manual social class, home overcrowding, and pollution exposure) and spirometric decline later in life; this was potentiated by smoking status (**Fig. 3**).[73]

Low socioeconomic status appears to be associated with an increased risk for developing COPD, but the exact components of poverty that contribute are not completely clear.[74] Consistent evidence indicates that indoor air pollution increases the risk of acute respiratory infections in childhood and the risk of developing COPD.[75] Roughly half the world's population and up to 90% of rural households in developing countries rely on unprocessed biomass fuels (wood, dung, and crop residues) burned indoor in open fires or stoves.[76] Hence, women and young children are most heavily exposed, and poverty remains a significant barrier to the adoption of cleaner fuels. Low socioeconomic status has also been linked to greater respiratory infections in childhood. In one study, factors in early life termed "childhood disadvantage factors" including maternal asthma, paternal asthma, childhood asthma, maternal smoking, and childhood respiratory infections were all associated with increased risk of developing COPD in adulthood.[77]

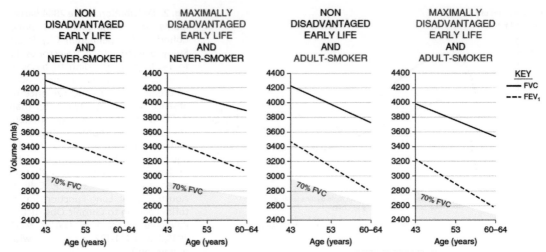

Fig. 3. Comparison of estimated pattern of FEV_1 decline in relation to FVC decline between ages 43 to 60 to 64 for men of average age and weight at age 43 and average birth weight according to adult smoking behavior and early life disadvantage. (*From* Allinson JP, Hardy R, Donaldson GC, et al. Combined Impact of Smoking and Early-Life Exposures on Adult Lung Function Trajectories. *Am J Respir Crit Care Med.* 2017;196(8):1021-1030; with permission.)

SUMMARY

The origins of COPD are clearly multifactorial. As many as half of individuals have low attained peak lung function in early adulthood with normal age-related lung function decline in adulthood suggesting early-life events are the major contributor to COPD development. Hence, in thinking about how we might prevent this disease, public health policies that improve prenatal care, reduce infant smoke exposure, and vaccination programs aimed at reducing respiratory infections in childhood will all be key. Although genetic susceptibility may account for as much as 30% of variation in risk for developing COPD, the attributable risk contribution from most individual genes outside of Alpha-1 antitrypsin to the development of COPD is likely quite small. Other host factors including female gender may be associated with increased disease susceptibility, both from tobacco smoke but also non–tobacco-related COPD. Occupational and environmental exposures also play a role, with estimates suggesting that exposures to vapors, gas, dust, or fumes contribute to the population burden of COPD by approximately 15%. Hence, public health measures to improve indoor and outdoor air quality will also be important in reducing the disease burden of COPD.

REFERENCES

1. Barnes PJ, Burney PG, Silverman EK, et al. Chronic obstructive pulmonary disease. Nat Rev Dis Primers 2015;1:15076.

2. Silverman EK, Sandhaus RA. Clinical practice. Alpha1-antitrypsin deficiency. N Engl J Med 2009; 360(26):2749–57.

3. Foreman MG, Wilson C, DeMeo DL, et al. Alpha-1 antitrypsin PiMZ genotype is associated with chronic obstructive pulmonary disease in two racial groups. Ann Am Thorac Soc 2017;14(8):1280–7.

4. Wilk JB, Chen TH, Gottlieb DJ, et al. A genome-wide association study of pulmonary function measures in the Framingham Heart Study. PLoS Genet 2009;5(3): e1000429.

5. Hancock DB, Eijgelsheim M, Wilk JB, et al. Meta-analyses of genome-wide association studies identify multiple loci associated with pulmonary function. Nat Genet 2010;42(1):45–52.

6. Pillai SG, Ge D, Zhu G, et al. A genome-wide association study in chronic obstructive pulmonary disease (COPD): identification of two major susceptibility loci. PLoS Genet 2009;5(3):e1000421.

7. Silverman EK. Genetics of COPD. Annu Rev Physiol 2020;82:413–31.

8. Yonchuk JG, Silverman EK, Bowler RP, et al. Circulating soluble receptor for advanced glycation end products (sRAGE) as a biomarker of emphysema and the RAGE axis in the lung. Am J Respir Crit Care Med 2015;192(7):785–92.

9. Oelsner EC, Ortega VE, Smith BM, et al. A Genetic risk score associated with chronic obstructive pulmonary disease susceptibility and lung structure on computed tomography. Am J Respir Crit Care Med 2019;200(6):721–31.

10. Ragland MF, Benway CJ, Lutz SM, et al. Genetic advances in chronic obstructive pulmonary disease.

Insights from COPDGene. Am J Respir Crit Care Med 2019;200(6):677–90.

11. Wain LV, Shrine N, Artigas MS, et al. Genome-wide association analyses for lung function and chronic obstructive pulmonary disease identify new loci and potential druggable targets. Nat Genet 2017; 49(3):416–25.

12. Sakornsakolpat P, Prokopenko D, Lamontagne M, et al. Genetic landscape of chronic obstructive pulmonary disease identifies heterogeneous cell-type and phenotype associations. Nat Genet 2019; 51(3):494–505.

13. Busch R, Cho MH, Silverman EK. Progress in disease progression genetics: dissecting the genetic origins of lung function decline in COPD. Thorax 2017;72(5):389–90.

14. Obeidat M, Nie Y, Fishbane N, et al. Integrative genomics of emphysema-associated genes reveals potential disease biomarkers. Am J Respir Cell Mol Biol 2017;57(4):411–8.

15. Han MK. Chronic obstructive pulmonary disease in women: a biologically focused review with a systematic search strategy. Int J Chron Obstruct Pulmon Dis 2020;15:711–21.

16. World Lung Foundation. The tobacco atlas 2015. Available at: http://www.tobaccoatlas.org/. Accessed December 17, 2015.

17. World Health Organization (WHO). Gender, health and tobacco. 2003. Available at: https://www.who.int/gender-equityrights/knowledge/gender_tobacco_leaflet/en/.

18. Salvi SS, Barnes PJ. Chronic obstructive pulmonary disease in non-smokers. Lancet 2009;374(9691): 733–43.

19. Rycroft CE, Heyes A, Lanza L, et al. Epidemiology of chronic obstructive pulmonary disease: a literature review. Int J Chron Obstruct Pulmon Dis 2012;7: 457–94.

20. World Health Organization (WHO). Empower women - combating tobacco industry marketing in the WHO European region 2010. Available at: http://www.euro.who.int/__data/assets/pdf_file/0014/128120/e9 3852.pdf. Accessed December 15, 2015.

21. Aryal S, Diaz-Guzman E, Mannino DM. Influence of sex on chronic obstructive pulmonary disease risk and treatment outcomes. Int J Chron Obstruct Pulmon Dis 2014;9:1145–54.

22. Goel S, Tripathy JP, Singh RJ, et al. Smoking trends among women in India: analysis of nationally representative surveys (1993-2009). South Asian J Cancer 2014;3(4):200–2.

23. Hitchman SC, Fong GT. Gender empowerment and female-to-male smoking prevalence ratios. Bull World Health Organ 2011;89(3):195–202.

24. Vozoris NT, Stanbrook MB. Smoking prevalence, behaviours, and cessation among individuals with COPD or asthma. Respir Med 2011;105(3):477–84.

25. 2001 Surgeon General's Report: Women and Smoking. Available at: https://www.cdc.gov/tobacco/data_statistics/sgr/2001/index.htm.

26. Han MK, Postma D, Mannino DM, et al. Gender and chronic obstructive pulmonary disease: why it matters. Am J Respir Crit Care Med 2007;176(12): 1179–84.

27. Jordan RE, Miller MR, Lam KB, et al. Sex, susceptibility to smoking and chronic obstructive pulmonary disease: the effect of different diagnostic criteria. Analysis of the Health Survey for England. Thorax 2012;67(7):600–5.

28. Rahmanian SD, Diaz PT, Wewers ME. Tobacco use and cessation among women: research and treatment-related issues. J Womens Health (Larchmt) 2011;20(3):349–57.

29. Sørheim IC, Johannessen A, Gulsvik A, et al. Gender differences in COPD: are women more susceptible to smoking effects than men? Thorax 2010;65(6): 480–5.

30. Hardin M, Foreman M, Dransfield MT, et al. Sex-specific features of emphysema among current and former smokers with COPD. Eur Respir J 2016; 47(1):104–12.

31. Prescott E, Bjerg AM, Andersen PK, et al. Gender difference in smoking effects on lung function and risk of hospitalization for COPD: results from a Danish longitudinal population study. Eur Respir J 1997;10(4):822–7.

32. Gan WQ, Man SF, Senthilselvan A, et al. Association between chronic obstructive pulmonary disease and systemic inflammation: a systematic review and a meta-analysis. Thorax 2004;59(7):574–80.

33. Dransfield MT, Davis JJ, Gerald LB, et al. Racial and gender differences in susceptibility to tobacco smoke among patients with chronic obstructive pulmonary disease. Respir Med 2006;100(6):1110–6.

34. Ben-Zaken Cohen S, Pare PD, Man SF, et al. The growing burden of chronic obstructive pulmonary disease and lung cancer in women: examining sex differences in cigarette smoke metabolism. Am J Respir Crit Care Med 2007;176(2):113–20.

35. Gan WQ, Man SF, Postma DS, et al. Female smokers beyond the perimenopausal period are at increased risk of chronic obstructive pulmonary disease: a systematic review and meta-analysis. Respir Res 2006; 7:52.

36. Amaral AFS, Strachan DP, Burney PGJ, et al. Female smokers are at greater risk of airflow obstruction than male smokers. UK biobank. Am J Respir Crit Care Med 2017;195(9):1226–35.

37. Bjornson W, Rand C, Connett JE, et al. Gender differences in smoking cessation after 3 years in the lung health study. Am J Public Health 1995;85(2): 223–30.

38. Silverman EK, Weiss ST, Drazen JM, et al. Gender-related differences in severe, early-onset chronic

obstructive pulmonary disease. Am J Respir Crit Care Med 2000;162(6):2152–8.

39. Patrick DL, Cheadle A, Thompson DC, et al. The validity of self-reported smoking: a review and meta-analysis. Am J Public Health 1994;84(7):1086–93.

40. Mollerup S, Berge G, Baera R, et al. Sex differences in risk of lung cancer: expression of genes in the PAH bioactivation pathway in relation to smoking and bulky DNA adducts. Int J Cancer 2006;119(4): 741–4.

41. Polverino M, Capuozzo A, Cicchitto G, et al. Smoking pattern in men and women: a possible contributor to gender differences in smoke-related lung diseases. Am J Respir Crit Care Med 2020. https://doi.org/10.1164/rccm.202004-1472LE.

42. Jain NK, Thakkar MS, Jain N, et al. Chronic obstructive pulmonary disease: does gender really matter? Lung India 2011;28(4):258–62.

43. Gordon SB, Bruce NG, Grigg J, et al. Respiratory risks from household air pollution in low and middle income countries. Lancet Respir Med 2014;2(10): 823–60.

44. Camp PG, Ramirez-Venegas A, Sansores RH, et al. COPD phenotypes in biomass smoke- versus tobacco smoke-exposed Mexican women. Eur Respir J 2014;43(3):725–34.

45. Bhome AB. COPD in India: iceberg or volcano? J Thorac Dis 2012;4(3):298–309.

46. KalagoudaMahishale V, Angadi N, Metgudmath V, et al. The prevalence of chronic obstructive pulmonary disease and the determinants of underdiagnosis in women exposed to biomass fuel in India- a cross section study. Chonnam Med J 2016;52(2): 117–22.

47. Tan WC, Sin DD, Bourbeau J, et al. Characteristics of COPD in never-smokers and ever-smokers in the general population: results from the CanCOLD study. Thorax 2015;70(9):822–9.

48. Rokoff LB, Koutrakis P, Garshick E, et al. Wood stove pollution in the developed world: a case to raise awareness among pediatricians. Curr Probl Pediatr Adolesc Health Care 2017;47(6):123–41.

49. Han MK. The "other" COPD. Eur Respir J 2014;43(3): 659–61.

50. Salvi SS, Brashier BB, Londhe J, et al. Phenotypic comparison between smoking and non-smoking chronic obstructive pulmonary disease. Respir Res 2020;21(1):50.

51. Blanc PD, Iribarren C, Trupin L, et al. Occupational exposures and the risk of COPD: dusty trades revisited. Thorax 2009;64(1):6–12.

52. Thurston GD, Balmes JR, Garcia E, et al. Outdoor air pollution and new-onset airway disease. An official American Thoracic Society workshop report. Ann Am Thorac Soc 2020;17(4):387–98.

53. Blanc PD, Eisner MD, Earnest G, et al. Further exploration of the links between occupational exposure

and chronic obstructive pulmonary disease. J Occup Environ Med 2009;51(7):804–10.

54. Roy S, Dasgupta A. A study on health status of women engaged in a home-based "Papad-making" industry in a slum area of Kolkata. Indian J Occup Environ Med 2008;12(1):33–6.

55. Marino E, Caruso M, Campagna D, et al. Impact of air quality on lung health: myth or reality? Ther Adv Chronic Dis 2015;6(5):286–98.

56. Fairbairn AS, Reid DD. Air pollution and other local factors in respiratory disease. Br J Prev Soc Med 1958;12(2):94–103.

57. Andersen ZJ, Hvidberg M, Jensen SS, et al. Chronic obstructive pulmonary disease and long-term exposure to traffic-related air pollution: a cohort study. Am J Respir Crit Care Med 2011; 183(4):455–61.

58. Fasola S, Maio S, Baldacci S, et al. Effects of particulate matter on the incidence of respiratory diseases in the pisan longitudinal study. Int J Environ Res Public Health 2020;17(7):2540.

59. Paulin LM, Gassett AJ, Alexis NE, et al. Association of long-term ambient ozone exposure with respiratory morbidity in smokers. JAMA Intern Med 2019. https://doi.org/10.1001/jamainternmed.2019.5498.

60. Lange P, Celli B, Agusti A, et al. Lung-function trajectories leading to chronic obstructive pulmonary disease. N Engl J Med 2015;373(2):111–22.

61. Postma DS, Bush A, van den Berge M. Risk factors and early origins of chronic obstructive pulmonary disease. Lancet 2015;385(9971):899–909.

62. Savran O, Ulrik CS. Early life insults as determinants of chronic obstructive pulmonary disease in adult life. Int J Chron Obstruct Pulmon Dis 2018;13: 683–93.

63. Barker DJ, Godfrey KM, Fall C, et al. Relation of birth weight and childhood respiratory infection to adult lung function and death from chronic obstructive airways disease. Br Med J 1991;303(6804):671–5.

64. Bui DS, Lodge CJ, Burgess JA, et al. Childhood predictors of lung function trajectories and future COPD risk: a prospective cohort study from the first to the sixth decade of life. Lancet Respir Med 2018;6(7): 535–44.

65. Grant T, Brigham EP, McCormack MC. Childhood origins of adult lung disease as opportunities for prevention. J Allergy Clin Immunol Pract 2020;8(3): 849–58.

66. Centers for Disease Control and Prevention. Pregnancy Risk Assessment Monitoring System, PRAMS, Prevalence of Selected Maternal and Child Health Indicators for all PRAMS sites, 2012-2015. 2015. Available at: https://www.cdc.gov/prams/index.htm.

67. Milner AD, Rao H, Greenough A. The effects of antenatal smoking on lung function and respiratory symptoms in infants and children. Early Hum Dev 2007;83(11):707–11.

68. Morales E, Garcia-Esteban R, de la Cruz OA, et al. Intrauterine and early postnatal exposure to outdoor air pollution and lung function at preschool age. Thorax 2015;70(1):64–73.

69. Urs R, Kotecha S, Hall GL, et al. Persistent and progressive long-term lung disease in survivors of preterm birth. Paediatr Respir Rev 2018;28:87–94.

70. Gough A, Linden M, Spence D, et al. Impaired lung function and health status in adult survivors of bronchopulmonary dysplasia. Eur Respir J 2014;43(3):808–16.

71. World Health Organization. Global Strategy for Women's, Children's and Adolescents' Health (2016–2030) 2018 monitoring report: current status and strategic priorities. 2018. Available at: https://www.who.int/life-course/partners/global-strategy/gswcah-2018-monitoring-report/en/.

72. Agusti A, Noell G, Brugada J, et al. Lung function in early adulthood and health in later life: a transgenerational cohort analysis. Lancet Respir Med 2017;5(12):935–45.

73. Allinson JP, Hardy R, Donaldson GC, et al. Combined impact of smoking and early-life exposures on adult lung function trajectories. Am J Respir Crit Care Med 2017;196(8):1021–30.

74. GOLD Science Committee. Global Strategy for the Diagnosis, Management and Prevention of COPD 2020 Report. Available at: https://goldcopd.org/wp-content/uploads/2019/12/GOLD-2020-FINAL-ver1.2-03Dec19_WMV.pdf.

75. Smith KR, Samet JM, Romieu I, et al. Indoor air pollution in developing countries and acute lower respiratory infections in children. Thorax 2000;55(6):518–32.

76. Bruce N, Perez-Padilla R, Albalak R. Indoor air pollution in developing countries: a major environmental and public health challenge. Bull World Health Organ 2000;78(9):1078–92.

77. Svanes C, Sunyer J, Plana E, et al. Early life origins of chronic obstructive pulmonary disease. Thorax 2010;65(1):14–20.

Alpha-1 Antitrypsin Deficiency Associated COPD

Charlie Strange, MD

KEYWORDS

- Emphysema • Alpha-1 • Antitrypsin • Protease • Antiprotease • Genetic

KEY POINTS

- Alpha-1 antitrypsin deficiency (AATD) diagnosis requires a test from all individuals with chronic obstructive pulmonary disease (COPD). Attempts to clinically characterize this genetic condition to decide who needs testing miss affected individuals.
- Airway disease in AATD can take the form of asthma, chronic bronchitis, or bronchiectasis.
- Augmentation therapy with plasma-derived alpha-1 protease inhibitor slows the progression of emphysema in randomized trials and is associated with strong signals of improved mortality in observational cohorts.
- Clinical liver disease occurs in approximately 10% of patients with AATD. Tests for cirrhosis should occur at least yearly in PiZZ individuals to recognize this complication.
- A diagnosis of AATD-associated COPD establishes a family at risk. Family testing for AATD is the most cost-effective and successful strategy to find patients who may benefit from lifestyle interventions or therapies.

INTRODUCTION

Alpha-1 antitrypsin (AAT) is the most abundant serine proteinase inhibitor in human plasma. When Laurell and Erikson[1] first noted the association between a deficiency of the protein (AAT deficiency [AATD]) and emphysema in 1963, they were likely unaware that interest in the mechanisms of chronic obstructive pulmonary disease (COPD) pathogenesis associated with AATD would continue for the next half century. Genetically determined deficiency of AAT is associated with emphysema, particularly in individuals who smoke cigarettes or are exposed to other inhaled particulates and/or fumes.[2,3] Features of this unique endotype of COPD continue to inform aspects of smoking-related COPD and suggest the pathway forward if cigarette cessation is ever eliminated as a public health risk. In AATD, COPD continues to progress with aging in the absence of smoking. As such, this disease helps answer questions on genetic risks, protease/antiprotease biology, and translation of these findings to the AATD patients in the clinic.

Alpha-1 Antitrypsin Synthesis and Regulation

AAT is a 52-kDa glycoprotein produced mainly in hepatocytes[4,5] but also synthesized by blood monocytes, macrophages, pulmonary alveolar cells, and other cells throughout the body.[6–11] Daily hepatic production of AAT of more than 30 mg/kg body weight results in high plasma concentrations, ranging from 90 mg/dL to 175 mg/dL that further increase during times of stress. Because of an acute-phase response, particularly after interleukin (IL)-6, IL-1, tumor necrosis factor α, or endotoxin,[12,13] AAT levels are higher during

Division of Pulmonary, Critical Care, Allergy and Sleep Medicine, Medical University of South Carolina, 96 Jonathan Lucas Street, MSC630, Charleston, SC 29425, USA
E-mail address: strangec@musc.edu

Clin Chest Med 41 (2020) 339–345
https://doi.org/10.1016/j.ccm.2020.05.003
0272-5231/20/© 2020 Elsevier Inc. All rights reserved.

times of infections and tissue inflammation, accounting for high concentrations in patients with normal genotypes in intensive care units. The tissue concentration of the protein is reduced to approximately 10% of the plasma levels in the fluid of the lower respiratory tract.[14,15] AAT also diffuses through endothelial and epithelial cell walls. AAT expression also is autoregulated with enhanced synthesis after exposure to neutrophil elastase (NE) either alone or complexed to AAT.[16]

Alpha-1 Antitrypsin Structure and Mechanisms of Protease Inhibitory Activity

Human AAT has a single polypeptide chain of 394 amino acid residues and 3 carbohydrate side chains.[17] The reactive site loop is susceptible to protease attack in which the reactive site loop migrates to form a stable complex between the inhibitor and the proteinase.[5,18] The inhibitory activity of AAT is strong for NE, proteinase 3, and other serine proteases. In addition, AAT also inhibits some cysteine proteinases, including caspase-3.[19,20] Complexes of AAT and the affected proteases can be measured in the lower airway, and signatures of cleavage products further inform the protease-antiprotease balance in the lung.[21,22] AAT, like other serpins, can be inactivated by oxidants and proteases that are not inhibitor targets. This occurs clinically in cigarette smoking, in which the AAT molecule can be cleaved by oxidant injury in the local environment of the lung. The genesis of the protease-antiprotease balance model of emphysema pathogenesis was initiated with the discovery of AATD but may play large roles in other forms of AAT replete COPD.

Genetic Modifications of the Alpha-1 Antitrypsin Molecule

The usual serum AAT concentrations are determined by the genetic alleles depicted in **Fig. 1**. Because of the variability of serum AAT concentrations every day due to stress, associations with human disease are best correlated with AAT gene mutations. The AAT molecule is produced on the SERPINA1 gene (OMIM: 107400), and approximately 130 pathogenic variations in human gene structure have been defined.[23] AAT nomenclature is unique, because the clinical disease states originally were defined by plasma protein determination rather than by sequencing. The protease inhibitor (Pi) system informs the AAT concentration as product of each of 2 alleles in a codominant fashion. For example, the variant PiMZ has 1 M allele (a normally functioning allele) and 1 Z mutation that produces low serum AAT

levels. The resulting serum level is intermediate between normal and severely deficient. Unlike most clinical diseases, the AATD deficiency states were called phenotypes. Recently, polymerase chain reaction (PCR) and gene sequencing have been used to probe blood DNA to define these phenotypes by specific gene presence. There are a few rare genetic variants that produce dysfunctional AAT proteins. PiF and PiI produce near-normal AAT concentrations, but the association constant with elastase is markedly reduced.[24] **Table 1** lists some common allelic variants of SERPINA1. Recently, buccal swab samples that test for 14 deficiency alleles are available.[25]

PiZ and PiS are the most common severe deficiency alleles. Recent evidence suggests that carriers of 1 S allele (PiMS) are functionally normal. In contrast, carriers of 1 Z allele (PiMZ) that make up 2% to 3% of the US population have a higher risk of COPD if they smoke compared with PiMM normals.[26] In addition, studies evaluating genes associated with progression of COPD have shown the PiMZ state to be independently correlated with disease progression.[27] Similar findings in smoking versus nonsmoking PiSZ individuals recently have been described.[28]

The Z variant produces a misfolded protein that cannot get out of the hepatic endoplasmic reticulum and causes polymers. In the homozygous condition (PiZZ), serum concentrations of AAT are approximately 10% to 15% of normal, and AAT accumulates in hepatocytes where it can cause cirrhosis. A variety of SERPINA1 gene variants (cumulatively called the null alleles) produce no appreciable AAT at the cellular level and, therefore, have no excess risk for clinical liver disease. Gene distribution studies have found PiZ alleles in almost every country of the world, although of lower frequency in Asian and African populations.[29]

The epidemiology of AATD suggests that between 47,000 and 100,000 PiZZ-affected individuals live in the United States.[30] At most, 10,000 to 15,000 individuals have been identified. The most commonly cited reason for the low diagnosis rate is failure to follow published guidelines that have been in place since 2003 to test every individual with COPD once in a lifetime[31] (**Box 1**). As a result of not testing, the diagnostic delay from onset of COPD diagnosis to a diagnosis of AATD approximates 7 years and was not getting better when last evaluated.[32]

The simplistic theory of AATD COPD pathogenesis suggests that the low total serum concentration of AAT is inadequate to protect against airway proteases, in particular NE produced by activated neutrophils from smoking.[14] This

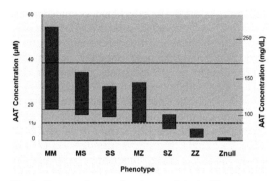

Fig. 1. Range of serum levels associated with common genotypes of AAT. One micromole approximately equals 5.2 mg/dL. (*Adapted from* Brantly M. Alpha 1-Antitrypsin Genotypes and Phenotypes. In: Crystal RD, ed. *Alpha 1-Antitrypsin.* Vol 88. New York: Marcel Dekker, Inc.; 1996:45-60; with permission.)

unopposed NE cleaves elastin, one of the supporting structures of the lung airway and parenchyma leading to emphysema and the collapse of airways characteristic of COPD with bronchiectasis and emphysema endotypes, respectively. A more nuanced pathogenesis supports the concept that circulating polymers of AAT from liver or from lung cells are chemotactic for neutrophils driving airway and lung injury.[33] Therefore, AAT polymers

may participate in the pathogenesis of COPD.[34,35] Furthermore, NE exosomes are generated from activated neutrophils that cannot be inhibited from the exosome membrane by AAT.[36] Whether these play a role in continued progression of emphysema while on augmentation therapy remains to be seen.

Clinical Lung Disease

In the years since the discovery of AATD, a variety of clinical lung diseases, including COPD with both emphysematous and chronic bronchitis phenotypes,[37] asthma, and bronchiectasis,[38] have been seen in patients with severe deficiency. Much of the work describing the natural history of AATD is derived from a study of 200,000 live births in Sweden between 1972-1974, in which 127 PiZZ infants were diagnosed. This birth cohort now is greater than 45 years of age with symptoms evident, particularly in smokers.[39] Nonsmoking individuals with AATD may get COPD but do so at an older age than smoking individuals. The life span of PiZZ individuals who do not smoke remains unknown although individuals are known who are greater than 90 years of age. Recent testing series suggest that the median age of diagnosis is 60 to 65 years, a decade prior to usual COPD diagnoses.

Table 1
The most common normal and deficiency alleles

		Exon	Comments
Normal alleles	M1 (Ala213)	III	Most common M allele
	M1 (Val213)	III	
	M2	II	
	M3	V	
	M4	II	
	M5	II	2 alleles, M5 berlin and M5 karlsruhe
	M6	II	
	L	II, III, V	2 alleles, L frankfurt and L offenbach
	V	II, V	3 alleles, V, V donauworth, and V munich
	X	III, V	2 alleles, X and X christchurch
	B	Unknown	B alhambra
	P	III, V	2 alleles, P st. louis and P albans
Deficiency alleles	Z	V	Most common severe deficiency gene
	S	III	Lesser degrees of deficiency than Z gene but more common
	M alleles	II, V	M herleen, M malton, M mineral springs, M procida, M bethesda, M palermo, and M nichinan
	W	V	
	I	II	Near-normal serum level with dysfunctional protein
	P	III	2 alleles, P lowell and P duarte
Dysfunctional allele	F	III	Low-normal serum level with dysfunctional protein
	Pittsburg	V	

Asthma is a clinically defined disease that may be more prevalent in PiMZ and PiZZ AATD.[39] Some studies have suggested that airway inflammation and clinical asthma diagnoses are simply the beginning symptoms of neutrophilic lung inflammation that advance to COPD. The excess incidence of allergic rhinitis in populations of MZ carriers and in PiZZ individuals,[40] however, suggests that asthma incidence may be independent of the COPD risk in AATD. Because most individuals with AATD present with wheezing and dyspnea as a first symptom and asthma is the most common misdiagnosis in AATD individuals, AAT testing once in a lifetime is recommended for all individuals with asthma whose spirometry fails to return to normal on appropriate treatment of asthma.[23]

COPD is common in AATD and almost universal after 5 years of cigarette smoking. Most of these individuals over the age of 40 have emphysema on a chest computed tomography (CT) that precedes spirometric obstruction. Emphysema, however, does not sufficiently dominate the clinical condition such that chronic bronchitis or asthma is rare.[37] Therefore, testing of all individuals regardless of COPD endotype is recommended. Nonsmokers tend to get radiographic emphysema after age 60 years.

Bronchiectasis, defined as permanent enlargement of 1 or more central airways, is increased in AATD. CT studies have suggested a prevalence of any airway being enlarged in 95% of PiZZ patients with clinically significant bronchiectasis found in 27%.[38] Bronchiectasis in AATD is associated with atypical mycobacterial infection, although it is not known whether this occurs due to colonization of bronchiectatic airways or defects in innate immunity from AATD.[41]

The only specific approved treatment of AATD is intravenous augmentation of plasma-derived AAT, first approved for severe deficiency of AATD in 1989. There now are many formulations of this pooled plasma-derived medication available in some countries. Randomized controlled studies have shown a slower decline in CT density over 2 years of administration compared with placebo.[42] Studies to date have not been powered to evaluate for exacerbation reduction or change in forced expiratory volume in the first second of expiration (FEV_1) decline.

There also is an important reduction in mortality seen in the National Institutes of Health National Heart, Lung, and Blood Institute observational registry that concluded in 1997. The mortality reduction was seen predominantly in the group receiving augmentation therapy with baseline FEV_1 less than 30%.[43] CT density decline independently has been correlated with mortality and quality of life in the ADAPT [Antitrypsin Deficiency Assessment and Programme for Treatment] Registry in the United Kingdom.[44,45]

Plasma-derived augmentation therapy usually is given intravenously, at a dose of 60 mg/kg/wk.[46] Studies administering the drug at 4-times the weekly dose every 4 weeks have been shown safe, but this large protein load leaves later timepoints with lower blood levels.[47] Ongoing studies continue to evaluate whether the 60 mg/kg/wk dose is suboptimal with regard to emphysema progression compared with doses of 120 mg/kg/wk.

Newer therapeutic options are in clinical trials. Low-molecular-weight compounds to improve intracellular folding of AAT have been developed that allow serum AAT levels to rise. Recombinant AAT with constructs that allow for longer serum half-life have been developed. Oral NE inhibitors remain in trials.

Other Aspects of Care

Because AATD is genetic in origin, identification of a deficient individual also identifies a family at risk.[48] This is a disease state that clinically presents most often in adulthood, but the risk factor modifications that diagnosis allows are lifelong. The Swedish birth cohort showed that diagnosed children were much more likely to be nonsmokers compared with the remainder of the age-matched

Swedish population.[49] Many investigators and patients have suggested that this reason is sufficient to put a test for AATD on infant genetic screening platforms, although comprehensive demonstration programs have not been done. Testing in a family is facilitated without cost through the Alpha-1 Foundation in the Alpha-1 Coded Testing Study. In this program, an online consent is followed by mailed testing materials that can facilitate testing of family members in distant sites from the index case.

Individuals diagnosed with AATD also need to be followed for clinical liver disease. Similar to lung disease, there are lifestyle modifications that improve the liver outcomes for these patients. Many of the 10% of individuals with clinical liver disease have the metabolic syndrome. As such, maintaining normal body weight is important.

In addition, therapies are available in clinical trials for AATD liver disease. Silencing RNA therapies are being developed that would send the serum level of AAT to lower values than normal because the mechanism is to shut off production of AAT in the hepatocyte. The hope is that less misfolded protein would lower the number and amount of AAT globules and AAT polymers. Therefore, liver injury might improve, analogous to cirrhosis from hepatitis C virus when the viral load is reduced. Unfortunately, there are no noninvasive tests to define with accuracy the amount of hepatic scar prior to the onset of portal hypertension. Therefore, there is much work being done to optimize imaging of the liver in AATD-affected patients. At a minimum, patients with COPD from AATD should have liver function assessed yearly after the age of 50 years. Patients with cirrhosis are at increased risk of hepatocellular carcinoma.

The last aspect of AATD that may be the most important is that this diagnosis allows a social networking opportunity with others with the disease that clearly has an impact on outcomes. The Alpha-1 Foundation is a patient-organized foundation that provides support and fosters research in AATD. AlphaNet is a disease management not-for-profit organization with a mission that includes disease management for affected individuals. The AlphaNet model places individuals who have AATD in place as peer coaches to improve the lives of other affected individuals. Every individual with AATD is invited to these programs.

SUMMARY

In summary, AATD is a rare genetic condition that results in COPD due to imbalances in protease-antiprotease protection in the lung. Recognition of the condition requires an inexpensive blood test for AAT concentration that should be obtained once in a lifetime from all individuals who have COPD, including those with clinical asthma when spirometry does not return to normal with therapy. Recognition of AATD improves a patient's environmental exposures to dust and fumes, improves smoking cessation efforts,[50] and allows access to AAT augmentation therapy and clinical trials for individuals severely deficient in AAT. Family screening is appropriate but commonly overlooked. Liver disease can be prospectively monitored to allow appropriate and timely interventions. The hope is that lessons learned from identifying and treating the population with AATD-associated COPD will help other genetic communities who are identified with COPD.

CONFLICT OF INTEREST

Dr C. Strange is a medical director of AlphaNet, a not-for-profit disease management company for AATD. Dr C. Strange consults on AATD with AstraZeneca, CSL Behring, Dicerna, Grifols, and Vertex. He has grants paid to the Medical University of South Carolina from Adverum, CSA Medical, CSL Behring, Grifols, MatRx, Novartis, Nuvaira, Pulmonx, Takeda, and Vertex.

REFERENCES

1. Laurell CB, Erickson S. The electrophoretic alpha-1-globulin pattern of serum in alpha-1-antitrypsin deficiency. Scand J Clin Lab Invest 1963;15:132–40.
2. Piitulainen E, Tornling G, Eriksson S. Environmental correlates of impaired lung function in non-smokers with severe alpha 1-antitrypsin deficiency (PiZZ). Thorax 1998;53(11):939–43.
3. Piitulainen E, Sveger T. Effect of environmental and clinical factors on lung function and respiratory symptoms in adolescents with alpha1-antitrypsin deficiency. Acta Paediatr 1998;87(11):1120–4.
4. Hutchison DC. Natural history of alpha-1-protease inhibitor deficiency. Am J Med 1988;84(6A):3–12.
5. Carrell RW, Jeppsson JO, Laurell CB, et al. Structure and variation of human alpha 1-antitrypsin. Nature 1982;298(5872):329–34.
6. Carlson JA, Rogers BB, Sifers RN, et al. Multiple tissues express alpha 1-antitrypsin in transgenic mice and man. J Clin Invest 1988;82(1):26–36.
7. Mornex JF, Chytil-Weir A, Martinet Y, et al. Expression of the alpha-1-antitrypsin gene in mononuclear phagocytes of normal and alpha-1-antitrypsin-deficient individuals. J Clin Invest 1986;77(6):1952–61.
8. Kalsheker N, Morley S, Morgan K. Gene regulation of the serine proteinase inhibitors alpha1-

antitrypsin and alpha1-antichymotrypsin. Biochem Soc Trans 2002;30(2):93–8.

9. Chowanadisai W, Lonnerdal B. Alpha(1)-antitrypsin and antichymotrypsin in human milk: origin, concentrations, and stability. Am J Clin Nutr 2002;76(4): 828–33.

10. Berman MB, Barber JC, Talamo RC, et al. Corneal ulceration and the serum antiproteases. I. Alpha 1-antitrypsin. Invest Ophthalmol 1973;12(10):759–70.

11. Boskovic G, Twining SS. Local control of alpha1-proteinase inhibitor levels: regulation of alpha1-proteinase inhibitor in the human cornea by growth factors and cytokines. Biochim Biophys Acta 1998; 1403(1):37–46.

12. Perlmutter DH, Punsal PI. Distinct and additive effects of elastase and endotoxin on expression of alpha 1 proteinase inhibitor in mononuclear phagocytes. J Biol Chem 1988;263(31):16499–503.

13. Knoell DL, Ralston DR, Coulter KR, et al. Alpha 1-antitrypsin and protease complexation is induced by lipopolysaccharide, interleukin-1beta, and tumor necrosis factor-alpha in monocytes. Am J Respir Crit Care Med 1998;157(1):246–55.

14. Morrison HM, Kramps JA, Burnett D, et al. Lung lavage fluid from patients with alpha 1-proteinase inhibitor deficiency or chronic obstructive bronchitis: anti-elastase function and cell profile. Clin Sci (Lond) 1987;72(3):373–81.

15. Soy D, de la Roza C, Lara B, et al. Alpha-1-antitrypsin deficiency: optimal therapeutic regimen based on population pharmacokinetics. Thorax 2006; 61(12):1059–64.

16. Perlmutter DH, Travis J, Punsal PI. Elastase regulates the synthesis of its inhibitor, alpha 1-proteinase inhibitor, and exaggerates the defect in homozygous PiZZ alpha 1 PI deficiency. J Clin Invest 1988;81(6): 1774–80.

17. Carrell RW, Jeppsson JO, Vaughan L, et al. Human alpha 1-antitrypsin: carbohydrate attachment and sequence homology. FEBS Lett 1981;135(2):301–3.

18. Wright HT, Scarsdale JN. Structural basis for serpin inhibitor activity. Proteins 1995;22(3):210–25.

19. Petrache I, Fijalkowska I, Zhen L, et al. A novel anti-apoptotic role for alpha1-antitrypsin in the prevention of pulmonary emphysema. Am J Respir Crit Care Med 2006;173(11):1222–8.

20. Petrache I, Fijalkowska I, Medler TR, et al. alpha-1 antitrypsin inhibits caspase-3 activity, preventing lung endothelial cell apoptosis. Am J Pathol 2006; 169(4):1155–66.

21. Carter RI, Ungurs MJ, Pillai A, et al. The relationship of the fibrinogen cleavage biomarker Aalpha-Val360 with Disease Severity and Activity in alpha1-antitrypsin deficiency. Chest 2015;148(2):382–8.

22. Newby PR, Crossley D, Crisford H, et al. A specific proteinase 3 activity footprint in alpha1-antitrypsin deficiency. ERJ Open Res 2019;5(3). 00095-2019.

23. American Thoracic Society, European Respiratory Society. American Thoracic Society/European Respiratory Society statement: standards for the diagnosis and management of individuals with alpha-1 antitrypsin deficiency. Am J Respir Crit Care Med 2003;168(7):818–900.

24. Okayama H, Brantly M, Holmes M, et al. Characterization of the molecular basis of the alpha 1-antitrypsin F allele. Am J Hum Genet 1991;48(6):1154–8.

25. Greulich T, Rodriguez-Frias F, Belmonte I, et al. Real world evaluation of a novel lateral flow assay (AlphaKit(R) QuickScreen) for the detection of alpha-1-antitrypsin deficiency. Respir Res 2018;19(1):151.

26. Molloy K, Hersh CP, Morris VB, et al. Clarification of the risk of chronic obstructive pulmonary disease in alpha1-antitrypsin deficiency PiMZ heterozygotes. Am J Respir Crit Care Med 2014;189(4):419–27.

27. Sandford AJ, Chagani T, Weir TD, et al. Susceptibility genes for rapid decline of lung function in the lung health study. Am J Respir Crit Care Med 2001;163(2):469–73.

28. Franciosi AN, Hobbs BD, McElvaney OJ, et al. Clarifying the risk of lung disease in SZ alpha1-antitrypsin deficiency. Am J Respir Crit Care Med 2020. https://doi.org/10.1164/rccm.202002-0262OC.

29. Hutchinson DC. Alpha-1 antitrypsin deficiency in Europe: geographicaal distribution of Pi types S and Z. Respir Med 1998;92:367–77.

30. de Serres FJ. Worldwide racial and ethnic distribution of alpha1-antitrypsin deficiency: summary of an analysis of published genetic epidemiologic surveys. Chest 2002;122(5):1818–29.

31. Sandhaus RA, Turino G, Brantly ML, et al. The diagnosis and management of alpha-1 antitrypsin deficiency in the adult. Chronic Obstr Pulm Dis 2016; 3(3):668–82.

32. Stoller JK, Sandhaus RA, Turino G, et al. Delay in diagnosis of alpha1-antitrypsin deficiency: a continuing problem. Chest 2005;128(4):1989–94.

33. Tan L, Dickens JA, Demeo DL, et al. Circulating polymers in alpha1-antitrypsin deficiency. Eur Respir J 2014;43(5):1501–4.

34. Mahadeva R, Atkinson C, Li Z, et al. Polymers of Z alpha1-antitrypsin co-localize with neutrophils in emphysematous alveoli and are chemotactic in vivo. Am J Pathol 2005;166(2):377–86.

35. Mulgrew AT, Taggart CC, Lawless MW, et al. Z alpha1-antitrypsin polymerizes in the lung and acts as a neutrophil chemoattractant. Chest 2004; 125(5):1952–7.

36. Genschmer KR, Russell DW, Lal C, et al. Activated PMN exosomes: pathogenic Entities causing matrix Destruction and disease in the lung. Cell 2019; 176(1–2):113–126 e115.

37. McElvaney NG, Stoller JK, Buist AS, et al. Baseline characteristics of enrollees in the National Heart, Lung and Blood Institute registry of alpha 1-

antitrypsin deficiency. Alpha 1-antitrypsin deficiency registry study group. Chest 1997;111(2):394–403.

38. Parr DG, Guest PG, Reynolds JH, et al. Prevalence and impact of bronchiectasis in alpha1-antitrypsin deficiency. Am J Respir Crit Care Med 2007; 176(12):1215–21.

39. Bernspang E, Sveger I, Piitulainen E. Respiratory symptoms and lung function in 30-year-old individuals with alpha-1-antitrypsin deficiency. Respir Med 2007;101(9):1971–6.

40. Eden E, Strange C, Holladay B, et al. Asthma and allergy in alpha-1 antitrypsin deficiency. Respir Med 2006;100(8):1384–91.

41. Adair-Kirk TL, Senior RM. Fragments of extracellular matrix as mediators of inflammation. Int J Biochem Cell Biol 2007;40(6–7):1101–10.

42. Chapman KR, Burdon JG, Piitulainen E, et al. Intravenous augmentation treatment and lung density in severe alpha1 antitrypsin deficiency (RAPID): a randomised, double-blind, placebo-controlled trial. Lancet 2015;386(9991):360–8.

43. Survival and FEV1 decline in individuals with severe deficiency of alpha1-antitrypsin. The alpha-1-antitrypsin deficiency registry study group. Am J Respir Crit Care Med 1998;158(1):49–59.

44. Dowson LJ, Guest PJ, Hill SL, et al. High-resolution computed tomography scanning in alpha1-antitrypsin deficiency: relationship to lung function and health status. Eur Respir J 2001;17(6): 1097–104.

45. Dawkins PA, Dowson LJ, Guest PJ, et al. Predictors of mortality in alpha1-antitrypsin deficiency. Thorax 2003;58(12):1020–6.

46. Wewers MD, Brantly ML, Casolaro MA, et al. Evaluation of tamoxifen as a therapy to augment alpha-1-antitrypsin concentrations in Z homozygous alpha-1-antitrypsin-deficient subjects. Am Rev Respir Dis 1987;135(2):401–2.

47. Hubbard RC, Sellers S, Czerski D, et al. Biochemical efficacy and safety of monthly augmentation therapy for alpha 1-antitrypsin deficiency. JAMA 1988; 260(9):1259–64.

48. Strange C, Dickson R, Carter C, et al. Genetic testing for alpha1-antitrypsin deficiency. Genet Med 2004;6(4):204–10.

49. Sveger T, Thelin T. A future for neonatal alpha1-antitrypsin screening? Acta Paediatr 2000;89(3): 259–61.

50. Carpenter MJ, Strange C, Jones Y, et al. Does genetic testing result in behavioral health change? Changes in smoking behavior following testing for alpha-1 antitrypsin deficiency. Ann Behav Med 2007;33(1):22–8.

Section II : Diagnosis and Assessment of COPD

Lung Function Testing in Chronic Obstructive Pulmonary Disease

J. Alberto Neder, MD, PhD, FRCP(C), FERS[a], Juan Pablo de-Torres, MD, PhD[a],
Kathryn M. Milne, MD FRCP(C)[a,b],
Denis E. O'Donnell, MD, FRCP(I), FRCP(C), FERS[a,*]

KEYWORDS

- Lung function • Dyspnea • COPD • Exertion • Diagnosis • Pulmonary function tests

KEY POINTS

- Expiratory airflow limitation is the defining physiologic abnormality of chronic obstructive pulmonary disease (COPD).
- Increase in resting lung volumes with further hyperinflation, when expiratory airflow limitation and increased ventilation are combined, has deleterious consequences for the sensory-perceptual and mechanical responses to physical activity.
- Lung function tests allow a detailed evaluation of the physiologic consequences of airway, alveolar, capillary, and respiratory muscle abnormalities induced by COPD.
- Physiologic parameters from pulmonary function tests are clinically relevant for diagnosis, assessment of disease severity, individualized management, and evaluation of the effect of treatment.
- Important complementary information can be obtained by integrated cardiopulmonary exercise testing, which includes noninvasive measurements of pulmonary gas exchange and lung mechanics, and exertional dyspnea ratings.

INTRODUCTION

Chronic obstructive pulmonary disease (COPD) is characterized by inflammatory injury of airways, lung parenchyma, and pulmonary vasculature secondary to noxious environmental exposures (eg, tobacco smoking, biomass, and fuel burning) in interaction with individual factors (eg, genetics, prematurity, small lung size).[1] A physiologic abnormality, poorly reversible expiratory airflow limitation on spirometry, is a key defining feature of the disease.[2] Most of the currently available pulmonary function tests (PFTs) were developed and clinically validated in patients with COPD.[3] In fact, no other chronic respiratory disease has been so thoroughly studied from the physiologic standpoint as COPD. Accordingly, PFTs remain central to the accurate diagnosis, assessment of disease severity, and evaluation of the effects of treatments in this highly prevalent disease (**Table 1**).[2] The current review discusses the practical applications of PFTs; thus, the authors specifically avoid detailed physiologic discussions, technical considerations, or epidemiologic implications of abnormal physiologic tests. They address specific scenarios in which PFTs can impact clinical decision making and help clinicians frame an individualized patient-centered approach to COPD management (**Box 1**).

[a] Division of Respiratory Medicine, Department of Medicine, Kingston Health Science Center, Queen's University, Richardson House, 102 Stuart Street, Kingston, Ontario K7L 2V6, Canada; [b] Clinician Investigator Program, Department of Medicine, University of British Columbia, Vancouver, British Columbia, Canada
* Corresponding author. Kingston Health Science Center, Queen's University, Richardson House, 102 Stuart Street, Kingston, Ontario K7L 2V6, Canada.
E-mail address: odonnell@queensu.ca

Clin Chest Med 41 (2020) 347–366
https://doi.org/10.1016/j.ccm.2020.06.004
0272-5231/20/© 2020 Elsevier Inc. All rights reserved.

chestmed.theclinics.com

Table 1
Summary of the expected results of pulmonary function tests in different clinical scenarios involving patients with chronic obstructive pulmonary disease

Test	Diagnostic Workup	Assessment of Disease Severity	Main Effects of BDs
Spirometry			
Key findings	• ↓ Post-BD FEV_1/FVC	• ↓ FEV_1	• ↑ FEV_1 used by regulatory bodies
Secondary findings	• ↓ $FEF_{25\%-75\%}$, ↓ $FEF_{25\%-75\%}/FVC$, ↓ FEV_1/FEV_6, ↓ FEV_3/FEV_6	• As disease progresses, ↓ FVC may reflect worsening gas trapping	• ↑ FVC and/or SVC may indicate less gas trapping
Lung volumes			
Key findings	• ↑ RV	• ↑ RV, ↓ IC (and ↓ IC/TLC)	• ↓ RV, ↑ IC (and ↑ IC/TLC)
Secondary findings	• ↑ FRC, ↑ TLC	• ↑ FRC, ↑ TLC	• ↓ FRC, ↓ TLC
Airway resistance			
Key findings	• ↑ sRaw	No current role	• ↓ sRaw
Small airway function			
SB N_2 washout	• ↑ phase III slope	No current role	• ↓ phase III slope
MB N_2 washout	• ↓ LCI, ↓ *Scond* and/or ↓ *Sacin*	No current role	• ↑ LCI, ↑ *Scond* and/or ↑ *Sacin*
FOT	• ↑ X_5	• ↑ X_5	• ↓ ΔX_{rs}
Arterial blood gases			
Key findings	Variable	• ↓ Pao_2, ↑ $Paco_2$	Variable
Gas transfer			
Key findings	• ↓ DL_{CO} and/or ↓ K_{CO}	• ↓ DL_{CO}	No current role
RM strength	No current role	• MIP may ↓ due to hyperinflation	• MIP may ↑ due to lung deflation
6-MWT	Variable	• ↓ 6-MWD. ↓ SpO_2	• 6-MWD may or not ↑
CPET			
Incremental	• ↓ ventilatory efficiency • ↑ operating lung volumes • ↑ dyspnea/WR and/or ventilation	• ↑ operating lung volumes • ↑ dyspnea/WR and ventilation	• ↓ operating lung volumes • ↓ dyspnea/WR and ventilation
Constant work rate	No current role	No current role	• ↑ Tlim • ↑ IC and ↓ dyspnea at isotime

Abbreviations: ↑, increased; ↓, decreased; 6-MWD, 6-min walking distance; CO, carbon monoxide; *K*, transfer coefficient; LCI, lung clearance index; MB, multiple breath; Pa, arterial partial pressure; RM, respiratory muscle; SB, single breath; *Scond*, ventilation heterogeneity in the acinar airways; *Scond*, ventilation heterogeneity in the conducting (preacinar) airways; SpO_2, oxygen saturation by pulse oximetry; sRaw, specific airway resistance; Tlim, time to exercise limitation; WR, work rate; X_5, reactance at 5 Hz; ΔX_{rs}, differences between inspiratory and expiratory phases of respiratory reactance.

> **Box 1**
> **Expiratory airflow limitation**
>
> A physiologic abnormality, poorly reversible expiratory airflow limitation on spirometry, is a key defining feature of COPD.

STRUCTURAL AND PHYSIOLOGIC BASIS OF RESPIRATORY DYSFUNCTION IN CHRONIC OBSTRUCTIVE PULMONARY DISEASE
Rest

The small airways (ie, <2 mm diameter, noncartilaginous bronchioles) constitute the initial locus of inflammation and increased airway resistance in COPD.[4] Several studies have shown evidence of active inflammation and obliteration of peripheral airways even in the earlier stages of the disease.[5] Loss of alveolar attachments as a result of emphysema contributes to greater collapsibility of small airways on expiration and increased resistance to airflow.[6] Airway narrowing owing to mucosal edema, mucus plugging, airway remodeling, and peribronchial fibrosis together with reduced lung elastic recoil predispose to dynamic airway closure.[4] It follows that even during spontaneous tidal breathing, many patients generate the maximal possible flow rates at that particular lung volume, a phenomenon termed expiratory flow limitation (EFL).[7]

The volume of air left in the lungs at the end of a quiet expiration is termed end-expiratory lung volume (EELV) and is used interchangeably with functional residual capacity (FRC). The relaxation volume (Vr) of the respiratory system refers to the equilibrium point where the algebraic sum of the outward recoil of the chest wall and the inward recoil of the lungs is zero.[8] Consequently, the alveolar and mouth pressure are also zero at end-expiration. In COPD, emphysema can result in increased compliance, such that EELV exceeds the Vr, often termed "static" or resting lung hyperinflation.[9] However, in patients with resting EFL, EELV is a dynamic variable that varies with the prevailing breathing pattern. In other words, EELV is dynamically as well as "statically" determined.[10] Thus, when breathing frequency increases, expiratory time is often insufficient to allow EELV to decline to the natural Vr, contributing to lung hyperinflation.[11] In such individuals with significant EFL and increased EELV at rest, alveolar and mouth pressure are still positive at the onset of inspiration.[9] Lung hyperinflation places the inspiratory muscles, particularly the diaphragm, at a significant mechanical disadvantage by shortening its fibers, thereby decreasing its force-

generating capacity.[12] Moreover, it forces tidal breathing to occur closer to total lung capacity (TLC) and the upper, nonlinear, poorly compliant, portion of the respiratory system's pressure-volume relaxation curve.[13] High inspiratory threshold (auto-positive end-expiratory pressure effect) and elastic loading of the functionally weakened inspiratory muscles require a greater inspiratory neural drive or electrical activation to generate a given force, a key mechanism of dyspnea in these patients (**Fig. 1**).[13,14]

The efficiency of pulmonary gas exchange in COPD is compromised by several mechanisms[2]:

- Inhomogeneity of alveolar ventilation (VA) distribution caused by vastly dissimilar mechanical time constants (product of resistance and compliance) for emptying of alveolar units in different lung regions;
- Regional lung hyperinflation with extrinsic compression of adjacent parenchyma, blood vessels, and small airways; and
- Heterogeneity of alveolar and vascular destruction owing to emphysema and vascular inflammation.

Overall, there is a trend for patients with predominant emphysema to show more extensive areas of high VA/capillary perfusion (Qc) ratios, whereas those with predominant chronic bronchitis may have low VA/Qc regions as a result of increased small airways resistance and mucus plugging.[15] However, it is clear that in many patients with COPD lacking specific phenotypical characteristics, VA/Qc abnormalities can be quite heterogenous.[16] Vascular injury may occur before, simultaneously, or after the described small airway abnormalities; increased intimal thickness owing to deposition of extracellular matrix proteins and muscle cell proliferation contributes to increased pulmonary vascular resistance.[17,18] Compensatory adaptations of the central respiratory controller can preserve arterial oxygenation and acid-base status in patients with less severe COPD.[19] However, these compensatory adjustments fail to varying degrees with disease progression. Thus, abnormalities in ventilatory control, critical respiratory muscle weakness, and the negative mechanical effects of lung hyperinflation culminate in decreased VA leading to variable degrees of hypoxemia and ultimately to CO_2 retention (**Box 2**).[14]

Exercise

Resting physiologic abnormalities are substantially amplified during the stress of exercise in patients with COPD.[2] Exercise intolerance in COPD,

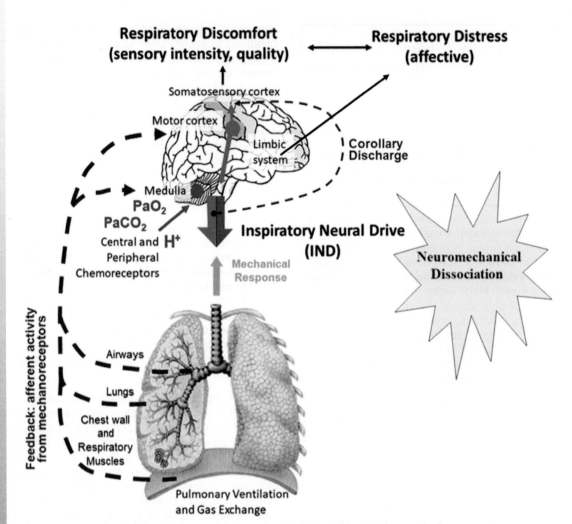

Fig. 1. Neuromechanical dissociation and dyspnea in COPD. Neural inputs that reach the somatosensory cortex and contribute to intensity and quality of dyspnea come from (i) increased central corollary discharge from brainstem and cortical motor centers; (ii) altered afferent information from receptors in the airways, lungs, locomotor, and respiratory muscles; and (iii) information from central and peripheral chemoreceptors regarding the adequacy of ventilation and gas exchange. When the mechanical/muscular response of the respiratory system is constrained in the face of increasing inspiratory neural drive (IND), the intensity of "respiratory discomfort" increases and the sense of "unsatisfied inspiration" dominates as neuromechanical dissociation occurs. Concomitant increased activation of limbic structures also likely contributes to "respiratory distress." [H$^+$], hydrogen ion concentration; Paco$_2$, partial pressure of arterial carbon dioxide; Pao$_2$, partial pressure of arterial oxygen. (*Adapted from* O'Donnell DE, Ora J, Webb KA, et al. Mechanisms of activity-related dyspnea in pulmonary diseases. Respir Physiol Neurobiol 2009;167(1):116-32; with permission.)

Box 2
Consequences of lung hyperinflation
Lung hyperinflation shortens the inspiratory muscles' fibers: high inspiratory threshold and elastic loading of the functionally weakened inspiratory muscles require a greater inspiratory neural drive to generate a given force, a key mechanism of dyspnea in COPD.

however, is characteristically multifactorial with the exact mechanisms varying widely across the spectrum of disease severity and among patients with similar degrees of resting respiratory impairment.[20] During exercise when ventilation increases, temporary and variable increase in EELV above its resting value occurs (dynamic lung hyperinflation [DH]), because of the combination of tachypnea and EFL.[21] DH is manifest as a progressive reduction of inspiratory capacity (IC) and inspiratory reserve volume (IRV) at relatively

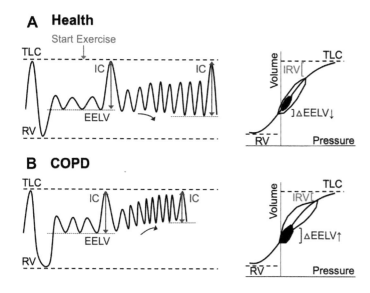

Fig. 2. Operating lung volumes at rest and during exercise (*left*) and the corresponding respiratory system pressure-volume relationship (*right*) in (*A*) a healthy subject and (*B*) a patient with COPD. In the healthy subject, EELV decreases during exercise, leading to a higher IC. In the COPD patient, EELV increases and IC is reduced. In COPD, the patient breathes at a higher, less compliant portion of the P-V curve where the work of breathing is increased. As a result, there is less "room" for VT expansion (lower IC) and a lower IRV is reached at lower exercise intensity. (*Adapted from* O'Donnell DE. Hyperinflation, dyspnea, and exercise intolerance in chronic obstructive pulmonary disease. Proc Am Thorac Soc. 2006;3(2):180-4; with permission.)

low exercise intensities in the setting of largely preserved TLC.[20] Acute-on-chronic lung hyperinflation during exercise amplifies elastic and inspiratory threshold loading of the already burdened inspiratory muscles and results in intolerable dyspnea and exercise limitation (**Fig. 2**).[14,22]

In patients with mild-to-moderate COPD, 1 consistent abnormality has been the finding of higher than normal ventilation ($\dot{V}E$)-carbon dioxide production ($\dot{V}CO_2$) relationship (ventilatory inefficiency) (**Fig. 3**) secondary to[23]

- Increased physiologic dead space (high dead space ventilation [VD]/tidal volume [VT] ratio); and/or
- Altered chemosensitivity with mild alveolar hyperventilation, potentially leading to a chronically reduced arterial partial pressure of CO_2 ($Paco_2$).

Preservation of the arterial partial pressure for oxygen (Pao_2) during exercise in these patients is a result of compensatory increases in inspiratory neural drive and $\dot{V}E$ to overcome a high VD/VT.[24] In addition, altered afferent feedback from ergoreceptors responding to early metabolic acidosis (deconditioning) or mechanical distortion in active peripheral muscles, together with increased sympathetic nervous system activation, can directly stimulate ventilation.[25] Increased return of poorly oxygenated mixed venous blood during exercise[26] (because of reduced O_2 delivery or increased extraction)[27] to areas of low VA/Qc in the lungs may precipitate (or worsen) arterial hypoxemia.[15]

DH and ventilatory inefficiency are not independent: high $\dot{V}E$-$\dot{V}CO_2$ and the consequent increased stimulus for inspiratory neural drive and ventilation accelerate the rate of DH leading to earlier attainment of critical inspiratory mechanical constraints because the end-inspiratory lung volume approaches, TLC and IRV disappear (**Fig. 4**).[28] Low IC decreases the reserve for VT expansion, which, in turn, tends to increase VD/VT, potentially compromising CO_2 elimination.[29] As COPD worsens, and the relative contribution of mechanical constraints to dyspnea and exercise

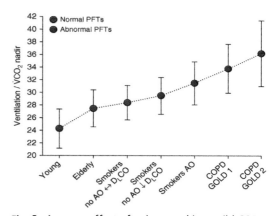

Fig. 3. Average effect of aging, smoking, mild COPD, and moderate COPD on $\dot{V}CO_2$ nadir, a metric of exercise ventilatory inefficiency. The modulating influence of airflow obstruction (AO) and decrements (*downward arrow*) in lung DL_{CO} in smokers are also shown. Values are mean ± standard deviation. GOLD, Global Initiative for Chronic Obstructive Lung Disease. (*From* Neder JA, Berton DC, Müller P de T, et al. Ventilatory Inefficiency and Exertional Dyspnea in Early Chronic Obstructive Pulmonary Disease. Ann Am Thorac Soc. 2017;14:S22-29; with permission.)

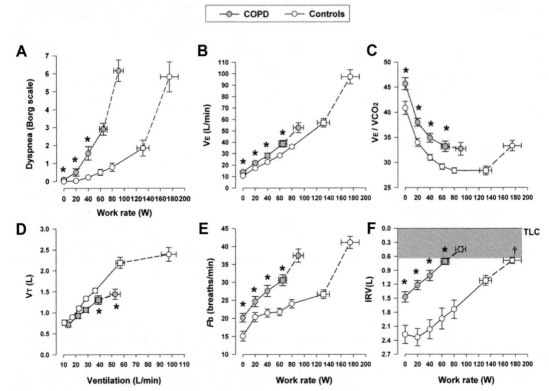

Fig. 4. Select panels from cardiopulmonary exercise tests in COPD (solid symbols) compared with healthy controls (open symbols). (*A*) Dyspnea intensity and (*B*) ventilatory response to exercise are higher in COPD stimulated in part by increased (*C*) ventilatory inefficiency. As mechanical constraints develop during exercise, a rapid shallow breathing pattern emerges in COPD (*D, E*) and critical reduction in IRV (*F*) occurs. Fb, breathing frequency; V$_E$, minute ventilation. * $p < 0.05$: patients versus controls. (*Adapted from* Faisal A, Alghamdi B, Ciavaglia CE, et al. Common mechanisms of dyspnea in chronic interstitial and obstructive lung disorders. Am J Respir Crit Care Med. 2016;193(3):299-309; with permission.)

intolerance increases markedly, deterioration of pulmonary gas exchange and acid-base balance increases metabolic demand in the setting of a reduced capacity of the respiratory system to adequately respond.[29]

Exertional dyspnea increases steeply during exercise as inspiratory neural drive progressively increases in the face of demand-capacity imbalance.[30] Thus, a high inspiratory neural drive in COPD patients stems from (see **Fig. 1**; **Box 3**)[31] the following:

- Increased efferent output from central chemo-sensitive receptors in the medulla responding

to altered afferent inputs owing to the effects of increased wasted ventilation, early metabolic acidosis, critical arterial O$_2$ desaturation, increased ergo-receptor activation, sympathetic nervous system overactivation, and altered cardiovascular afferent activity; and/or
- Increased cortical motor command output owing to increased respiratory muscle loading and functional weakness secondary to accelerated dynamic mechanical abnormalities.

LUNG FUNCTION TESTS IN THE DIAGNOSTIC ASSESSMENT OF CHRONIC OBSTRUCTIVE PULMONARY DISEASE

The prevalence of COPD varies widely across the globe. Underdiagnosis and overdiagnosis have been estimated between 10% and 95% and 5% and 60%, respectively.[32,33] These discrepancies are largely ascribed to differences in defining criteria for poorly reversible airflow obstruction within the framework of COPD diagnosis.

Box 3
Dynamic hyperinflation

Acute-on-chronic lung hyperinflation during exercise amplifies elastic and inspiratory threshold loading of the already burdened inspiratory muscles and results in intolerable exertional dyspnea and exercise limitation.

Current Controversies in Defining Airflow Limitation

Forced expiratory volume in 1 second/forced vital capacity cutoff

During a forced expiratory maneuver from TLC to residual volume (RV), the largest fraction of exhaled volume (forced vital capacity, FVC) occurs at the earliest phase of expiration (ie, forced expiratory volume in 1 second, FEV_1) with the subsequent exhaled volume decreasing with increased time of the expiratory maneuver.[34] It follows that the FEV_1/FVC ratio is greater than 0.5 in most normal healthy individuals.[35] Complicating the use of the FEV_1/FVC ratio thresholds in the diagnosis of COPD are the naturally occurring changes in pulmonary function with age.[36] With aging, loss of lung elastic recoil occurs, resulting in a decreasing FEV_1/FVC ratio.[37] Thus, whereas ratios near 0.85 are seen in normal children, values less than 0.6 might lie within the expected range in the very old. Ratios ≥ 0.7 are observed in most middle-aged subjects (**Fig. 5**).[35] Expiratory airflow limitation arises in COPD when the pathologic loss of lung elastic recoil and/or small airway obstruction and increased airway collapsibility on expiration slows the rate of lung emptying (see *Structural and physiologic basis of respiratory dysfunction in chronic obstructive pulmonary disease: Rest*); consequently, flows are reduced for a given volume.[4] It follows that an FEV_1 lower than expected for FVC after bronchodilator (BD) and a FEV_1/FVC ratio below a critical defined threshold are thought to reflect the presence of airflow limitation in these subjects.[1,38]

Persistent airflow limitation has been defined by a post-BD FEV_1/FVC ratio less than 0.7[1] or below the lower limit of normal (LLN).[36] The fixed ratio cutoff, however, can lead to overdiagnosis of COPD in the elderly, particularly when an FEV_1/FVC ratio is interpreted without the important context of respiratory symptoms and exposures to risk factors. Conversely, underdiagnosis of COPD can occur in younger individuals (<40–45 years).[39] The LLN has a more solid statistical rationale, although its use remains largely restricted to epidemiologic research rather than clinical practice.[36] The wide confidence interval for FEV_1/FVC ratio increases the likelihood of underdiagnosis of COPD, particularly in the elderly and symptomatic smokers.[40] The topic of spirometric criteria for COPD diagnosis remains highly controversial with an almost similar number of articles supporting each of these competing definitions.[33,40] Of note, a recent study found evidence that a sizable fraction of smokers with FEV1/FVC ratio in-between the LLN and 0.7 present with exercise abnormalities consistent with COPD (see Structural and physiologic basis of respiratory dysfunction in chronic obstructive pulmonary disease: Exercise),[41]

It should be noted that, in practice, many smokers with FEV_1/FVC ratio ≥ 0.7 report respiratory symptoms and present with structural changes (emphysema and airway wall thickening)[42] similar to their counterparts with lower fixed-ratio values.[43] Some of these patients with maintained FEV_1/FVC ratios have a low FEV_1, a pattern recently named preserved ratio impaired spirometry (PRISm),[44] and others did not (ie, abnormalities found exclusively on imaging but not on spirometry). The pseudorestrictive, "nonspecific" pattern (if associated with preserved TLC) was originally described by Hyatt and coworkers[45] many years ago. In these patients, low FEV_1 is fundamentally related to a low FVC, which, in turn, may reflect the constraining effects of obesity and other possible comorbidities (heart failure, diabetes)[44] in addition to decreased VC resulting from increased RV and early airway closure.[46] Because of dynamic collapse of small airways during a forced expiratory maneuver, FVC might underestimate VC; consequently, the low denominator would lead to a normal FEV_1/FVC ratio despite the presence of significant airway disease.[47] Indeed, slow vital capacity (SVC) has been found to enhance the yield of spirometry in detecting mild airflow obstruction

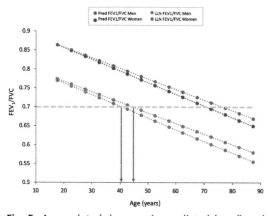

Fig. 5. Age- related decrease in predicted (pred) and LLN for FEV_1/FVC ratio in men and women. Note that a sizable fraction of normal subjects older than 50 may present with FEV_1/FVC greater than 0.70. (*Adapted from* Tan WC, Bourbeau J, Hernandez P, et al. Canadian prediction equations of spirometric lung function for caucasian adults 20 to 90 years of age: results from the Canadian Obstructive Lung Disease (COLD) study and the Lung Health Canadian Environment (LHCE) study. Can Respir J. 2011;18(6):321-6; with permission.)

in younger and obese subjects; however, a low FEV_1/SVC ratio but preserved FEV_1/FVC ratio may represent a false positive for airflow limitation in the elderly.[48] The diagnostic role of a low $FEV_1/$ forced inspiratory VC ratio also remains elusive and warrants study in larger prospective studies.[49]

Because of concerns related to diagnostic stability of a single measurement of the post-BD FEV_1/FVC ratio, there is some evidence that spirometry should be repeated on a separate occasion if the value is between 0.6 and 0.8.[50] Specifically, if the initial post-BD FEV_1/FVC ratio is less than 0.6, it is very unlikely to increase greater than 0.7 spontaneously, whereas values greater than 0.8 are unlikely to decrease to less than 0.7.[50] These assertions, however, should be tempered with practicalities: (a) repeating spirometry on a short-term basis is not a trivial task in most health care systems and (b) the risk of false positive or false negative results of any diagnostic test is always judged by the physician on an individual basis: clinical history, dyspnea severity, and likelihood of an alternative diagnosis in those at risk for COPD (**Box 4**).

Alternatives to forced expiratory volume in 1 second/forced vital capacity in detecting and defining airflow limitation

As mentioned, the FEV_1/FVC ratio may remain within the normal range even after considerable small airway pathologic condition has occurred.[51] It has been argued that defining a fixed time denominator "to correct" FEV_1 would decrease variability of the ratio. The FEV_6 maneuver, for example, is more easily performed than FVC for patients with severe COPD[52]; however, FEV_6 is expected to be a larger fraction of any imposed expiratory time duration during the test shorter than that required for full expiration. Thus, FEV_1/FEV_6 may be within the normal range in patients with particularly slow rates of lung emptying.[53(p6)]

Mid-FVC expiratory airflow (forced expiratory flow between 25% and 75% [$FEF_{25-75\%}$]) is

frequently reduced when FEV_1 is lower than predicted and adds little new information.[3] Nevertheless, a sizable fraction of symptomatic smokers/ex-smokers with structural evidence of COPD on computed tomography (CT) has a low $FEF_{25\%-75\%}$ despite a preserved FEV_1.[54] Critics of using $FEF_{25\%-75\%}$ to detect clinically significant airflow obstruction argue that its high variability precludes a meaningful interpretation[55]; moreover, a low $FEF_{25\%-75\%}$ might merely reflect an equally reduced FVC. $FEF_{25\%-75\%}$ divided by FVC corresponds to effort-independent expiratory airflow adjusted for lung volume. Thus, a low $FEF_{25\%-75\%}/FVC$ ratio reflects a lower elastic recoil or reduced small airway size for a given lung volume,[56] being potentially more useful than $FEF_{25\%-75\%}$ alone. FEV_3 has been proposed as superior to FEV_1 in detecting small airways dysfunction while avoiding the limitations of $FEF_{25\%-75\%}$. In fact, some studies reported that a greater number of smokers showing FEV_3/FEV_6 below the LLN had preserved FEV_1/FEV_6 ratio.[57] However, the clinical importance of these newer indices to improve the diagnostic yield of spirometry (without increasing false-positive results) in individual patients remains unclear.[50]

Tests of small airway function

A small proportion of the total lower airway resistance is attributable to small airways less than 2 mm in diameter.[6] As discussed in *Structural and physiologic basis of respiratory dysfunction in chronic obstructive pulmonary disease*, there is robust evidence that structural abnormalities of these small airways largely precede emphysema and the phenotypical exteriorization of COPD.[5] Functional (and anatomic) assessment of the so-called quiet zone,[58] however, is fraught with complexities; thus, disease can progress over many years without being noticed by traditional PFTs or even high-resolution CT. Single-breath (phase III slope)[59] and multiple-breath nitrogen washout (lung clearing index)[60] probes ventilation distribution homogeneity. The latter test, in particular, may provide further information on the possible mechanisms behind abnormal ventilation distribution and the relative location of underlying pathologic processes, for example, ventilation heterogeneity in conducting airways and the small airways in acinar regions.[61] The forced oscillation technique (FOT) is a promising tool because it is performed without the need of a voluntary effort as is the case of the FVC maneuver, and thus it can be performed in children and individuals incapable of performing most lung function testing. FOT provides measurement of resistance and reactance of the respiratory system, allowing

---

Box 4
Forced spirometry on the diagnosis of chronic obstructive pulmonary disease

FEV_1/FVC less than 0.7 can lead to overdiagnosis of COPD in the elderly, particularly when interpreted without consideration of respiratory symptoms and exposures to risk factors. Conversely, the wide confidence interval for FEV_1/FVC increases the likelihood of underdiagnosis based on the LLN, particularly in the elderly and symptomatic smokers.

derivation of the frequency dependence of resistance, that is, nonuniformity of mechanical time constants for emptying because of regional variation in compliance and resistance.[62] These tests have shown acceptable reproducibility and responsiveness to interventions in population-based studies[63]; moreover, they do correlate to some extent with the severity of dyspnea[64] and changes in clinical status, for example, acute COPD exacerbation.[65] Additional studies are necessary to provide population normative reference values for the various parameters measured in these tests in order to determine their utility in COPD diagnosis and in phenotyping of symptomatic smokers who do not meet current spirometric criteria. Thus, their usefulness beyond traditional PFTs in the management of individual patients remains unclear: at this point in time, FOT seems the most promising test for use in the clinical arena (see **Table 1**).[63]

The added value of lung volumes, airway resistance, and lung diffusing capacity for carbon monoxide

There is growing recognition that spirometry alone is insufficient to diagnose and phenotype COPD.[66] There has been significant investment and development of quantitative CT imaging and biomarkers in COPD diagnosis[66]; however, beyond spirometry, additional easily available PFTs can provide information helpful in COPD diagnosis that is complementary to changes visualized on imaging.[67] In several circumstances, assessment of resting or "static" lung volumes and lung diffusing capacity for carbon monoxide (DL_{CO}) provides critical information to increase or decrease the probability of COPD:

- In smokers suspected of having COPD with equivocal findings on spirometry (eg, $0.7 < FEV_1/FVC$ ratio $> LLN$, PRISm criteria),[68] a high pretest probability of COPD, high RV greater than 120% predicted (absolute pulmonary gas trapping), RV/TLC ratio greater than 0.40 (relative gas trapping), and/or FRC >120% predicted (lung hyperinflation) might help to confirm the presence of COPD. These cutoffs are arbitrary, which nevertheless provide insight into the nature of underlying physiologic impairment beyond simple spirometry.[19]
- Conversely, absence of any of these findings decreases the probability of COPD in a non-obese subject.[69]
- In those showing low FEV_1/FVC ratio and low FVC, assessment of lung volumes might clarify whether the reduced FVC is related to a low

ceiling ($\downarrow$ TLC indicating associated restriction) or a high floor ($\uparrow$ RV), the latter finding further corroborating the diagnosis of COPD.[19]
- Although airway resistance is a highly variable measurement with large reference limits, it may provide evidence to suggest COPD in equivocal cases.[70]
- Regardless of FEV_1 or FEV_1/FVC ratio, a low DL_{CO} (indicating disruption of the alveolar/capillary interface or maldistribution of VA) is expected to occur in a subject with predominance of emphysema over chronic bronchitis, provided recent smoking (increased carboxyhemoglobin [Hb-CO]) and confounders (eg, anemia, pulmonary vascular disease, early interstitial lung disease) are not present (**Fig. 6**).[71,72]

Despite early enthusiasm, relating DL_{CO} to lung diffusing capacity (DL) for nitric oxide to separate out the relative contribution of the "membrane" and "hematic" components of alveolar gas transfer[73] has not gained clinical popularity in the assessment of patients with COPD (**Box 5**).[74]

LUNG FUNCTION TESTS IN THE ASSESSMENT OF DISEASE SEVERITY

Assessment of disease severity in COPD is, in part, complicated by heterogeneous COPD phenotypes from a physiologic and symptom and structural (imaging) perspective. Understanding how structure-function-symptom linkages vary in COPD remains an area of ongoing and future research. The challenges remain to capture, in a succinct and clinically meaningful way, the various combinations of imaging, physiologic and symptom burden patterns, and their relative importance. In light of these exciting challenges, the authors review the contribution of physiologic tests, including measures of airflow, lung volumes, gas exchange, respiratory muscle function, and integrated cardiopulmonary exercise testing (CPET) in assessing disease severity.

Spirometry, Lung Volumes, and Airway Resistance

FEV_1 has long been considered the most important measurement of COPD severity.[75] Although this simplified approach may work to some extent at a population level, and in situations whereby access to full PFTs is limited, it can also be misleading from a clinical standpoint. Indeed, FEV_1 alone gives little insight into the nature and degree of heterogeneous physiologic impairment in the individual. Moreover, it does not relate well to the severity of clinical (eg, symptoms,

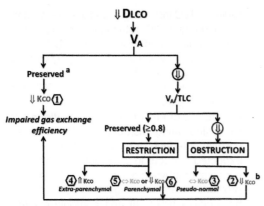

Fig. 6. A simplified algorithm to further interpret the meaning of a low ($\Downarrow$) lung DL_{CO} (< LLN) taking into consideration the caveats outlined in the text. If the accessible alveolar volume (VA) is preserved ($\Leftrightarrow$), the DL_{CO}/VA ratio (K_{CO}) will be low, that is, there is impaired gas exchange efficiency due to pulmonary vascular disease, right-to-left shunt or mild emphysema, and others (*scenario 1*). If VA is reduced, the next step is to check whether the VA/TLC ratio is low due to ventilation maldistribution secondary to an obstructive airway disease. A low VA/TLC may "normalize" K_{CO}, precluding any further interpretation of this index (*scenario 3*). However, if K_{CO} is reduced *despite* a low VA/TLC, there is impaired gas exchange efficiency (eg, extensive emphysema) (*scenario 2*). Conversely, if VA/TLC is preserved, a high ($\Uparrow$) K_{CO} here signals extraparenchymal restriction (*scenario 4*), that is, capillary volume is relatively greater than alveolar volume (eg, neuromuscular, pleural, and chest wall diseases). Parenchymal restriction (eg, interstitial lung disease) may be associated with either preserved K_{CO} (*scenario 5*) or a low K_{CO} (*scenario 6*). Whereas *scenario 5* does not allow further mechanistic elaboration (because of the trend of a low VA to normalize K_{CO}), *scenario 6* also indicates impaired pulmonary gas exchange efficiency. [a] A normal VA may coexist with airflow obstruction in a patient with mild airflow limitation in whom the distributive abnormalities are not severe enough to decrease VA/TLC less than 0.8. [b] VA may still lie in the normal range despite a low VA/TLC in a severely hyperinflated patient (high TLC). (*From* Neder JA, Berton DC, Muller PT, O'Donnell DE. Incorporating lung diffusing capacity for carbon monoxide in clinical decision making in chest medicine. Clin Chest Med. 2019;40(2):285-305; with permission.)

Box 5
The value of additional physiological testing

Beyond spirometry, additional easily available PFTs (resting or "static" lung volumes and DL_{CO}) can provide information helpful in COPD diagnosis and complementary to changes visualized on imaging.

---

exacerbation burden) and structural abnormalities (eg, emphysema, airways disease and vascular attenuation on CT) in individual patients.[76] Nevertheless, severe to very severe decrements in FEV_1 are somewhat useful to predict negative functional outcomes, including exertional hypoxemia, and to a lesser extent, activity-related dyspnea. There have been new attempts to classify the severity of FEV_1 using additional statistical criteria (z scores)[77]; however, these cutoffs have not yet been clinically validated in patients with COPD. In contrast, there is solid evidence that functional derangements and clinical outcomes (eg, mortality, cardiocirculatory impairment, exercise tolerance, dyspnea) are more closely related to lung hyperinflation, reduced IC (and IC/TLC ratio),[78] and low DL_{CO} and are superior to FEV_1 in estimating the burden of disease.[21] In fact, there is a large variability of these abnormalities at a given FEV_1, providing a rationale for its poor performance in gauging disease severity. There is little evidence that specific airway resistance provides additional information to spirometry and lung volumes in determining the severity of COPD.[63]

Gas Exchange: DL_{CO} and Arterial Blood Gases

There is well-established evidence that a low single-breath DL_{CO} is a key correlate of exertional dyspnea and reduced exercise capacity across the spectrum of COPD severity.[71,72,79] Importantly, this is true regardless of the underlying mechanism, that is, either a slow rate of gas transfer or a low alveolar volume.[80] The former scenario indicates reduced anatomic and/or functional surface area for alveolar-capillary gas exchange (eg, emphysema, pulmonary vascular disease), high Hb-CO (heavy smoking), and/or anemia, all causes of poor exercise tolerance. Conversely, a low VA points to poor ventilation distribution, an important predictor of impaired gas exchange efficiency in COPD.[81]

A major point of confusion about DL_{CO} interpretation in COPD, however, arises from the misconception that a "preserved" DL_{CO}/VA (diffusing coefficient, K_{CO}) provides evidence that intrapulmonary gas exchange efficiency is normal. This common mistake is the result of the lack of recognition that K_{CO} may lie within its (large) reference ranges provided that VA substantially underestimates TLC, which occurs when VA/TLC is less than 0.8. In other words, a low VA/TLC ratio implies that a sizable fraction of aerated alveoli (measured by TLC) was not properly exposed to the inert gas used in the DL_{CO} measurement.[81,82] This caveat has led some experts to even declare that "K_{CO} is a flawed index," which should be excluded from

PFTs reports.[83] However, if the PFT interpreter (and the requesting physician) is aware of this source of confusion, this variable can help in the clinical interpretation of DL_{CO} (see **Fig. 6**).[84,85] For instance, a low K_{CO} *despite* a low VA/TLC ratio (which would otherwise conspire to normalize K_{CO}) signals extensive destruction/reduction of the functioning alveolar-capillary membrane, usually extensive emphysema in patients with COPD.[85] If the emphysema burden is deemed only "mild" or absent (and the patient is not anemic or has recently smoked before testing), further investigations are warranted to provide a reasonable explanation for this finding, such as pulmonary vascular disease and right-to-left shunt.[86,87]

Resting hypoxemia is a well-established marker of more advanced COPD.[88] Whether this is also true for exercise-induced hypoxemia remains highly controversial.[89] Regardless of its cause (usually mechanical),[29,90] persistent hypercapnia also signals severe to very severe COPD, particularly if there is long-standing compensated hypercapnic respiratory failure. Sleep-disordered breathing, a common comorbidity of COPD, may be associated with increased $Paco_2$ regardless of the severity of the disease as assessed by PFTs.[91] Conversely, some patients with coexistent heart failure may in fact be hypocapnic despite fairly severe COPD, an important correlate of exertional dyspnea (**Box 6**).[92]

Respiratory Muscle Function

Maximal (static) inspiratory pressure (MIP) and sniff inspiratory pressure decrease as COPD progresses.[93] However, this is largely proportional to the degree of lung hyperinflation and therefore represents functional (not intrinsic) respiratory muscle weakness, and the expected decrease in pressure-generating capacity when the inspiratory maneuver starts from a higher lung volume.[94] There is a theoretic rationale supporting the concept that isolated inspiratory muscle weakness indicates systemic consequences of COPD (myopathy, sarcopenia).[95] Nevertheless, there is no clear evidence that there is an independent role of these static respiratory muscle maximal pressure measurements to gauge disease severity. However, maximal pressure measurements may be relevant when

selecting patients for consideration of specific inspiratory muscle training.[96,97]

Exercise

Walking tests

Field exercise tests are poorly informative when interrogating mechanisms of exercise limitation in COPD. Nevertheless, the distance covered in the 6-minute walking test (6MWT) does correlate with disease severity; it may clinically help detect oxygen desaturation during exercise and has been successfully incorporated in popular multiparametric prognostic indices that relate well to important outcomes, such as exacerbations and risk of death.[98] Shuttle walking tests[99] and newer, simplified tests of functional capacity[100,101] in addition to 6MWT have largely surpassed laboratory CPET because of their convenience, simplicity, and low cost. However, as discussed later, CPET provides important clinical physiologic insights, particularly in patients with unremarkable spirometry, who report disproportionate dyspnea and exercise intolerance.[102]

Cardiopulmonary exercise testing

There is a widespread notion that incremental CPET in COPD does not add clinically useful information to resting PFTs because the test would merely confirm the expected pattern of mechanical-ventilatory limitation. Although this is likely to be the case in patients with advanced COPD, this oversimplification discounts that CPET provides valuable information in many clinically important circumstances[102]:

- Uncovering ventilatory limitation contributing to poor exercise performance in patients with only mild to moderate airflow limitation at rest, who in the absence of this important information may otherwise be labeled as simply deconditioned;
- Exposing the reasons for disproportionate dyspnea in those with unremarkable resting PFTs; and
- Determining the relative contribution of comorbidities (including obesity and skeletal muscle deconditioning) in limiting exercise in individual patients.

A detailed account of the expected CPET responses is beyond the scope of this review and is comprehensively discussed elsewhere.[103,104] In any circumstance, measurement of ventilatory efficiency ($\dot{V}E-\dot{V}CO_2$), operating lung volumes (EELV and end-inspiratory lung volume), and dyspnea ratings during CPET is very informative (see **Fig. 4**).[102] Schematically, excessive ventilation to

---

Box 6
Low lung diffusing capacity for carbon monoxide

There is well-established evidence that a low DL_{CO} is a key correlate of exertional dyspnea and reduced exercise capacity across the spectrum of COPD severity.

overcome an enlarged dead space largely explains patient's shortness of breath in the earlier phases of the disease.[105] In these subjects, increased dyspnea is roughly commensurate with heightened ventilatory stress, reflecting increased motor command output from cortical and bulbo-pontine respiratory centers (see **Fig. 1**). Thereafter, there is a progressive increase in the contribution of inspiratory mechanical constraints and a growing disparity between increasing inspiratory neural drive and blunted VT expansion leading to additional unpleasant respiratory sensations frequently described as "I cannot get enough air in."[22,23] As inspiratory constraints become critical, VT plateaus and dyspnea increase out of proportion to ventilation.[31] Peripheral muscular mechanisms (eg, ergoreceptor activation) are pervasive across the spectrum of disease severity,[106] whereas cardiocirculatory mechanisms owing to negative cardiopulmonary interactions may play a secondary role in severe COPD patients.[107]

Advances in CPET protocols and interpretation algorithms in COPD have enhanced their clinical utility. The traditional approach to dichotomize patients as ventilatory limited versus nonlimited based solely on the so-called breathing reserve ([(1 − $\dot{V}$Emax/MVV ratio) × 100] >85%)[108] frequently misses the key contribution of mechanical constraints and critical reduction of the IRV to the emergence of limiting dyspnea and exercise intolerance (see **Fig. 4**).[109] Contrary to popular belief, DH (inferred by a progressive decrease in IC) is not essential for attainment of critical inspiratory constraints[110] because patients with low resting IC (and high VT/IC ratio >0.7) soon reach critical minimal IRV with only minor expansion of VT as ventilation begins to increase in early exercise.[111]

Complicating interpretation of indices of cardiovascular function during CPET in patients with COPD is the frequent occurrence of cardiac comorbidities and medications that impact the cardiovascular response to exercise.[112] Interpretation of dysfunction based on cardioacceleration might be misleading if heart rate (HR) is under pharmacologic control or there is chronotropic incompetence.[112] A low peak O_2 pulse (O_2 uptake/HR ratio)[113] may reflect early exercise cessation (due to dyspnea) before this variable reaches its asymptotic value,[103] that is, this does not necessarily imply an abnormally low stroke volume.

Consideration should also be given to the exercise modality used during CPET and its resulting impact on test results. Although cycle-based tests are useful for most CPET applications, increased leg discomfort at higher exercise intensities may be reported as the dominant exercise-limiting symptom. Focus on leg discomfort at peak exercise may obscure the important contribution of "central" respiratory mechanisms to significant dyspnea evident at submaximal levels of exercise.[114] In fact, treadmill CPET should be preferred to uncover the severity of exercise-related hypoxemia (**Box 7**).[115]

LUNG FUNCTION TESTS IN THE INDICATION FOR AND RESPONSES TO INTERVENTIONS
Bronchodilator Therapy

The current criteria for a significant "flow" response to inhaled BD (ΔFEV_1 = 0.2 L and 12% increase from pre-BD baseline)[3] are highly controversial for several reasons:

- The likelihood of a positive response as expressed as a percentage change is inversely related to the baseline value, whereas the opposite is true for an absolute response[116];
- Whatever the criteria, lack of FEV_1 response in a given test is poorly predictive of long-term clinical response and vice versa[117];
- In patients with severe COPD and resting lung hyperinflation, clinically significant reduction in lung volumes (RV and FRC) can occur in the absence of improvement in FEV_1. In COPD patients, improvement in FEV_1 close to 20% of baseline often reflects a proportional "volume" response. In such individuals pre-BD and post-BD FEV_1/FVC do not change appreciably because changes in FEV_1 reflect lung volume recruitment.[118] This volume response to BDs leads to improvement in exertional dyspnea by effectively expanding IRV allowing VT to be positioned at a more compliant portion of the respiratory system's pressure-volume curve.[119] An increase in IC by approximately 0.2 L corresponds with clinically meaningful improvements in exercise endurance time during constant work rate cycle exercise.[118,120,121] Failure to consider lung

---

Box 7
Cardiopulmonary exercise testing

CPET may uncover critical mechanical-ventilatory abnormalities in patients with only mild to moderate airflow limitation, expose the reasons for disproportionate dyspnea in those with unremarkable PFTs, and determine the relative contribution of comorbidities (including obesity and skeletal muscle deconditioning) in limiting exercise tolerance.

deflation effects may underestimate BD efficacy in some individuals.[118]

- A large isolated improvement in FEV_1 ("flow" response) is suggestive of asthma. However, a large increase in FEV_1 (eg, >0.4 L) may occur secondary to an increase in FVC, which may also occur in COPD. Frequent overlooking of this phenomenon may have artificially increased the prevalence of the so-called asthma-COPD overlap.[122] In practice, normalization of spirometry from baseline obstruction provides strong evidence *against* COPD. In the right clinical context, this might suggest asthma. Any other scenario is equivocal in differentiation of asthma from COPD. Albeit largely ignored, the ΔFEV_1 expressed as a percent predicted criterion for reversibility[123] has a sounder rationale because it diminishes the confounding influence of baseline FEV_1.[124,125]

It should also be recognized that the clinician relies on subjective response of the individual patient (dyspnea relief) and not on arbitrary improvements in FEV_1 to guide pharmacotherapy.[49] In any case, for those who derive symptomatic benefit (dyspnea relief and improved exercise endurance), there is evidence that BDs work primarily on the "slow" compartment of alveolar units with slow mechanical time constants for emptying, leading to lung deflation.[118] As discussed above, FEV_1 response can be independent of changes in key lung volumes and capacities, such as RV, FRC, and IC. The same line of reasoning applies to mid-volume expiratory flow rates. Thus, if FVC does not change appreciably, FEV_1 and mid-volume flow rates might remain relatively unaltered after effective treatment.[125] Conversely, a positive "flow" response might be rather inconsequential to a patient's dyspnea. Simple resting IC is particularly relevant because it establishes the limits for VT expansion and therefore time to critical mechanical constraints during exercise in patients with EFL.[118] The corollary is that improvement in resting IC following BD can delay the onset of critical mechanical constraints and the associated intolerable dyspnea during exercise.[118] Interestingly, TLC may decrease slightly (by approximately 0.1 L) after BD in some patients, and this means an underestimation of the decrease in EELV by the same amount.[120] Specific airway resistance may decrease in isolation after inhaled BD, but this seems poorly related to symptomatic improvement.[63]

An official statement of the European Respiratory Society summarized extensive evidence that high-intensity constant work-rate (endurance)

tests are more responsive than incremental exercise tests and 6MWTs to detect the effects of BDs in patients with COPD.[99] It is specifically emphasized that the former tests need to be standardized to reduce interindividual variability. In this context, a pragmatic approach has been recently found useful. Thus, if a first test performed at 75% peak is associated with an endurance time less than 3 minutes, the test should be repeated on the same day at 60% peak; conversely, if the former test lasts more than 8 minutes, the test should be repeated (also on the same day) at 90% peak.[126] Important physiologic information and responsiveness can be obtained from isotime measurements, particularly IC and dyspnea (**Box 8**).[127]

Nonpharmacologic Interventions

PFTs might help, in addition to specific clinical and structural features, to select the ideal candidate for the following surgical interventions:

- An FEV_1 less than 35% predicted, severe gas trapping, large difference between TLC measured by body plethysmography and gas dilution methods, normal or near normal DL_{CO}, and normal arterial blood gases are useful to predict which patients might derive higher symptomatic benefit from giant bullectomy.[128]
- Post-BD FEV_1 between 30% and 45% predicted, RV >150% predicted, TLC >100% predicted jointly help in identifying candidates for lung volume reduction surgery[129]; conversely, the risk of death increases in those with FEV_1 and DL_{CO} less than 20% predicted.[130]
- Patients with thoracic hyperinflation (TLC >100% predicted), severe gas trapping (RV >180% to 200% predicted), and DL_{CO} $\geq$20% predicted are more likely to report benefit after bronchoscopic LVR (endobronchial valves).[131–133]

Box 8
Lung volumes response to inhaled BDs

In patients with resting lung hyperinflation, clinically significant reduction in lung volumes (RV and FRC) with BDs can occur in the absence of improvement in FEV_1. Increase in resting IC is particularly relevant because it can delay the onset of critical mechanical constraints and the associated intolerable dyspnea during exercise.

- Lung transplant might be better suited to patients showing FEV_1 less than 25% predicted. Conversely, more impaired gas exchange (hypoxemia, hypercapnia, DL_{CO} <20% predicted) are predictors of complications after lung transplantation.[134]
- Identification of patients presenting with inspiratory muscle weakness (eg, MIP <70% predicted) might prompt inspiratory muscle training in dyspneic, maximally treated patients.[95] Interestingly, there is emerging evidence that this is the case regardless of the underlying mechanism, that is, functional (volume mediated) or intrinsic weakness. In this context, dyspnea relief may occur in conjunction with reduced activation of the diaphragm relative to maximum.[96]

BALANCED RECOMMENDATIONS

Despite challenges in defining diagnosis and severity of COPD, the physiologic abnormalities underpinning COPD are well established and provide meaningful insight for clinicians. The future challenge that exists is how the diverse pathophysiology of COPD can be measured as a composite index and related to advances in imaging and cellular biology.[66] Layered with this are the implications of defining "abnormal" lung function and the not insignificant discrepancies in availability and access to spirometry as well as more detailed physiologic tests.

Diagnosis of Chronic Obstructive Pulmonary Disease

It is unlikely that the fixed ratio versus the LLN dispute to confirm a diagnosis of COPD will ever be settled.[135] The simplest explanation is that FEV_1/FVC ratio (or any other ratio expressing flow-volume relationships) is not a discrete dichotomous variable.[136] Whatever the chosen cutoff, the likelihood of COPD is higher the lower the FEV_1 and concordance between FEV_1/FVC fixed ratio and less LLN criteria increases the likelihood of accurate COPD diagnosis in those at risk.[137] One should be cautious about diagnostic criteria for COPD based solely on a single PFT test.[50] Thus, the interpretation of FEV_1/FVC should follow a Bayesian approach, taking into consideration the pretest probability of COPD. In this context, it should be recognized that pulmonologists usually have clinical information relevant to the diagnosis of COPD (burden of risk factors, symptoms, lung volumes, DL_{CO}, chest imaging), which is not readily available to the epidemiologist or the frontline caregiver on an individual basis. Chest medicine specialists, in particular, assess smokers with at greater risk for COPD. Thus, the posttest probability of COPD based on fixed ratio criteria is inherently higher in this circumstance. This approach however has limitations because physicians in primary care may not have access to the same information on physiologic impairment that can be used to inform likelihood of COPD diagnosis. It is therefore incumbent on physicians reporting PFTs to succinctly summarize observed PFT patterns and the importance of interpretation within the clinical context. A pragmatic, clinically oriented approach for an integrated interpretation of PFTs vis-à-vis diagnosis of COPD is depicted in **Fig. 7**.

Assessment of Disease Severity

The initial assessment of COPD severity should, whenever feasible, include not only "basic" PFTs

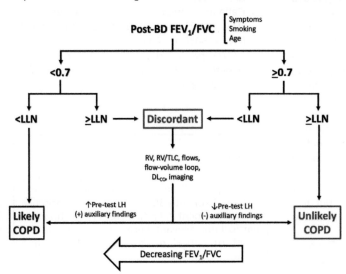

Fig. 7. A pragmatic approach for spirometry interpretation in a patient at risk for COPD, which considers the uncertainties surrounding the interpretation of "discordance" in post-BD FEV_1/FVC ratio between 0.7 and the LLN. See text for further elaboration. LH, likelihood.

(forced and slow expiratory maneuver pre-BD and post-BD) but also selected "advanced" PFTs (IC, body plethysmography, and DL_{CO} measurements). Arterial blood gases are not mandatory, unless there is a high suspicion of hypoxemia (reduced arterial O_2 saturation) or hypercapnia. Newer PFTs are currently being systematically evaluated (eg, forced oscillation, DL for nitric oxide, multiple-breath N_2 washout) and show promise. CPET is particularly valuable to better understand dyspnea and exercise intolerance when spirometry is largely preserved.

Recommendations regarding optimal frequency of PFT follow-up are more controversial. If the patient is clinically stable, there little justification to repeat full PFTs on a yearly basis: spirometry pre-BD and post-BD is probably sufficient for most subjects. Currently, annual PFTs are the only means the authors have of identifying the subpopulation of patients with COPD whose pulmonary function is rapidly declining. Changes in clinical status (particularly worsening dyspnea) may prompt repetition of more complex tests, and CPET frequently proves clinically valuable in this circumstance, particularly when changes in resting PFTs are unremarkable.

Predictors of Response to and the Effects of Interventions

In the clinical management of individual patients, improvement in symptoms is certainly more relevant than PFT results in a chronic, incurable disease such as COPD. However, in some circumstances, such as a patient with complex dyspnea and multiple comorbidities undergoing several treatments, detecting a positive objective effect manifest as reduced airway obstruction or lung deflation after BD therapy, provides reassurance. The authors should never assume that progressively increasing dyspnea is always the result of worsening airway obstruction, which will respond to BD therapy: dyspnea is generally multifactorial in COPD. Although endorsing the above-mentioned recommendations on the use of PFTs to predict a positive response to nonpharmacologic interventions (see *Nonpharmacologic interventions*), the authors recognize that they are likely to change in tandem with technical and technological advances.

SUMMARY

Most physicians still rely on PFTs, in addition to symptoms and exacerbation burden, to guide management in individual COPD patients. Thus, it is regrettable that time-honored PFTs have progressively been abandoned beyond spirometry for diagnosis, comprehensive assessment of disease severity, and evaluation of the effects of interventions. Contrary to other chronic degenerative diseases in which more complex functional tests linking structure and function have recently been emphasized, heart failure being perhaps the best example,[138] a simplified approach to COPD has been increasingly adopted.[66] Advances in quantified imaging over the past decade in COPD have been impressive and the stage is now set to undertake a more profound interrogation of structure-function correlations than ever before. Detailed, combined, physiologic, and structural measurements in well-characterized populations at risk for COPD may uncover distinct phenotypes to guide biologists in their quest to better understand the heterogenous pathologic underpinnings of this complex disease.[139]

DISCLOSURE

The authors have no conflict of interest to disclose relative to the subject matter or materials discussed in this article.

REFERENCES

1. GOLD Executive Committee. Global strategy for the diagnosis, management and prevention of chronic obstructive pulmonary disease: 2019 report. Available at: www.goldcopd.org.
2. O'Donnell DE, Laveneziana P, Webb K, et al. Chronic obstructive pulmonary disease: clinical integrative physiology. Clin Chest Med 2014; 35(1):51–69.
3. Pellegrino R, Viegi G, Brusasco V, et al. Interpretative strategies for lung function tests. Eur Respir J 2005;26(5):948–68.
4. Hogg JC. Pathophysiology of airflow limitation in chronic obstructive pulmonary disease. Lancet 2004;364(9435):709–21.
5. Hogg JC, Paré PD, Hackett T-L. The contribution of small airway obstruction to the pathogenesis of chronic obstructive pulmonary disease. Physiol Rev 2017;97(2):529–52.
6. Macklem PT. The physiology of small airways. Am J Respir Crit Care Med 1998;157(5 Pt 2):S181–3.
7. Calverley PMA, Koulouris NG. Flow limitation and dynamic hyperinflation: key concepts in modern respiratory physiology. Eur Respir J 2005;25(1): 186–99.
8. Gibson GJ. Lung volumes and elasticity. Clin Chest Med 2001;22(4):623–35, vii.
9. Macklem PT. The pathophysiology of chronic bronchitis and emphysema. Med Clin North Am 1973; 57(3):669–70.

10. Calverley PMA. Dynamic hyperinflation: is it worth measuring? Proc Am Thorac Soc 2006;3(3): 239–44.

11. Aldrich TK, Hendler JM, Vizioli LD, et al. Intrinsic positive end-expiratory pressure in ambulatory patients with airways obstruction. Am Rev Respir Dis 1993;147(4):845–9.

12. Celli BR. Respiratory muscle function. Clin Chest Med 1986;7(4):567–84.

13. Gibson GJ, Pride NB. Lung distensibility. The static pressure-volume curve of the lungs and its use in clinical assessment. Br J Dis Chest 1976;70(3): 143–84.

14. O'Donnell DE, Webb KA. The major limitation to exercise performance in COPD is dynamic hyperinflation. J Appl Physiol (1985) 2008;105(2):753–5 [discussion 755–7].

15. Wagner PD. Gas exchange in chronic pulmonary disease. Clin Physiol 1985;5(Suppl 3):9–17.

16. Rodríguez-Roisin R, Drakulovic M, Rodríguez DA, et al. Ventilation-perfusion imbalance and chronic obstructive pulmonary disease staging severity. J Appl Physiol (1985) 2009;106(6):1902–8.

17. Barberà JA, Riverola A, Roca J, et al. Pulmonary vascular abnormalities and ventilation-perfusion relationships in mild chronic obstructive pulmonary disease. Am J Respir Crit Care Med 1994;149(2 Pt 1):423–9.

18. Liebow AA. Pulmonary emphysema with special reference to vascular changes. Am Rev Respir Dis 1959;80(1, Part 2):67–93.

19. O'Donnell DE, Neder JA, Elbehairy AF. Physiological impairment in mild COPD. Respirology 2016; 21(2):211–23.

20. O'Donnell DE, Elbehairy AF, Berton DC, et al. Advances in the evaluation of respiratory pathophysiology during exercise in chronic lung diseases. Front Physiol 2017;8:82.

21. Langer D, Ciavaglia CE, Neder JA, et al. Lung hyperinflation in chronic obstructive pulmonary disease: mechanisms, clinical implications and treatment. Expert Rev Respir Med 2014;1–19. https://doi.org/10.1586/17476348.2014.949676.

22. O'Donnell DE, Elbehairy AF, Webb KA, et al, Canadian Respiratory Research Network. The link between reduced inspiratory capacity and exercise intolerance in chronic obstructive pulmonary disease. Ann Am Thorac Soc 2017;14(Supplement_1):S30–9.

23. Neder JA, Arbex FF, Alencar MCN, et al. Exercise ventilatory inefficiency in mild to end-stage COPD. Eur Respir J 2015;45(2):377–87.

24. Neder JA, Berton DC, Arbex FF, et al. Physiological and clinical relevance of exercise ventilatory efficiency in COPD. Eur Respir J 2017;49(3):1602036.

25. Casaburi R, Patessio A, Ioli F, et al. Reductions in exercise lactic acidosis and ventilation as a result of exercise training in patients with obstructive lung disease. Am Rev Respir Dis 1991;143(1): 9–18.

26. Minh VD, Lee HM, Dolan GF, et al. Hypoxemia during exercise in patients with chronic obstructive pulmonary disease. Am Rev Respir Dis 1979; 120(4):787–94.

27. Chiappa GR, Borghi-Silva A, Ferreira LF, et al. Kinetics of muscle deoxygenation are accelerated at the onset of heavy-intensity exercise in patients with COPD: relationship to central cardiovascular dynamics. J Appl Physiol (1985) 2008;104(5): 1341–50.

28. Neder JA, Berton DC, Marillier M, et al, Canadian Respiratory Research Network. The role of evaluating inspiratory constraints and ventilatory inefficiency in the investigation of dyspnea of unclear etiology. Respir Med 2019;158:6–13.

29. O'Donnell DE, D'Arsigny C, Fitzpatrick M, et al. Exercise hypercapnia in advanced chronic obstructive pulmonary disease: the role of lung hyperinflation. Am J Respir Crit Care Med 2002; 166(5):663–8.

30. O'Donnell DE, Neder JA. The enigma of dyspnoea in COPD: a physiological perspective. Respirology 2020;25(2):134–6.

31. O'Donnell DE, Milne KM, James MD, et al. Dyspnea in COPD: new mechanistic insights and management implications. Adv Ther 2019. https://doi.org/10.1007/s12325-019-01128-9.

32. Buist AS, McBurnie MA, Vollmer WM, et al. International variation in the prevalence of COPD (the BOLD Study): a population-based prevalence study. Lancet 2007;370(9589):741–50.

33. Ho T, Cusack RP, Chaudhary N, et al. Under- and over-diagnosis of COPD: a global perspective. Breathe (Sheff) 2019;15(1):24–35.

34. Gaensler EA. Air velocity index; a numerical expression of the functionally effective portion of ventilation. Am Rev Tuberc 1950;62(1-A):17–28.

35. Quanjer PH, Brazzale DJ, Boros PW, et al. Implications of adopting the global lungs initiative 2012 all-age reference equations for spirometry. Eur Respir J 2013;42(4):1046–54.

36. Quanjer PH, Stanojevic S, Cole TJ, et al. Multi-ethnic reference values for spirometry for the 3-95-yr age range: the global lung function 2012 equations. Eur Respir J 2012;40(6):1324–43.

37. Auerbach O, Hammond EC, Garfinkel L, et al. Relation of smoking and age to emphysema. Whole-lung section study. N Engl J Med 1972;286(16):853–7.

38. Gaensler EA. Analysis of the ventilatory defect by timed capacity measurements. Am Rev Tuberc 1951;64(3):256–78.

39. Swanney MP, Ruppel G, Enright PL, et al. Using the lower limit of normal for the FEV1/FVC ratio reduces

the misclassification of airway obstruction. Thorax 2008;63(12):1046–51.

40. Diab N, Gershon AS, Sin DD, et al. Underdiagnosis and overdiagnosis of chronic obstructive pulmonary disease. Am J Respir Crit Care Med 2018; 198(9):1130–9.

41. Neder JA, Milne KM, Berton DC, de-Torres JP, Jensen D, Tan WC, Bourbeau J, O'Donnell DE; Canadian Respiratory Research Network (CRRN) and the Canadian Cohort of Obstructive Lung Disease (CanCOLD) Collaborative Research Group. Exercise Tolerance According to the Definition of Airflow Obstruction in Smokers. Am J Respir Crit Care Med. 2020 Apr 28. doi: 10.1164/rccm.202002-0298LE.

42. Alcaide AB, Sanchez-Salcedo P, Bastarrika G, et al. Clinical features of smokers with radiological emphysema but without airway limitation. Chest 2016. https://doi.org/10.1016/j.chest.2016.10.044.

43. Regan EA, Lynch DA, Curran-Everett D, et al. Clinical and radiologic disease in smokers with normal spirometry. JAMA Intern Med 2015;175(9): 1539–49.

44. Wan ES, Hokanson JE, Murphy JR, et al. Clinical and radiographic predictors of GOLD-unclassified smokers in the COPDGene study. Am J Respir Crit Care Med 2011;184(1):57–63.

45. Hyatt RE, Cowl CT, Bjoraker JA, et al. Conditions associated with an abnormal nonspecific pattern of pulmonary function tests. Chest 2009;135(2): 419–24.

46. Park SS. Effect of effort versus volume on forced expiratory flow measurement. Am Rev Respir Dis 1988;138(4):1002–5.

47. Fortis S, Corazalla EO, Wang Q, et al. The difference between slow and forced vital capacity increases with increasing body mass index: a paradoxical difference in low and normal body mass indices. Respir Care 2015;60(1):113–8.

48. Saint-Pierre M, Ladha J, Berton DC, et al. Is the slow vital capacity clinically useful to uncover airflow limitation in subjects with preserved FEV1/FVC ratio? Chest 2019. https://doi.org/10.1016/j.chest.2019.02.001.

49. Sakhamuri S, Seemungal T. COPD: gaps in the GOLD recommendations and related imperative research needs. COPD 2020;1–3. https://doi.org/10.1080/15412555.2019.1708297.

50. Aaron SD, Tan WC, Bourbeau J, et al. Diagnostic instability and reversals of chronic obstructive pulmonary disease diagnosis in individuals with mild to moderate airflow obstruction. Am J Respir Crit Care Med 2017;196(3):306–14.

51. Stănescu D. Small airways obstruction syndrome. Chest 1999;116(1):231–3.

52. Llordés M, Zurdo E, Jaén Á, et al. Which is the best screening strategy for COPD among smokers in primary care? COPD 2017;14(1):43–51.

53. Jing J-Y, Huang T-C, Cui W, et al. Should FEV1/FEV6 replace FEV1/FVC ratio to detect airway obstruction? A metaanalysis. Chest 2009;135(4): 991–8.

54. Bhatt SP, Soler X, Wang X, et al. Association between functional small airways disease and FEV1 decline in COPD. Am J Respir Crit Care Med 2016. https://doi.org/10.1164/rccm.201511-2219OC.

55. Hansen JE, Sun X-G, Wasserman K. Discriminating measures and normal values for expiratory obstruction. Chest 2006;129(2):369–77.

56. Mead J. Dysanapsis in normal lungs assessed by the relationship between maximal flow, static recoil, and vital capacity. Am Rev Respir Dis 1980;121(2): 339–42.

57. Dilektasli AG, Porszasz J, Casaburi R, et al. A novel spirometric measure identifies mild COPD unidentified by standard criteria. Chest 2016;150(5): 1080–90.

58. Mead J. The lung's "quiet zone. N Engl J Med 1970;282(23):1318–9.

59. Cosio M, Ghezzo H, Hogg JC, et al. The relations between structural changes in small airways and pulmonary-function tests. N Engl J Med 1978; 298(23):1277–81.

60. Robinson PD, Latzin P, Verbanck S, et al. Consensus statement for inert gas washout measurement using multiple- and single-breath tests. Eur Respir J 2013;41(3):507–22.

61. Verbanck S, Schuermans D, Van Muylem A, et al. Ventilation distribution during histamine provocation. J Appl Physiol (1985) 1997;83(6): 1907–16.

62. Oostveen E, MacLeod D, Lorino H, et al. The forced oscillation technique in clinical practice: methodology, recommendations and future developments. Eur Respir J 2003;22(6):1026–41.

63. Kaminsky DA. What does airway resistance tell us about lung function? Respir Care 2012;57(1): 85–96 [discussion: 96–9].

64. Mahut B, Caumont-Prim A, Plantier L, et al. Relationships between respiratory and airway resistances and activity-related dyspnea in patients with chronic obstructive pulmonary disease. Int J Chron Obstruct Pulmon Dis 2012;7:165–71.

65. Yamagami H, Tanaka A, Kishino Y, et al. Association between respiratory impedance measured by forced oscillation technique and exacerbations in patients with COPD. Int J Chron Obstruct Pulmon Dis 2018;13:79–89.

66. Lowe KE, Regan EA, Anzueto A, et al. COPDGene® 2019: redefining the diagnosis of

chronic obstructive pulmonary disease. Chronic Obstr Pulm Dis 2019;6(5):384–99.

67. Pompe E, Strand M, van Rikxoort EM, et al. Five-year progression of emphysema and air trapping at CT in smokers with and those without chronic obstructive pulmonary disease: results from the COPDGene study. Radiology 2020;191429. https://doi.org/10.1148/radiol.2020191429.

68. Adibi A, Sadatsafavi M. Looking at the COPD spectrum through "PRISm. Eur Respir J 2020;55(1). https://doi.org/10.1183/13993003.02217-2019.

69. O'Donnell DE, Ciavaglia CE, Neder JA. When obesity and chronic obstructive pulmonary disease collide. Physiological and clinical consequences. Ann Am Thorac Soc 2014;11(4):635–44.

70. Knudson RJ, Burrows B. Early detection of obstructive lung diseases. Med Clin North Am 1973;57(3): 681–90.

71. Elbehairy AF, Guenette JA, Faisal A, et al. Mechanisms of exertional dyspnoea in symptomatic smokers without COPD. Eur Respir J 2016;48(3): 694–705.

72. Elbehairy AF, O'Donnell CD, Abd Elhameed A, et al. Low resting diffusion capacity, dyspnea, and exercise intolerance in chronic obstructive pulmonary disease. J Appl Physiol (1985) 2019; 127(4):1107–16.

73. Hughes JMB, Pride NB. Examination of the carbon monoxide diffusing capacity (DL(CO)) in relation to its KCO and VA components. Am J Respir Crit Care Med 2012;186(2):132–9.

74. Hughes JMB, Dinh-Xuan AT. The DLNO/DLCO ratio: physiological significance and clinical implications. Respir Physiol Neurobiol 2017;241: 17–22.

75. Fletcher C, Peto R. The natural history of chronic airflow obstruction. Br Med J 1977;1(6077):1645–8.

76. Barnes PJ, Burney PGJ, Silverman EK, et al. Chronic obstructive pulmonary disease. Nat Rev Dis Primers 2015;1:15076.

77. Quanjer PH, Pretto JJ, Brazzale DJ, et al. Grading the severity of airways obstruction: new wine in new bottles. Eur Respir J 2014;43(2):505–12.

78. Casanova C, Cote C, de Torres JP, et al. Inspiratory-to-total lung capacity ratio predicts mortality in patients with chronic obstructive pulmonary disease. Am J Respir Crit Care Med 2005;171(6): 591–7.

79. Elbehairy AF, Ciavaglia CE, Webb KA, et al. Pulmonary gas exchange abnormalities in mild chronic obstructive pulmonary disease. Implications for dyspnea and exercise intolerance. Am J Respir Crit Care Med 2015;191(12):1384–94.

80. Hughes JMB. The single breath transfer factor (Tl,co) and the transfer coefficient (Kco): a window onto the pulmonary microcirculation. Clin Physiol Funct Imaging 2003;23(2):63–71.

81. Neder JA, O'Donnell CDJ, Cory J, et al. Ventilation distribution heterogeneity at rest as a marker of exercise impairment in mild-to-advanced COPD. COPD 2015;12(3):249–56.

82. Davis C, Sheikh K, Pike D, et al. Ventilation heterogeneity in never-smokers and COPD: comparison of pulmonary functional magnetic resonance imaging with the poorly communicating fraction derived from plethysmography. Acad Radiol 2016;23(4): 398–405.

83. Cotes JE. Carbon monoxide transfer coefficient KCO (TL/VA): a flawed index. Eur Respir J 2001; 18(5):893–4.

84. Hughes JM, Pride NB. In defence of the carbon monoxide transfer coefficient Kco (TL/VA). Eur Respir J 2001;17(2):168–74.

85. Neder JA, Marillier M, Bernard A-C, et al. Transfer coefficient of the lung for carbon monoxide and the accessible alveolar volume: clinically useful if used wisely. Breathe (Sheff) 2019;15(1):69–76.

86. Neder JA, Berton DC, Muller PT, et al. Incorporating lung diffusing capacity for carbon monoxide in clinical decision making in chest medicine. Clin Chest Med 2019;40(2):285–305.

87. Neder JA, Berton DC, O'Donnell DE. Why we should never ignore an "isolated" low lung diffusing capacity. J Bras Pneumol 2019;45(4):e20190241.

88. Tiep BL. Long-term home oxygen therapy. Clin Chest Med 1990;11(3):505–21.

89. Branson RD. Oxygen therapy in COPD. Respir Care 2018;63(6):734–48.

90. Haluszka J, Chartrand DA, Grassino AE, et al. Intrinsic PEEP and arterial PCO2 in stable patients with chronic obstructive pulmonary disease. Am Rev Respir Dis 1990;141(5 Pt 1):1194–7.

91. McNicholas WT, Verbraecken J, Marin JM. Sleep disorders in COPD: the forgotten dimension. Eur Respir Rev 2013;22(129):365–75.

92. Rocha A, Arbex FF, Sperandio PA, et al. Excess ventilation in COPD-heart failure overlap: implications for dyspnea and exercise intolerance. Am J Respir Crit Care Med 2017. https://doi.org/10.1164/rccm.201704-0675OC.

93. Gibson GJ, Clark E, Pride NB. Static transdiaphragmatic pressures in normal subjects and in patients with chronic hyperinflation. Am Rev Respir Dis 1981;124(6):685–9.

94. Decramer M. Effects of hyperinflation on the respiratory muscles. Eur Respir J 1989;2(4):299–302.

95. Charususin N, Dacha S, Gosselink R, et al. Respiratory muscle function and exercise limitation in patients with chronic obstructive pulmonary disease: a review. Expert Rev Respir Med 2018;12(1): 67–79.

96. Langer D, Ciavaglia CE, Faisal A, et al. Inspiratory muscle training reduces diaphragm activation and dyspnea during exercise in COPD. J Appl Physiol

(1985) 2018. https://doi.org/10.1152/japplphysiol.01078.2017.

97. Charususin N, Gosselink R, Decramer M, et al. Randomised controlled trial of adjunctive inspiratory muscle training for patients with COPD. Thorax 2018;73(10):942–50.

98. Divo M, Cote C, de Torres JP, et al. Comorbidities and risk of mortality in patients with chronic obstructive pulmonary disease. Am J Respir Crit Care Med 2012;186(2):155–61.

99. Puente-Maestu L, Palange P, Casaburi R, et al. Use of exercise testing in the evaluation of interventional efficacy: an official ERS statement. Eur Respir J 2016;47(2):429–60.

100. Yoshida C, Ichiyasu H, Ideguchi H, et al. Four-meter gait speed predicts daily physical activity in patients with chronic respiratory diseases. Respir Investig 2019;57(4):368–75.

101. Vaidya T, Chambellan A, de Bisschop C. Sit-to-stand tests for COPD: a literature review. Respir Med 2017;128:70–7.

102. O'Donnell DE, Elbehairy AF, Faisal A, et al. Exertional dyspnoea in COPD: the clinical utility of cardiopulmonary exercise testing. Eur Respir Rev 2016;25(141):333–47.

103. Neder JA, Berton DC, Rocha A, et al. Abnormal patterns of response to incremental CPET. In: Palange P, Laveneziana P, Neder JA, et al, editors. 2018 Clinical exercise testing, vol. 80. European Respiratory Society Journals; 2018. p. 34–58. European Respiratory Monograph.

104. O'Donnell DE, James MD, Milne KM, et al. The pathophysiology of dyspnea and exercise intolerance in chronic obstructive pulmonary disease. Clin Chest Med 2019;40(2):343–66.

105. Neder JA, Berton DC, Müller P de T, et al. Ventilatory inefficiency and exertional dyspnea in early chronic obstructive pulmonary disease. Ann Am Thorac Soc 2017. https://doi.org/10.1513/AnnalsATS.201612-1033FR.

106. Maltais F, Decramer M, Casaburi R, et al. An official American Thoracic Society/European Respiratory Society statement: update on limb muscle dysfunction in chronic obstructive pulmonary disease. Am J Respir Crit Care Med 2014;189(9):e15–62.

107. Neder JA, Rocha A, Berton DC, et al. Clinical and physiologic implications of negative cardiopulmonary interactions in coexisting chronic obstructive pulmonary disease-heart failure. Clin Chest Med 2019;40(2):421–38.

108. American Thoracic Society, American College of Chest Physicians. ATS/ACCP statement on cardiopulmonary exercise testing. Am J Respir Crit Care Med 2003;167(2):211–77.

109. Neder JA, Berton DC, Marillier M, et al, Canadian Respiratory Research Network. Inspiratory constraints and ventilatory inefficiency are superior to breathing reserve in the assessment of exertional dyspnea in COPD. COPD 2019;16(2):174–81.

110. Guenette JA, Webb KA, O'Donnell DE. Does dynamic hyperinflation contribute to dyspnoea during exercise in patients with COPD? Eur Respir J 2012;40(2):322–9.

111. O'Donnell DE, Guenette JA, Maltais F, et al. Decline of resting inspiratory capacity in COPD: the impact on breathing pattern, dyspnea, and ventilatory capacity during exercise. Chest 2012;141(3):753–62.

112. Neder JA, Laveneziana P, Ward SA, et al. CPET in clinical practice. Recent advances, current challenges and future directions. In: Palange P, Laveneziana P, Neder JA, et al, editors. 2018 Clinical exercise testing, vol. 80. European Respiratory Society Journals; 2018. p. x–xxv. European Respiratory Monograph.

113. Montes de Oca M, Rassulo J, Celli BR. Respiratory muscle and cardiopulmonary function during exercise in very severe COPD. Am J Respir Crit Care Med 1996;154(5):1284–9.

114. Saey D, Debigare R, LeBlanc P, et al. Contractile leg fatigue after cycle exercise: a factor limiting exercise in patients with chronic obstructive pulmonary disease. Am J Respir Crit Care Med 2003;168(4):425–30.

115. Andrianopoulos V, Franssen FME, Peeters JPI, et al. Exercise-induced oxygen desaturation in COPD patients without resting hypoxemia. Respir Physiol Neurobiol 2014;190:40–6.

116. Hansen JE, Sun XG, Adame D, et al. Argument for changing criteria for bronchodilator responsiveness. Respir Med 2008;102(12):1777–83.

117. Shim C. Response to bronchodilators. Clin Chest Med 1989;10(2):155–64.

118. O'Donnell DE. Assessment of bronchodilator efficacy in symptomatic COPD: is spirometry useful? Chest 2000;117(2 Suppl):42S–7S.

119. Mead J. Respiration: pulmonary mechanics. Annu Rev Physiol 1973;35:169–92.

120. Newton MF, O'Donnell DE, Forkert L. Response of lung volumes to inhaled salbutamol in a large population of patients with severe hyperinflation. Chest 2002;121(4):1042–50.

121. Calzetta L, Rogliani P, Matera MG, et al. A systematic review with meta-analysis of dual bronchodilation with LAMA/LABA for the treatment of stable chronic obstructive pulmonary disease. Chest 2016. https://doi.org/10.1016/j.chest.2016.02.646.

122. Sin DD, Miravitlles M, Mannino DM, et al. What is asthma-COPD overlap syndrome? Towards a consensus definition from a round table discussion. Eur Respir J 2016;48(3):664–73.

123. Brand PL, Quanjer PH, Postma DS, et al. Interpretation of bronchodilator response in patients with

obstructive airways disease. The Dutch Chronic Non-Specific Lung Disease (CNSLD) Study Group. Thorax 1992;47(6):429–36.

124. Tuomisto LE, Ilmarinen P, Lehtimäki L, et al. Immediate bronchodilator response in FEV1 as a diagnostic criterion for adult asthma. Eur Respir J 2019;53(2). https://doi.org/10.1183/13993003.00904-2018.

125. Quanjer PH, Ruppel GL, Langhammer A, et al. Bronchodilator response in FVC is larger and more relevant than in FEV1 in severe airflow obstruction. Chest 2017;151(5):1088–98.

126. Degani-Costa LH, O'Donnell DE, Webb K, et al. A simplified approach to select exercise endurance intensity for interventional studies in COPD. COPD 2018. https://doi.org/10.1080/15412555.2018.1428944.

127. Guenette JA, Chin RC, Cory JM, et al. Inspiratory capacity during exercise: measurement, analysis, and interpretation. Pulm Med 2013;2013:956081.

128. Benditt JO. Surgical options for patients with COPD: sorting out the choices. Respir Care 2006;51(2):173–82.

129. Caviezel C, Schneiter D, Opitz I, et al. Lung volume reduction surgery beyond the NETT selection criteria. J Thorac Dis 2018;10(Suppl 23):S2748–53.

130. National Emphysema Treatment Trial Research Group, Fishman A, Fessler H, et al. Patients at high risk of death after lung-volume-reduction surgery. N Engl J Med 2001;345(15):1075–83.

131. Criner GJ, Belt P, Sternberg AL, et al. Effects of lung volume reduction surgery on gas exchange and breathing pattern during maximum exercise. Chest 2009;135(5):1268–79.

132. Kemp SV, Slebos D-J, Kirk A, et al. A multicenter randomized controlled trial of zephyr endobronchial valve treatment in heterogeneous emphysema (TRANSFORM). Am J Respir Crit Care Med 2017;196(12):1535–43.

133. Criner GJ, Sue R, Wright S, et al. A multicenter randomized controlled trial of Zephyr endobronchial valve treatment in heterogeneous emphysema (LIBERATE). Am J Respir Crit Care Med 2018;198(9):1151–64.

134. Weill D, Benden C, Corris PA, et al. A consensus document for the selection of lung transplant candidates: 2014–an update from the Pulmonary Transplantation Council of the International Society for Heart and Lung Transplantation. J Heart Lung Transplant 2015;34(1):1–15.

135. Miller MR, Pedersen OF, Pellegrino R, et al. Debating the definition of airflow obstruction: time to move on? Eur Respir J 2009;34(3):527–8.

136. Reyes-García A, Torre-Bouscoulet L, Pérez-Padilla R. Controversies and limitations in the diagnosis of chronic obstructive pulmonary disease. Rev Invest Clin 2019;71(1):28–35.

137. van Dijk W, Tan W, Li P, et al. Clinical relevance of fixed ratio vs lower limit of normal of FEV1/FVC in COPD: patient-reported outcomes from the CanCOLD cohort. Ann Fam Med 2015;13(1):41–8.

138. Neder JA, Rocha A, Alencar MCN, et al. Current challenges in managing comorbid heart failure and COPD. Expert Rev Cardiovasc Ther 2018;16(9):653–73.

139. O'Donnell DE, Neder JA. Why clinical physiology remains vital in the modern era. Clin Chest Med 2019;40(2). xiii–xiv.

Assessing Symptom Burden

Claus F. Vogelmeier, MD*, Peter Alter, MD

KEYWORDS

- COPD • Assessment • Dyspnea • Health status • mMRC scale • COPD assessment test

KEY POINTS

- Symptoms are key drivers to consider the diagnosis of chronic obstructive pulmonary disease (COPD).
- Assessment of symptoms together with exacerbation history is the basis of treatment decisions.
- Symptoms can be evaluated by the use of dyspnea scores, health status questionnaires, and multi-dimensional scoring systems.
- According to the Global Obstructive Lung Disease recommendations, the modified Medical Research Council Score and the COPD Assessment Test are the preferred choice to evaluate the presence and significance of symptoms.

INTRODUCTION

Chronic obstructive pulmonary disease (COPD) is a chronic disease whereby symptoms are the main driver for patients to seek medical attention. The symptoms can be multifaceted and range from subtle to very severe. In fact, many patients are diagnosed while they experience the first exacerbation, when for the first time, the patient may report dyspnea as the predominant symptom causing his medical problem. Cough or phlegm production may also accompany dyspnea as an important health problem, but patients usually consider these symptoms natural consequences of smoking or working in polluted environments, being reported by up to 30% of patients.[1] Fatigue, weight loss, and anorexia may be observed in more severe forms of the disease.[2,3] Symptoms may vary from day to day, at different times of the day,[4] and may precede the development of airflow limitation. They impact physical activity and health status,[5–7] and severe dyspnea has a similar impact on the time to hospitalization and risk of death as frequent COPD exacerbations have.[8] It follows that identification and quantification of dyspnea is an important element in the medical history of any persons suspected of having a respiratory disease.

As stated in the Global Obstructive Lung Disease (GOLD) document, COPD should be considered in any patient with respiratory symptoms and/or a history of exposure to risk factors. Although a spirometry showing airflow limitation is required to confirm the diagnosis of COPD,[1] symptoms and risk factors may be present without significant airflow limitation. Interestingly, those individuals may be receiving long-term treatment with respiratory medications and report events that are rated as exacerbations, and some may show structural lung changes on chest imaging (emphysema, gas trapping, airway wall thickening)[9,10] with "normal" spirometric values. In these individuals, the detection of dyspnea, cough, and/or sputum increases the risk of future development of airflow limitation; however, its management remains unknown, but it is reasonable to emphasize preventive measures. Particularly important is the issue that dyspnea itself is not a specific symptom of COPD. Relevant differential diagnoses like heart failure may be associated with similar complaints.

Department of Internal Medicine, Pulmonary and Critical Care Medicine, University Medical Center Giessen and Marburg, Philipps-Universität Marburg (UMR), Baldingerstrasse, Marburg 35043, Germany
* Corresponding author.
E-mail address: Claus.Vogelmeier@med.uni-marburg.de

Clin Chest Med 41 (2020) 367–373
https://doi.org/10.1016/j.ccm.2020.06.005
0272-5231/20/© 2020 Elsevier Inc. All rights reserved.

In addition, patients with COPD frequently exhibit comorbidities[11] that may modify and/or amplify the respiratory symptoms the identification of which and their management will improve the outcome of those patients.

ASSESSMENT OF SYMPTOMS

The "ABCD" assessment tool of the 2011 GOLD update was a major step forward from the simple spirometric grading system of the earlier versions of GOLD because it incorporated patient-reported outcomes and highlighted the importance of exacerbation prevention in the management of COPD.[12] The current GOLD assessment highlights the importance of symptoms and exacerbation risk in guiding therapies, reinforcing the concept that symptom quantification is of high importance in patients suspected or diagnosed as suffering from COPD.

Therefore, it may be preferable not to just ask the patient the generic question of "how are you doing," but also to use a more formalized approach. Generally speaking, there are 3 methods currently used in symptom quantification: scoring the intensity of dyspnea, evaluating health status, and finally, using multidimensional scoring systems. **Table 1** summarizes some of the features of currently used tests, all of which have been reviewed in detail by Glaab and colleagues.[13]

All scales mentioned rely on the basic presumption that there exists a generally valid minimal important difference (MID) that is suitable for categorization independent of the individual patient's status. However, the authors would like to point out that this conceptualization is based on the hypothesis that differences are linear, whereas most biological systems appear to have nonlinear relationships. Moreover, there is some disagreement in the literature regarding the MIDs for certain scales.[14] In addition, the published data addressing the use of these scales represent group comparison. Thus, the reported changes of scores show that they are responsive on a group level, whereas in clinical practice the authors are looking for an assessment tool that allows individual comparisons.

ASSESSMENT OF DYSPNEA
Baseline Dyspnea Index/Transition Dyspnea Index

The Baseline Dyspnea Index and Transition Dyspnea Index (BDI/TDI) were designed to measure multiple dimensions of breathlessness (functional impairment, magnitude of task, and magnitude of effort) in relation to the level of activity. Symptoms are evaluated at a specific time point (usually baseline, BDI), and the change over time (TDI) is

Table 1
Scales for measuring dyspnea and health status in patients with chronic obstructive pulmonary disease

Dyspnea				
	Scale	Stimulus	Items	Administration
BDI/TDI	Multidimensional	Everyday activities	8/9	Interview/self-administered
Borg	Unidimensional	Exertion	1	Self-administered
MRC/mMRC	Unidimensional	Everyday activities	1	Self-administered
Health status				
	Instrument	Domains	Items	Administration
SF-36	Generic	Physical and social function, mental health, energy/vitality, health perception, physical and mental role limitation, pain	36	Self-administered
SGRQ	Disease-specific	Symptoms, activities, psychosocial impact	50	Self-administered
CRQ	Disease-specific	Dyspnea, emotional function, fatigue, mastery	20	Interview
CCQ	Disease-specific	Symptoms, functional state, mental state	10	Self-administered
CAT	Disease-specific	Unidimensional	8	Self-administered

For details and references, see text.
Data from Glaab T, Vogelmeier C, Buhl R. Outcome measures in chronic obstructive pulmonary disease (COPD): strengths and limitations. Respir Res. 2010;11:79.

quantified.[15] In the original version, BDI and TDI are obtained during an interview by an experienced observer with open-ended questions regarding breathlessness during everyday activities. If the patient's recall of the baseline state (BDI) is limited, the measured change is not reliable (recall bias).

A self-administered computerized (SAC) version of the BDI/TDI has been developed to remove any interviewer bias and to provide direct patient-reported ratings of dyspnea.[16] The SAC BDI/TDI has already been used in clinical trials,[17] and an MID has been derived (1 unit difference between BDI and TDI), but this was mainly based on retrospective analyses of published data.[18]

Borg Scale

The CR-10 or Borg scale has been designed to measure exertional dyspnea in COPD patients.[19,20] The 10-point category ratio scale is easy to use. Nevertheless, detailed instructions are mandatory.[21] Based on retrospective analysis, an MID for the Borg scale in the range of 1 unit has been suggested.[22] It has widely been used in studies evaluating the effect of interventions on exercise endurance using constant load cardiopulmonary exercise testing.

Medical Research Council or Modified Medical Research Council Scale

The MRC scale was developed as a simple and standardized method to quantify dyspnea in relation to a function in COPD patients.[23] It is a 5-point scale whereby the patient is asked about dyspnea in relation to a specific level of activity. A modified version of this scale is used today (mMRC), which has simplified statements, such as "people" instead of "men." The grade of dyspnea is given from 1 to 5 (MRC) or 0 to 4 (mMRC). An MID has not been established, but 1 study has shown an increased risk of death for each unit increase in the scale. The method has been used in clinical studies[24,25] and in clinical practice primarily in many countries. Avoidance of exercise may induce underestimation of dyspnea (underestimation bias).[26] The MRC and mMRC are considered to be relatively insensitive to changes, for example, following interventions,[27,28] and its validation has been based on relatively few clinical studies.[24]

ASSESSMENT OF HEALTH STATUS

Although quality of life is a unique feature of a specific individual, health status represents a standardized quantification of the impact of a disease.[29] Health status is assessed using questionnaires.

Medical Outcomes Study Short Form-36

The medical outcomes study short form-36 (SF-36) is not a disease-specific, but a generic health survey.[30] It is designed for self-assessment of psychic, physical, and social features. Although it has 36 items, it is easy to use. The SF-36 seems to be less responsive than COPD-specific instruments.

St. George's Respiratory Questionnaire

The St. George's respiratory questionnaire (SGRQ) was developed to analyze health status in patients with respiratory disease, for example, COPD or asthma.[31] Later, a COPD-specific version was published.[32] The SGRQ has 3 domains: symptoms (frequency and severity), activity (effects on and adjustment of everyday activities), and psychosocial impact. The total score has a maximum of 100 points, with values ranging from 0 to 100. The higher the number, the more impact the disease has. The MID has been thought to be 4 points.[33]

The SGRQ represents the standard method for evaluation of health status in clinical trials. Nevertheless, it has some limitations: nonpole questions may induce a trend bias (first possible answer is usually "yes" and indicates worse health status). Besides, a missing answer is processed as if the patient had answered "no."[34] SGRQ scores are not independent of sex, age, education, and comorbidities.[35] Finally, the SGRQ has 50 items. Therefore, it is not feasible to be used in daily clinical practice.

Chronic Respiratory Disease Questionnaire

The chronic respiratory disease questionnaire (CRQ) evaluates physical-functional and emotional limitations owing to chronic lung diseases like COPD.[36] It covers dyspnea, fatigue, emotion, and mastery. The patient is asked to recall the 5 most important activities that caused breathlessness over the past 2 weeks. An MID of 0.5 has been calculated.[37] Because of its design that is based on individual assessment, it is not interchangeable with other disease-specific instruments.

Clinical Chronic Obstructive Pulmonary Disease Questionnaire

The clinical COPD questionnaire (CCQ) was developed to measure symptoms and the functional state in daily clinical practice. It is self-administered, has 10 items, and covers 3 domains (symptoms, functional, and mental state). It has been validated and is considered to be responsive to changes of the patient's situation.[38] An MID of 0.4 was calculated.[39]

CHRONIC OBSTRUCTIVE PULMONARY DISEASE ASSESSMENT TEST

The COPD Assessment Test (CAT) was developed to measure symptoms and functional state in daily life.[40,41] Besides, it may also be informative regarding comorbidities.[42] It is self-administered and contains 8 items. The CAT is validated, available in many languages, and easy to use. It has been shown to be responsive to rehabilitation[43] and exacerbations.[44] A good correlation between CAT and SGRQ has been reported.[40] Based on 1 study, CAT and CCQ have similar psychometric properties and are both valid and reliable questionnaires to assess health status in COPD patients.[45] The MID is 2 points.[46]

MULTIDIMENSIONAL SCORING SYSTEMS

There are several multidimensional scoring systems available, for example, ADO (age, dyspnea, obstruction),[47] DOSE (dyspnea, obstruction, smoking, exacerbations),[48] and body mass index, obstruction, dyspnea, and exercise capacity (BODE).[49]

The BODE index is so far the only multidimensional scoring system that has gained broader acceptance. It was developed as a prognostic marker for COPD. Included are nutritional state (Body mass index), airflow limitation (Obstruction; forced expiratory volume in 1 second, FEV_1), breathlessness (mMRC Dyspnea scale), and Exercise capacity (distance walked in 6 minutes). The BODE index has been used in interventional studies investigating effects of lung volume reduction surgery,[50] pulmonary rehabilitation,[51] and physical training.[52] The BODE index integrates subjective and objective measurements, including evaluation of exercise capacity. Its prognostic power to predict mortality and exacerbations in severe to very severe COPD is superior to the individual components.[53]

The BODE index has been optimized to predict 1-year mortality. Parameters that determine long-term survival may differ from those that predict shorter-term survival. Besides, the focus was on patients with severe and very severe airflow limitation. Thus, its validity in patients with less severe disease needs to be established. Finally, the measurement of the 6-minute walking distance requires a certain infrastructure that is not readily available in many clinics.[54]

Considering the pros and cons of all mentioned ways to assess symptoms, GOLD recommends primarily the mMRC and the CAT because of its practical implications.[1] Some of the features in both scores are shown in **Table 2**.

THRESHOLDS FOR SYMPTOM ASSESSMENT

For the SGRQ, a threshold of 25 has been established based on the findings that scores less than 25 are uncommon in COPD patients,[55] and scores greater than 25 are very unusual in healthy individuals.[56,57] An SGRQ cutoff of 25 has been related to a CAT score of 10.[58] Regarding mMRC, a threshold of greater than or equal to 2 versus smaller than 2 is used because it is at that threshold that significant increases in risk of death have been described.[1]

After the ABCD assessment system had been introduced, some discussion developed concerning the strengths and shortcomings of this concept.[59] Intensely debated was the fact that mortality was similar (and intermediate) in groups B and C. This finding may be due to comorbidities in group B that contribute to symptom load and mortality. In any case, the ABCD system (neither in its original form including FEV_1 for risk assessment of exacerbations nor in its current form

Table 2	
Measuring dyspnea and health status in patients with chronic obstructive pulmonary disease	
(A) mMRC	
Concept	Scale, simple and standardized
Methods	Selection of grade (0–4)
Strengths	Easy to use, applicable in primary care
Limitations	Relatively insensitive to change
(B) CAT	
Concept	Measure symptoms and functional status in daily practice
Methods	8 items, scale 0 to 40
Strengths	Validated, responsive, good correlation to SGRQ, applicable in primary care
Limitations	Needs scoring

Features of the scales that are recommended by the GOLD: (A) mMRC scale, (B) CAT.
Data from Refs.[13,40–43]

whereby risk of exacerbation is based on exacerbation history only) was meant to be a perfect predictor of mortality. Instead, it is a simple tool that may facilitate treatment strategies that are (better) tailored to the patient's needs.

CONFLICT OF INTEREST STATEMENT

C.F. Vogelmeier reports grants from German Federal Ministry of Education and Research (BMBF) Competence Network Asthma and COPD (ASCONET). C.F. Vogelmeier gave presentations at symposia and/or served on scientific advisory boards sponsored by AstraZeneca, Boehringer Ingelheim, CSL Behring, Chiesi, GlaxoSmithKline, Grifols, Menarini, Novartis, Nuvaira, OmniaMed, and MedUpdate. P. Alter reports grants from German Federal Ministry of Education and Research (BMBF) Competence Network Asthma and COPD (ASCONET), grants from AstraZeneca GmbH, grants and nonfinancial support from Bayer Schering Pharma AG, grants, personal fees, and nonfinancial support from Boehringer Ingelheim Pharma GmbH & Co. KG, grants and nonfinancial support from Chiesi GmbH, grants from GlaxoSmithKline, grants from Grifols Deutschland GmbH, grants from MSD Sharp & Dohme GmbH, grants and personal fees from Mundipharma GmbH, grants, personal fees, and nonfinancial support from Novartis Deutschland GmbH, grants from Pfizer Pharma GmbH and Takeda Pharma Vertrieb GmbH & Co. KG outside the submitted work. There is no conflict of interest with regard to this work.

REFERENCES

1. Vogelmeier CF, Criner GJ, Martinez FJ, et al. Global strategy for the diagnosis, management, and prevention of chronic obstructive lung disease 2017 report. GOLD executive summary. Am J Respir Crit Care Med 2017;195:557–82.

2. von Haehling S, Anker SD. Cachexia as a major underestimated and unmet medical need: facts and numbers. J Cachexia Sarcopenia Muscle 2010;1:1–5.

3. Schols AM, Soeters PB, Dingemans AM, et al. Prevalence and characteristics of nutritional depletion in patients with stable COPD eligible for pulmonary rehabilitation. Am Rev Respir Dis 1993;147:1151–6.

4. Kessler R, Partridge MR, Miravitlles M, et al. Symptom variability in patients with severe COPD: a pan-European cross-sectional study. Eur Respir J 2011;37:264–72.

5. Doyle T, Palmer S, Johnson J, et al. Association of anxiety and depression with pulmonary-specific symptoms in chronic obstructive pulmonary disease. Int J Psychiatry Med 2013;45:189–202.

6. Miravitlles M, Worth H, Soler Cataluña JJ, et al. Observational study to characterise 24-hour COPD symptoms and their relationship with patient-reported outcomes: results from the ASSESS study. Respir Res 2014;15:122.

7. Lange P, Marott JL, Vestbo J, et al. Prevalence of night-time dyspnoea in COPD and its implications for prognosis. Eur Respir J 2014;43:1590–8.

8. Calverley PM, Tetzlaff K, Dusser D, et al. Determinants of exacerbation risk in patients with COPD in the TIOSPIR study. Int J Chron Obstruct Pulmon Dis 2017;12:3391–405.

9. Regan EA, Lynch DA, Curran-Everett D, et al, Genetic Epidemiology of COPD (COPDGene) Investigators. Clinical and radiologic disease in smokers with normal spirometry. JAMA Intern Med 2015; 175:1539–49.

10. Woodruff PG, Barr RG, Bleecker E, et al. Clinical significance of symptoms in smokers with preserved pulmonary function. N Engl J Med 2016;374: 1811–21.

11. Vanfleteren LE, Spruit MA, Groenen M, et al. Clusters of comorbidities based on validated objective measurements and systemic inflammation in patients with chronic obstructive pulmonary disease. Am J Respir Crit Care Med 2013;187:728–35.

12. Vestbo J, Hurd SS, Agustí AG, et al. Global strategy for the diagnosis, management, and prevention of chronic obstructive pulmonary disease: GOLD executive summary. Am J Respir Crit Care Med 2013;187:347–65.

13. Glaab T, Vogelmeier C, Buhl R. Outcome measures in chronic obstructive pulmonary disease (COPD): strengths and limitations. Respir Res 2010;11:79.

14. Alma H, de Jong C, Tsiligianni I, et al. Clinically relevant differences in COPD health status: systematic review and triangulation. Eur Respir J 2018;52 [pii: 1800412].

15. Mahler DA, Weinberg DH, Wells CK, et al. The measurement of dyspnea. Contents, interobserver agreement, and physiologic correlates of two new clinical indexes. Chest 1984;85:751–8.

16. Mahler DA, Ward J, Fierro-Carrion G, et al. Development of self-administered versions of modified baseline and transition dyspnea indexes in COPD. COPD 2004;1:165–72.

17. Mahler DA, Decramer M, D'Urzo A, et al. Dual bronchodilation with QVA149 reduces patient-reported dyspnoea in COPD: the BLAZE study. Eur Respir J 2014;43:1599–609.

18. Mahler DA, Witek TJ. The MCID of the transition dyspnea index is a total score of one unit. COPD 2005; 2:99–103.

19. Borg G. Psychophysical bases of perceived exertion. Med Sci Sports Exerc 1982;14:377–81.

20. Borg G. Psychophysical scaling with applications in physical work and the perception of exertion. Scand J Work Environ Health 1990;16(Suppl1):55–8.

21. Mador MJ, Rodis A, Magalang UJ. Reproducibility of Borg scale measurements of dyspnea during exercise in patients with COPD. Chest 1995;107: 1590–7.

22. Cazzola M, MacNee W, Martinez FJ, et al. American Thoracic Society/European Respiratory Society Task Force on outcomes of COPD: outcomes for COPD pharmacological trials: from lung function to biomarkers. Eur Respir J 2008;31:416–69.

23. Fletcher CM, Elmes PC, Fairbairn AS, et al. The significance of respiratory symptoms and the diagnosis of chronic bronchitis in a working population. BMJ 1959;5147:257–66.

24. de Torres JP, Pinto-Plata V, Ingenito E, et al. Power of outcome measurements to detect clinically significant changes in pulmonary rehabilitation of patients with COPD. Chest 2002;121:1092–8.

25. Bourbeau J, Ford G, Zackon H, et al. Impact on patients' health status following early identification of a COPD exacerbation. Eur Respir J 2007;30: 907–13.

26. Rennard S, Decramer M, Calverley PM, et al. Impact of COPD in North America and Europe in 2000: subjects' perspective of confronting COPD international survey. Eur Respir J 2002;20:799–805.

27. Mahler DA. Measurement of dyspnea: clinical ratings. In: Mahler DA, editor. Dyspnea: mechanisms, measurement and management. 2nd edition. New York: Taylor and Francis; 2005. p. 147–64.

28. Haughney J, Gruffydd-Jones K. Patient-centred outcomes in primary care management of COPD - what do recent clinical trial data tell us? Prim Care Respir J 2004;13.105 07.

29. Jones PW. Health status and the spiral of decline. COPD 2009;6:59–63.

30. Ware JE Jr, Gandek B. Overview of the SF-36 health survey and the International Quality of Life Assessment (IQOLA) project. J Clin Epidemiol 1998;51: 903–12.

31. Jones PW, Quirk FH, Baveystock CM, et al. A self-complete measure of health status for chronic airflow limitation. The St. George's Respiratory Questionnaire. Am Rev Respir Dis 1992;145:1321–7.

32. Meguro M, Barley EA, Spencer S, et al. Development and validation of an improved, COPD-specific version of the St. George respiratory questionnaire. Chest 2007;132:456–63.

33. Jones PW. Interpreting thresholds for a clinically significant changes in health status in asthma and COPD. Eur Respir J 2002;19:398–404.

34. Mühlig S, Petermann F. Illness specific data collection on quality of life of patients with asthma and chronic obstructive bronchitis. Rehabilitation 1998; 37:25–38.

35. Ferrer M, Villasante C, Alonso J, et al. Interpretation of quality of life scores from the St george's respiratory questionnaire. Eur Respir J 2002;19:405–13.

36. Guyatt GH, Berman LB, Townsend M, et al. A measure of quality of life for clinical trials in chronic lung disease. Thorax 1987;42:773–8.

37. Schünemann HJ, Puhan M, Goldstein R, et al. Measurement properties and interpretability of the chronic respiratory disease questionnaire (CRQ). COPD 2005;2:81–9.

38. van der Molen T, Willemse BW, Schokker S, et al. Development, validity and responsiveness of the clinical COPD questionnaire. Health Qual Life Outcomes 2003;28:1–13.

39. Kon SS, Dilaver D, Mittal M, et al. The Clinical COPD Questionnaire: response to pulmonary rehabilitation and minimal clinically important difference. Thorax 2014;69:793–8.

40. Jones PW, Harding G, Berry P, et al. Development and first validation of the COPD assessment test. Eur Respir J 2009;34:648–54.

41. Jones PW, Brusselle G, Dal Negro RW, et al. Properties of the COPD assessment test in a cross-sectional European study. Eur Respir J 2011;38:29–35.

42. Marietta von Siemens S, Alter P, Lutter JI, et al. CAT score single item analysis in patients with COPD: results from COSYCONET. Respir Med 2019;159: 105810.

43. Jones PW, Harding G, Wiklund I, et al. Tests of the responsiveness of the COPD assessment test following acute exacerbation and pulmonary rehabilitation. Chest 2012;142:134–40.

44. Mackay AJ, Donaldson GC, Patel AR, et al. Usefulness of the chronic obstructive pulmonary disease assessment test to evaluate severity of COPD exacerbations. Am J Respir Crit Care Med 2012;185: 1218–24.

45. Tsiligianni IG, van der Molen T, Moraitaki D, et al. Assessing health status in COPD. A head-to-head comparison between the COPD assessment test (CAT) and the clinical COPD questionnaire (CCQ). BMC Pulm Med 2012;12:20.

46. Kon SS, Canavan JL, Jones SE, et al. Minimum clinically important difference for the COPD Assessment Test: a prospective analysis. Lancet Respir Med 2014;2:195–203.

47. Puhan MA, Garcia-Aymerich J, Frey M, et al. Expansion of the prognostic assessment of patients with chronic obstructive pulmonary disease: the updated BODE index and the ADO index. Lancet 2009;374:704–11.

48. Jones RC, Donaldson GC, Chavannes NH, et al. Derivation and validation of a composite index of severity in chronic obstructive pulmonary disease: the DOSE Index. Am J Respir Crit Care Med 2009; 180:1189–95.

49. Celli BR, Cote CG, Marin JM, et al. The body-mass index, airflow obstruction, dyspnea, and exercise

capacity index in chronic obstructive pulmonary disease. N Engl J Med 2004;350:1005–12.

50. Martinez FJ, Han MK, Andrei AC, et al. National Emphysema Treatment Trial Research Group. Longitudinal change in the BODE index predicts mortality in severe emphysema. Am J Respir Crit Care Med 2008;178:491–9.

51. Cote CG, Celli BR. Pulmonary rehabilitation and the BODE index in COPD. Eur Respir J 2005;26:630–6.

52. Nasis IG, Vogiatzis I, Stratakos G, et al. Effects of interval-load versus constant-load training on the BODE index in COPD patients. Respir Med 2009;103:1392–8.

53. Marin JM, Carrizo SJ, Casanova C, et al. Prediction of risk of COPD exacerbations by the BODE index. Respir Med 2009;103:373–8.

54. ATS statement: guidelines for the six-minute walk test. ATS Committee on Proficiency Standards for Clinical Pulmonary Function Laboratories. Am J Respir Crit Care Med 2002;166:111–7.

55. Agusti A, Calverley PM, Celli B, et al. Evaluation of COPD Longitudinally to Identify Predictive Surrogate Endpoints (ECLIPSE) investigators. Characterisation of COPD heterogeneity in the ECLIPSE cohort. Respir Res 2010;11:122.

56. Nishimura K, Mitsuma S, Kobayashi A, et al. COPD and disease-specific health status in a working population. Respir Res 2013;14:61.

57. Miravitlles M, Soriano JB, Garcia-Rio F, et al. Prevalence of COPD in Spain: impact of undiagnosed COPD on quality of life and daily life activities. Thorax 2009;64:863–8.

58. Jones PW, Tabberer M, Chen WH. Creating scenarios of the impact of COPD and their relationship to COPD Assessment Test (CAT™) scores. BMC Pulm Med 2011;11:42.

59. Agusti A, Hurd S, Jones P, et al. FAQs about the GOLD 2011 assessment proposal of COPD: a comparative analysis of four different cohorts. Eur Respir J 2013;42:1391–401.

Computerized Chest Imaging in the Diagnosis and Assessment of the Patient with Chronic Obstructive Pulmonary Disease

Carrie L. Pistenmaa, MD*, George R. Washko, MD, MSc

KEYWORDS

- Chronic obstructive pulmonary disease • Lung • Imaging • Computed tomography • Parenchyma
- Vasculature • Comorbidity

KEY POINTS

- Computed tomography provides information relevant to parenchymal, airway, vascular, and extrapulmonary manifestations of chronic obstructive pulmonary disease (COPD).
- Currently, the primary clinical application of imaging in COPD is to evaluate emphysema in candidates for surgical or bronchoscopic lung volume reduction.
- At the time of diagnosis and in management of COPD, imaging is also utilized to look for alternative or additional causes of dyspnea and cough.
- There has been a lag between research investigation and clinical applications of imaging in COPD; however, promising studies are ongoing with near-term potential to impact disease diagnosis, prognosis, and therapy.

INTRODUCTION

Computed tomography (CT) has been extensively leveraged in research investigations of chronic obstructive pulmonary disease (COPD). Computer-aided tools can provide objective characterization of lung disease, yet advances in clinical care lag behind discoveries made in research. Although this phenomenon is generally true of all medical conditions, the gulf between imaging-based research and COPD treatment is striking. This article provides an overview of the advances made in COPD-based image processing over the past 4 decades, describes the current standard of practice for COPD care, and then provides a brief description of the path forward where the two may meet.

BACKGROUND

Lung Parenchyma

CT was introduced into clinical care in the 1980s, and since that time there have been extensive efforts to identify and quantify features that may be

Competing interests: C.L. Pistenmaa received research grants from the Alpha-1 Foundation and Boehringer Ingelheim. G.R. Washko received research grants from Boehringer Ingelheim, BTG Interventional Medicine and Janssen Pharmaceuticals, and personal fees from Boehringer Ingelheim, PulmonX, Janssen Pharmaceuticals, GlaxoSmithKline, Novartis, and Vertex and is a cofounder and co-owner of Quantitative Imaging Solutions, a company that provides image-based consulting and develops software to enable data sharing.
Funded by: NIHHYB. Grant number(s): K23 HL141651; R01 HL116473.
Division of Pulmonary and Critical Care, Brigham and Women's Hospital, Harvard Medical School, 75 Francis Street, Boston, MA 02115, USA
* Corresponding author.
E-mail address: cpistenmaa@bwh.harvard.edu

Clin Chest Med 41 (2020) 375–381
https://doi.org/10.1016/j.ccm.2020.06.012

used to improve understanding of chronic respiratory conditions such as COPD. One of the pathologic bases for COPD is emphysematous destruction of the lung parenchyma. This process, defined as abnormal and permanent dilation of the distal airspaces due to destruction of alveolar walls, results in reduced lung elastic recoil leading to hyperinflation, expiratory airflow obstruction, and breathlessness.[1] On CT, emphysema appears as holes in the lung that can be readily quantified by measuring the density or attenuation (in Hounsfield units, HU) of the parenchyma.[2–4] While normal lung tissue may have an attenuation of approximately −856 HU, emphysema has attenuation values less than −910 to −960 HU depending on the parameters used for image acquisition and reconstruction. Thus, an HU threshold can be selected that differentiates nonemphysematous and emphysematous lung, and the percent of low attenuation areas (LAA%: volume of low attenuating lung/total lung volume*100) can be calculated as the proportion of emphysematous lung tissue (**Fig. 1**).[3] A second way to objectively quantify emphysema is by calculating the HU value that demarcates the lowest 15% of the lung histogram from the remaining 85%, called the percent density (PD) 15.[5] Both of these measures from the density histogram are obtained at suspended full

inspiration, and a limitation of the test is suboptimal inspiration during the CT scan. One way to overcome this limitation is to adjust PD15 for differences in lung volume,[6] although as hyperinflation is part of the disease process in COPD, it is possible this may cause some overcorrection in some cases.

The initial efforts to objectify emphysema were performed with density mask or densitometric analyses, which demonstrated that there was a direct relationship between the degree of emphysema evident on CT and both the severity of lung disease and histopathologically determined degree of airspace dilation.[3,4] Multiple subsequent investigations have replicated these findings, and densitometry has become the standard method for quantifying airspace dilation in clinical, epidemiologic, genetic, and therapeutic investigation. The evolution of computational capacity has fostered the growth of more advanced postprocessing machine learning and deep learning techniques. These algorithms have several advantages over conventional densitometry, as they incorporate information on the distribution of emphysema within the lung and quantifying the admixture of centrilobular, paraseptal, and panlobular emphysema present in an individual.

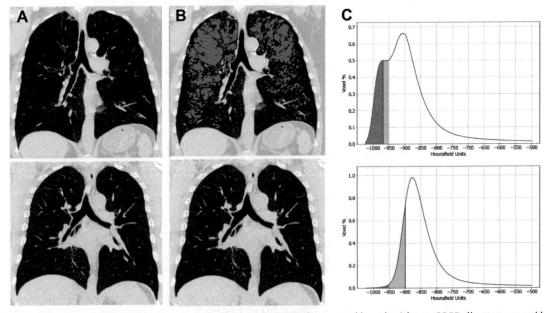

Fig. 1. Imaging of emphysema for an individual with COPD (*top panels*) and without COPD (*bottom panels*) showing (*A*) coronal CT image, (*B*) coronal CT image with blue shading to indicate low attenuation areas (LAA, or emphysema-like lung) with attenuation of no more than −950 HU and (*C*) lung density distribution of all voxels for each CT showing the percent LAA (shaded *blue*) and density at the lower 15th percentile (PD15, shaded *red*), y-axis is the percent density at each HU. (*Top panel*: %LAA 23.9, PD15 -968 HU. *Bottom panel*: %LAA 0.5, PD15 -898 HU.)

CT-based investigation has also demonstrated that the lung manifests divergent responses to noxious insults such as chronic tobacco smoke exposure. Smokers may appear resilient to the injurious effects of tobacco smoke or may develop emphysema and even pulmonary fibrosis. Recent investigation suggests approximately 6% to 8% of smokers over the age of 50 have some degree of interstitial remodeling of the lung parenchyma.[7] These processes have collectively been termed interstitial lung abnormalities (ILAs) and have been shown to have similar genetic associations as advanced pulmonary fibrosis. The presence of ILA is independently associated with all-cause and respiratory-specific mortality in population-based studies.[8–10] Extensive work is ongoing to determine which subset of these ILAs progress to classic interstitial lung disease and potentially when to initiate antifibrotic therapy.

AIRWAYS

A second area of focused investigation in smokers is the CT-based assessment of airway disease. Studies using these techniques initially reported that smokers with thicker airway walls on CT scan were more likely to have more compromised lung function.[11,12] Histopathologic studies have repeatedly demonstrated that remodeling of the small airways is the primary event in the development of expiratory airflow obstruction in smokers.[13,14] Using retrograde catheterization and explanted human lungs, Hogg and colleagues[15] demonstrated that those airways less than 2 mm in diameter were the site of greatest resistance to airflow in COPD. Subsequent work has explored the pathologic changes to the airways and discovered that not only does the remodeling process manifest as inflammation, fibrosis, and mural plugging, but these processes may culminate in destruction and ultimately an absence of these small airways.[16] More recent work has demonstrated that the reduction in numbers of terminal bronchioles was highly correlated with disease stage but was also associated with reductions of the more proximal airway count collected from clinical CT scanning, suggesting that objective assessments of the airways on conventional CT may provide insight into the distal lung.[17]

BEYOND LUNG PARENCHYMA AND AIRWAYS

Another quantitative method for assessing the airways on CT is parametric response mapping (PRM).[18] This technique utilizes the difference in lung density between inspiratory and expiratory scans to calculate gas trapping caused by small airway disease. Small airway obstruction does not allow full deflation of the lung parenchyma; this results in a lower attenuation of these areas on expiration when compared with lung parenchyma supplied by normal airways. PRM has been used extensively in the clinical characterization of COPD and has been recently validated against micro-CT based assessments of distal lung architecture.[19]

The increasing utilization of imaging in COPD and the multidisciplinary approaches to research have accelerated the refinement of techniques focused on the parenchyma and airways while facilitating the collection of imaging data that have provided more full characterization of the breadth of thoracic pathology evident in smokers. Examples of this work include morphologic assessments of the pulmonary vasculature, both the intraparenchymal vessels and central pulmonary artery and aorta. Vascular measures, including arterial and venous segmentation on CT, can be used to identify people at greatest risk for disease progression, improve the understanding of the interdependence of heart and lung, and be used to predict acute respiratory exacerbations and response to therapeutic interventions such as bronchoscopic lung volume reduction (**Fig. 2**).[20–23]

CT is also being leveraged to expand appreciation of the extracardiopulmonary effects of COPD. Examples of this include detailed assessments of body composition and the recognition that sarcopenia is a major contributor to the morbidity and mortality of COPD and even smokers with normal lung function.[24,25] Similarly, objective assessments of volumetric bone mineral density demonstrated that the pathologic loss of bone density is highly prevalent in smokers, even those without COPD.[26] Further, contrary to standard screening practices, these losses and subsequent vertebral compression fractures are equally if not more common in men than women.[26]

The next section of this document provides a description of the current use of imaging in the clinical care of patients with COPD in the ambulatory setting. It will become quickly evident to the reader that much of what was just described, the advanced postprocessing techniques enabling detection and quantification of parenchymal, airway, cardiovascular and metabolic conditions in COPD, are not utilized in clinical practice. The reasons for this are detailed after the section describing the current use of imaging in the clinical care of COPD in the ambulatory setting.

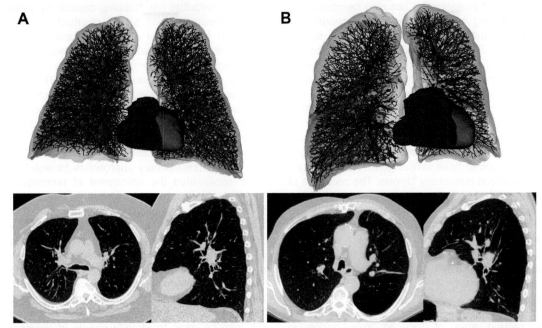

Fig. 2. Imaging from individuals without vascular pruning (*left*) and with vascular pruning (*right*) showing (*A*) reconstructed CT imaging of pulmonary vasculature, segmented into arteries (*blue*) and veins (*red*) and (*B*) axial and sagittal CT images from the same individuals. (*Left*: forced expiratory volume in the first second of expiration [FEV1] 1.3 L, FEV1/forced vital capacity [FVC] 0.38, %LAA 19.9, PD15 -959 HU. *Right*: FEV1 1.2 L, FEV1/FVC 0.34, % LAA 18.7, PD15 -955.)

CLINICAL UTILIZATION OF IMAGING IN CHRONIC OBSTRUCTIVE PULMONARY DISEASE

COPD should be considered in any patient with chronic dyspnea or productive cough, or those with recurrent exacerbations of these symptoms, particularly in the context of risk factors such as family history, tobacco smoke, or other inhalational exposures.[27] Imaging is not considered in the diagnosis of COPD, which requires the finding of an incompletely reversible obstructive deficit on spirometry. However, in clinical practice, chest imaging is often helpful to exclude other causes of cough or dyspnea, such as lung cancer, tuberculosis, bronchiectasis, interstitial lung disease, or pulmonary embolism.

In established COPD, imaging is used as needed to evaluate for coexisting pulmonary processes. Because COPD is so common, it has considerable overlap with other pulmonary diseases, particularly bronchiectasis, interstitial lung disease, and vascular abnormalities, including pulmonary embolism and pulmonary hypertension. In the authors' opinion, further evaluation is warranted when patients have disproportionate symptoms, more advanced disease than expected given their age and exposure history, when a restrictive deficit is also present on pulmonary function testing, or after recurrence of respiratory events.

Disproportionate symptoms refer to dyspnea that is disproportionate to the functional impairment observed in pulmonary function testing in obstructed patients, particularly if the symptom does not respond to bronchodilator therapy, or a cough that is more tenacious and purulent than usually seen, suggestive of bronchiectasis. More advanced disease than expected includes younger patients (those younger than 50) and those with minimal smoking history or other known exposures. On spirometry, a low vital forced vital capacity in COPD may be caused by gas trapping, but a true restrictive deficit by lung volumes may indicate coexisting interstitial lung disease. A significantly reduced DLCO without extensive emphysema or air trapping may indicate coexisting pulmonary vascular disease. Repeated hospitalizations or respiratory events may also indicate an additional process such as bronchiectasis. Thus, although CT is not routinely performed in COPD and may not alter treatment, there are many scenarios in which it is helpful to evaluate for coexisting diseases.

In severe COPD, chest imaging is recommended to evaluate for the distribution of emphysema as part of an assessment for lung volume reduction by surgical or bronchoscopic approach. Lung volume reduction surgery is one of the few treatments with proven mortality benefit in COPD, in selected patients.[28] Newer bronchoscopic approaches to lung volume reduction have also proven to be of clinical benefit in advanced emphysema, and longer term studies are ongoing.[29,30] Thus, patients with significant hyperinflation should be referred to an experienced hospital center with both thoracic surgery and interventional pulmonary expertise in order to determine the treatment options available.

THE PATH FORWARD

The gulf between the ability to objectively characterize the multifaceted nature of COPD on thoracic CT and what is used for the clinical management of COPD is clear. There are several reasons for this, which can be largely ascribed to the understandable lag between enhanced understanding of disease and the development of new therapies for that disease. The years spanning the 1980s to 2000s were characterized by the belief that objective metrics of emphysema and airway disease would allow clinicians to understand disease and optimize therapy. Although the heterogeneity of COPD quickly became visually apparent with the advent of CT, this enhanced understanding has as of yet had minimal impact on clinical practice. Short- and long-acting bronchodilators and anti-inflammatory agents, the long-standing backbone of COPD treatment, require little to no radiologic insight to initiate or monitor the effects of therapy. Improvements in symptoms, lung function or both were and are still deemed a success. Advances in CT technology over the past 40 years have also improved image resolution while lowering radiation exposure, and the risk-benefit profile makes them more palatable for research and increasing clinical applications.

Pharmaceutical companies are now developing therapies targeting the pathologic basis of disease and attempting to slow the progression of emphysema, all of which are of great interest. Although the relationship between emphysema and reduced lung function suggests that one could simply use lung function as the primary outcome, the sample sizes and study duration required to impact on lung function are prohibitive, and given the heterogeneity of disease and its progression, there is reason to believe that some interventions may work on only the airways or emphysema, not both simultaneously. CT is being used to detect patients most likely to respond to such treatment (ie, those with some degree of existing emphysema). The technique is also being used to monitor their response to treatment in placebo-controlled studies. The abundance of cross-sectional and longitudinal imaging and clinical data collected over the past 40 years has begun to foster a level of comfort in the biomedical community about using imaging to identify potential new therapies and has provided the foundation to prepare and submit an application to the US Food and Drug Administration (FDA) to qualify CT measures of emphysema progression as an endpoint for clinical investigation. This work is being led by the COPD Biomarkers Qualification Consortium similar to what has been done for other biomarkers like fibrinogen.[31]

There is another pragmatic utilization of CT data that can have immediate clinical implications related to disease diagnosis. Thoracic CT scans are among the most common types of imaging obtained during routine clinical care. The indications for such testing are broad and include acute-onset dyspnea or pleuritic chest discomfort. Such tests often rule out processes such as thromboembolism but are less often leveraged for more comprehensive assessments of lung heath and the presence of characteristics suggestive of chronic lung disease. As described earlier, there are multiple radiologic features evident on thoracic CT that may be used to detect and stratify smoking-related lung disease. The presence of emphysema, parenchymal fibrosis, or bronchiectatic dilation of the airways all merit further evaluation in patients with and without COPD. These features are also sometimes evident in the lung bases and thus can be an incidental finding on abdominal CT as well.

The first step in optimizing the clinical use of existing CT data is making sure that these features are noted by the interpreting radiologist and recorded in their report in a standardized fashion. Particularly with the evolution of smart electronic medical record systems, such documentation can then trigger further clinical evaluation such as a detailed review of exposure history, family history, spirometry, and even referral to a respiratory specialist depending upon practice location and physician availability. Even in the absence of obstructive or restrictive physiology, emphysema, fibrosis, and bronchiectasis are associated with a poorer prognosis and warrant clinical evaluation and often times therapeutic intervention. Although uncommon, emphysema in younger or nonsmoking patients should raise the possible diagnosis of alpha-1 antitrypsin deficiency, a diagnosis that has important implications for disease prevention (including in potentially affected family members) and therapy. There are also new promising therapies for fibrosis, but patients who are undiagnosed cannot access such care.

The goals of imaging-based detection of parenchymal and airway abnormalities are early diagnosis and intervention leading to disease prevention. If the goal is to identify treatments that work in early disease, research efforts must include those patients who do not yet meet the spirometric definition of COPD but who are at high risk. It is hoped that at some point, one will not wait for a patient to develop expiratory airflow obstruction before initiating therapies that may improve symptoms or reduce the risk of future respiratory events and hospitalization in chronic lung disease. CT imaging provides an important tool that can identify these patients, and one can expect that it will be increasingly incorporated into routine clinical care.

SUMMARY

CT imaging has been extensively utilized in research, as it provides qualitative and quantitative information relevant to parenchymal, airway, vascular, and extrapulmonary manifestations of COPD. However, there has been a delay in translating this knowledge to the bedside, as the current clinical application is primarily in evaluating the extent of emphysema in candidates for surgical or bronchoscopic lung volume reduction. Imaging is also helpful in evaluating for alternate or additional causes of dyspnea and/or cough, including coexisting diseases such as bronchiectasis, interstitial lung disease, lung cancer, pulmonary embolism, and pulmonary hypertension. Although much work remains, the authors believe imaging has the near-term potential to lead to earlier diagnosis, better disease prognostication, and more individualized therapeutic intervention.

REFERENCES

1. Snider GL. Emphysema: the first two centuries–and beyond. A historical overview, with suggestions for future research: part 1. Am Rev Respir Dis 1992; 146(5 Pt 1):1334–44.
2. Hayhurst MD, MacNee W, Flenley DC, et al. Diagnosis of pulmonary emphysema by computerised tomography. Lancet 1984;2(8398):320–2.
3. Muller NL, Staples CA, Miller RR, et al. "Density mask." An objective method to quantitate emphysema using computed tomography. Chest 1988; 94(4):782–7.
4. Kinsella M, Muller NL, Abboud RT, et al. Quantitation of emphysema by computed tomography using a "density mask" program and correlation with pulmonary function tests. Chest 1990;97(2):315–21.
5. Parr DG, Sevenoaks M, Deng C, et al. Detection of emphysema progression in alpha 1-antitrypsin deficiency using CT densitometry; methodological advances. Respir Res 2008;9:21.
6. Stoel BC, Putter H, Bakker ME, et al. Volume correction in computed tomography densitometry for follow-up studies on pulmonary emphysema. Proc Am Thorac Soc 2008;5(9):919–24.
7. Washko GR, Hunninghake GM, Fernandez IE, et al. Lung volumes and emphysema in smokers with interstitial lung abnormalities. N Engl J Med 2011; 364(10):897–906.
8. Hunninghake GM, Hatabu H, Okajima Y, et al. MUC5B promoter polymorphism and interstitial lung abnormalities. N Engl J Med 2013;368(23): 2192–200.
9. Doyle TJ, Washko GR, Fernandez IE, et al. Interstitial lung abnormalities and reduced exercise capacity. Am J Respir Crit Care Med 2012;185(7):756–62.
10. Putman RK, Hatabu H, Araki T, et al. Association between interstitial lung abnormalities and all-cause mortality. JAMA 2016;315(7):672–81.
11. Nakano Y, Muro S, Sakai H, et al. Computed tomographic measurements of airway dimensions and emphysema in smokers. Correlation with lung function. Am J Respir Crit Care Med 2000;162(3 Pt 1): 1102–8.
12. Hasegawa M, Nasuhara Y, Onodera Y, et al. Airflow limitation and airway dimensions in chronic obstructive pulmonary disease. Am J Respir Crit Care Med 2006;173(12):1309–15.
13. Cosio M, Ghezzo H, Hogg JC, et al. The relations between structural changes in small airways and pulmonary-function tests. N Engl J Med 1978; 298(23):1277–81.
14. Niewoehner DE, Kleinerman J, Rice DB. Pathologic changes in the peripheral airways of young cigarette smokers. N Engl J Med 1974;291(15):755–8.
15. Hogg JC, Macklem PT, Thurlbeck WM. Site and nature of airway obstruction in chronic obstructive lung disease. N Engl J Med 1968;278(25):1355–60.
16. Hogg JC, Chu F, Utokaparch S, et al. The nature of small-airway obstruction in chronic obstructive pulmonary disease. N Engl J Med 2004;350(26): 2645–53.
17. McDonough JE, Yuan R, Suzuki M, et al. Small-airway obstruction and emphysema in chronic obstructive pulmonary disease. N Engl J Med 2011;365(17):1567–75.
18. Galban CJ, Han MK, Boes JL, et al. Computed tomography-based biomarker provides unique signature for diagnosis of COPD phenotypes and disease progression. Nat Med 2012;18(11): 1711–5.
19. Vasilescu DM, Martinez FJ, Marchetti N, et al. Noninvasive imaging biomarker identifies small airway damage in severe chronic obstructive pulmonary

disease. Am J Respir Crit Care Med 2019;200(5): 575–81.

20. Wells JM, Washko GR, Han MK, et al. Pulmonary arterial enlargement and acute exacerbations of COPD. N Engl J Med 2012;367(10):913–21.

21. Estepar RS, Kinney GL, Black-Shinn JL, et al. Computed tomographic measures of pulmonary vascular morphology in smokers and their clinical implications. Am J Respir Crit Care Med 2013; 188(2):231–9.

22. Washko GR, Nardelli P, Ash SY, et al. Arterial vascular pruning, right ventricular size, and clinical outcomes in chronic obstructive pulmonary disease. A longitudinal observational study. Am J Respir Crit Care Med 2019;200(4):454–61.

23. Schuhmann M, Raffy P, Yin Y, et al. Computed to-mography predictors of response to endobronchial valve lung reduction treatment. Comparison with Chartis. Am J Respir Crit Care Med 2015;191(7): 767–74.

24. Marquis K, Debigare R, Lacasse Y, et al. Midthigh muscle cross-sectional area is a better predictor of mortality than body mass index in patients with chronic obstructive pulmonary disease. Am J Respir Crit Care Med 2002;166(6):809–13.

25. Diaz AA, Martinez CH, Harmouche R, et al. Pectora-lis muscle area and mortality in smokers without airflow obstruction. Respir Res 2018;19(1):62.

26. Jaramillo JD, Wilson C, Stinson DS, et al. Reduced Bone Density and vertebral fractures in smokers. men and COPD patients at increased risk. Ann Am Thorac Soc 2015;12(5):648–56.

27. Singh D, Agusti A, Anzueto A, et al. Global strategy for the diagnosis, management, and prevention of chronic obstructive lung disease: the GOLD science committee report 2019. Eur Respir J 2019;53(5): 1900164.

28. Fishman A, Martinez F, Naunheim K, et al. A randomized trial comparing lung-volume-reduction surgery with medical therapy for severe emphysema. N Engl J Med 2003;348(21):2059–73.

29. Klooster K, ten Hacken NH, Hartman JE, et al. Endo-bronchial valves for emphysema without interlobar collateral ventilation. N Engl J Med 2015;373(24): 2325–35.

30. Criner GJ, Delage A, Voelker K, et al. Improving lung function in severe heterogenous emphysema with the spiration valve system (EMPROVE). a multi-center, open-label randomized controlled clinical trial. Am J Respir Crit Care Med 2019;200(11): 1354–62.

31. Miller BE, Tal-Singer R, Rennard SI, et al. Plasma fibrinogen qualification as a drug development tool in chronic obstructive pulmonary disease. perspec-tive of the chronic obstructive pulmonary disease biomarker qualification consortium. Am J Respir Crit Care Med 2016;193(6):607–13.

Biomarkers in Chronic Obstructive Pulmonary Disease
The Gateway to Precision Medicine

Stephen Milne, BBiomedSc, MBBS, FRACP, PhD[a,b,*],
Don D. Sin, MD, MPH, FRCP(C)[a]

KEYWORDS

- Chronic obstructive pulmonary disease • Biomarkers • Precision medicine

KEY POINTS

- Chronic obstructive pulmonary disease (COPD) is a heterogeneous disease, and better targeted therapy is warranted.
- Biomarkers may be categorized by their primary role or purpose: susceptibility, diagnostic, prognostic, or therapeutic.
- Biomarkers that predict a therapeutic response may be used to guide treatment and form part of the precision medicine paradigm.
- Plasma fibrinogen, which predicts high risk of acute exacerbations, currently is the only biomarker approved by the Food and Drug Administration for use in COPD.
- There are any number of associations between potential biomarkers and COPD outcomes, but few meet the characteristics of a good biomarker.

INTRODUCTION

Chronic obstructive pulmonary disease (COPD) is a progressive disease of the lung characterized by irreversible airflow obstruction, persistent airway inflammation, and recurrent acute exacerbations. There is considerable heterogeneity in the susceptibility, inflammatory profiles, clinical presentations, long-term trajectories, and treatment responses among people with COPD. It, therefore, is not surprising that a 1-size-fits-all approach to managing COPD has led to limited progress in modifying the natural history of this disease. Biomarkers may have a role in dissecting this heterogeneity, from aiding diagnosis and early disease detection through to risk assessment and targeted treatment. This review outlines the characteristics of useful biomarkers while highlighting some of the challenges of biomarker research in a complex disease, such as COPD.

THE MOVE TOWARD PRECISION MEDICINE

Randomized controlled trials, which sit at the pinnacle of the evidence-based medicine pyramid, aim to minimize the effects of interindividual variability by randomly allocating large numbers of people to 2 or more groups distinguishable only by the intervention they receive (eg, treatment or placebo). The reported trial outcomes, therefore, represent the average response to an intervention among an average group of patients. Considerable heterogeneity of treatment response, however, is likely to exist within the allocated groups. In order to maximize benefit and minimize harm for

[a] Centre for Heart Lung Innovation and Division of Respiratory Medicine, University of British Columbia, Room 166, St Paul's Hospital, 1081 Burrard St, Vancouver, British Columbia V6Z 1Y6, Canada; [b] Faculty of Medicine and Health, University of Sydney, Camperdown, New South Wales 2006, Australia
* Corresponding author. Centre for Heart Lung Innovation, St Paul's Hospital, Room 166, 1081 Burrard Street, Vancouver, British Columbia V6Z 1Y6, Canada.
E-mail address: Stephen.milne@hli.ubc.ca

Clin Chest Med 41 (2020) 383–394
https://doi.org/10.1016/j.ccm.2020.06.001

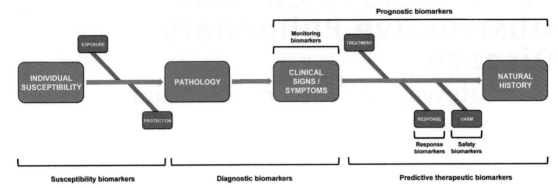

Fig. 1. Categories of biomarkers.

the individual, a more targeted approach clearly is necessary.

The National Institutes of Health (NIH) define precision medicine as "an approach to disease prevention and treatment that takes into account individual variability in genes, environment and lifestyle."[1] Under the precision medicine paradigm, heterogeneity is not minimized or ignored but instead is harnessed or embraced in order to provide a more targeted approach to patient care. Such an approach may maximize not only the benefit:risk ratio (which is an implicit part of precision medicine) but also the benefit:cost ratio. Targeting treatment toward patients who will gain the most benefit is necessary if health care systems are to be sustainable. Biomarkers, which help facilitate better-targeted therapy, will play a crucial role in the transition to a precision medicine future (**Fig. 1**).

WHAT IS (AND WHAT IS NOT) A BIOMARKER?
A Broad Definition of Biomarkers

The NIH defines a biomarker as "a characteristic that is objectively measured and evaluated as an indicator of normal biological processes, pathogenic processes, or pharmacologic responses to a therapeutic intervention."[2] This broad definition is attractive because it does not prescribe what form a biomarker must take. That is, a biomarker is not restricted to molecules or cells but can be any measurable quality—as long as it meets the criteria of being objective and is demonstrably related to biological processes. Biomarkers of relevance to the respiratory system, therefore, may include cellular, molecular, or microbiological measurements from biological samples (blood, sputum, and bronchoalveolar lavage); physiologic measurements (arterial blood gases, pulse oximetry, and lung function tests); medical imaging (computed tomography [CT] and magnetic resonance imaging [MRI]); and clinical prediction rules.

Categories of Biomarkers

Rather than grouping biomarkers by the type or source of the measurement, it is more useful to consider them based on their purpose or utility (**Fig. 2**, **Table 1**). This provides a useful framework for identifying gaps in knowledge in any given disease and for structuring biomarker research.

What Makes a Good Biomarker?

Within a broad conceptual framework of biomarkers, where virtually any objectively measured characteristic could meet the definition, it is pertinent to consider why some biomarkers might be considered useful, whereas many are not.

- Biological plausibility—there should be a strong, consistent, and independent relationship between the biomarker and the disease, either its pathology/physiology or its associated clinical outcomes. Although there need not be evidence of a direct, causal link between a biomarker and the disease, it should at least be plausible that the biomarker is reflecting the disease pathophysiology.
- Test performance—biomarker measurements may take many forms, but the test should be reliable and repeatable, with high sensitivity and specificity for the outcome.
- Confounders—the biomarker association with disease or treatment outcomes should be free from confounding influences unrelated to the disease itself. Known confounders (eg, active cigarette smoking) may be adjusted for in statistical models.
- Treatment outcomes—for a response biomarker, the measured change in the biomarker should be related directly to a change in clinical state. For a predictive biomarker, the predicted response should be a measurable and clinically relevant outcome,

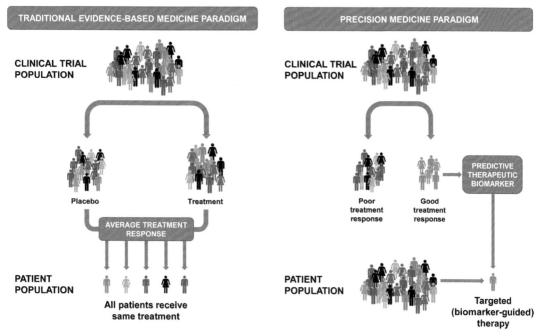

Fig. 2. Biomarker-guided therapy under the precision medicine paradigm. Under the traditional evidence-based medicine paradigm (*left panel*), variation among individuals in clinical trial populations is controlled for by randomization. An average treatment response is determined and applied to a heterogeneous patient population leading to heterogeneous treatment responses. Under the precision medicine paradigm (*right panel*), heterogeneity of treatment responses in clinical trials is investigated and predictive biomarkers developed. These then are used to identify individuals among a heterogeneous patient population who are most likely to respond to the treatment.

taking into account the minimal clinically important difference.

- Simplicity—in many cases, biomarkers may act as surrogates of pathology and thus avoid invasive diagnostic testing. A biomarker may not be useful in practice, however, if its measurement is excessively complicated or equally invasive. An ideal biomarker would be easy to obtain, measure, and interpret and would carry some meaning to a clinician.

THE CURRENT (AND FUTURE) LANDSCAPE OF BIOMARKERS IN CHRONIC OBSTRUCTIVE LUNG DISEASE

Only 1 biomarker—fibrinogen—so far has been approved under the US Food and Drug Administration (FDA) Biomarker Qualification Program.[3] This program applies rigorous standards to the evaluation of biomarker candidates for a specific context of use. Fibrinogen, therefore, is discussed on its own. For the remainder of this section, other biomarker candidates are discussed, including why they may or may not be considered useful. Our aim is to provide examples that illustrate some of the more novel - and challenging -

aspects of biomarker development in COPD, without necessarily endorsing individual biomarker candidates.

Plasma Fibrinogen: The Early Qualifier

Fibrinogen is a plasma glycoprotein that is an essential part of the blood coagulation cascade and is an acute phase reactant.[4] One of the first reported associations between plasma fibrinogen and COPD was by Alessandri and colleagues,[5] who found that plasma levels were increased in COPD patients, independent of smoking. Subsequently, large general population studies showed that higher plasma fibrinogen was associated with lower percentage of predicted forced expiratory volume in 1 second (FEV_1),[6] faster rate of FEV_1 decline over time,[6] and incident COPD.[7] Given the nonspecific nature of increased plasma fibrinogen, however, it was unlikely to ever be established as a diagnostic biomarker capable of identifying at-risk individuals within a general population.

Plasma fibrinogen is more useful as a prognostic biomarker. It is increased in COPD patients with a high rate of moderate and severe exacerbations,[8] and high levels are associated with increased risk of death.[9] High plasma fibrinogen, therefore, is

Table 1
Categories and examples of established and novel potential biomarkers in chronic obstructive pulmonary disease

Category	Description	Potential Applications	Established Biomarkers or Most Viable Candidates	Examples	
				Associated but Less Viable Candidates	Promising Novel Candidates
Susceptibility biomarkers	Indicate the likelihood of developing a disease in individuals who do not yet show pathologic changes or clinical signs/symptoms	Aggressive surveillance Targeted preventative strategies Enrichment of cohort studies/clinical trials of preventative interventions		Genetics SERPINA1 mutations	Genetics GWSs (weighted score of many SNPs with small individual effect sizes)[19] Imaging Anatomic variants or developmentally determined structural changes[21,22]
Diagnostic biomarkers	Assists diagnosis in individuals who already have pathology or clinical signs/symptoms of the disease	Surrogate tests to avoid complex/invasive diagnostic tests (eg, surgical biopsy) Increasing diagnostic certainty Early-stage disease detection Phenotyping/endotyping Surrogate for disease severity Monitoring disease progression over time	Physiology Reduced FEV$_1$/FVC ratio (gold standard diagnostic test, but still a biomarker of the underlying pathology)	Physiology Reduced DLCO[26] Increased RV/TLC ratio[27]	Physiology VH (MBNW)[30] Respiratory impedance (oscillometry)[30] Imaging Airspace enlargement (increased ADC) on 3He MRI[33] Thoracic CT changes (eg, density distribution)[34]

	Definition	Clinical uses			
Prognostic biomarkers	Indicate the likelihood of a particular event, outcome or trajectory in a person who already has the disease	Identify individuals at high risk of adverse outcomes—initiate aggressive treatment; Enrichment of clinical trials with high-risk subjects	Blood: Increased fibrinogen (exacerbation risk)[12a]; Physiology: Severely reduced FEV$_1$ (mortality)[49]; Objective clinical predictors BODE index (mortality)[50]	Blood: Reduced CC-16 (FEV$_1$ decline)[11,37,39]; Reduced SP-D (FEV$_1$ decline)[38]; sRAGE (FEV$_1$ decline)[40]; Eosinophil count (exacerbation risk)[43,44]	Blood: Reduced IgG (exacerbations)[46]; Physiology: Day-to-day variability in impedance on oscillometry (imminent exacerbation risk)[47]; Objective clinical predictors Comprehensive clinical calculators (lung function decline, exacerbation risk)[42]; Microbiology: Sputum microbiome (mortality after exacerbation)[52]
Therapeutic biomarkers	Identify individuals in whom a biological response has occurred after a treatment/intervention (response biomarker) or those who are likely to respond favorably/unfavorably to a treatment (predictive biomarker)	Determine the success of treatment; Targeted therapy—maximize benefit:harm ratio; Optimize cost-effectiveness	Blood: High eosinophil count (predictive of response to ICS therapy)[57,58]; Imaging: Upper lobe emphysema on CT (predicts success of LVRS/ELVR)[62,63]; Fissure completeness (predicts success of ELVR)[63–66]		Physiology: Increased impedance on oscillometry (predicts deflation/release of trapped gas after bronchodilator)[55]

Abbreviations: 3He, helium-3; ELVR, endoscopic lung volume reduction; FVC, forced vital capacity; LVRS, lung volume reduction surgery; SNP, single-nucleotide polymorphism.

[a] Plasma fibrinogen is the only CODP biomarker currently approved under the US FDA Biomarker Qualification Program.

Data from Refs. 1,11,12,19,21,22,26,27,30,33,34,37–40,42–44,46,47,49,50,52,55,57,58,62–66

considered predictive of these clinically relevant outcomes, although the effect size is small in comparison to that of a history of prior exacerbation, which remains the strongest predictor of exacerbation risk.[10] In contrast to the findings in the general population, it has not been reliably associated with FEV_1 decline in COPD cohorts.[11]

In light of these findings, the FDA has approved plasma fibrinogen as an "enrichment biomarker for clinical trials" that can be used to select participants at high risk of frequent exacerbations and morality, thus increasing statistical power.[12] For example, the FDA analysis suggests that enrichment based on a high plasma fibrinogen level could reduce the required sample size by 12%.[13] The recommendation comes, however, with several caveats, including[13] a specified threshold for fibrinogen-high participants (350 mg/dL), the use of a single type of assay (K-Assay, Kamiya Biomedical Company, Seattle, WA, USA), and that it should be used only as a complement for other clinical assessments of risk.

Potential Susceptibility Biomarkers for Chronic Obstructive Lung Disease

The recognition that up to one-third of all COPD occurs in never-smokers[14] has heightened interest in the genetic susceptibility to COPD. Genomic markers of COPD susceptibility are attractive because the genome is fixed over a lifetime; it is not altered by environmental exposures known to be associated with COPD but does give rise to important gene-environment interactions.[15,16] The only consistent monogenic association with COPD is mutation in the *SERPINA1* gene causing alpha-1 antitrypsin deficiency, which is the subject of a dedicated review in this issue of *Clinics*. The heterogeneous clinical expression of *SERPINA1* mutations, however, limits its viability as a genetic susceptibility biomarker of COPD in general populations.[17]

Hundreds of other genetic loci have been linked to adult lung function in genome-wide association studies (GWAS). Few of the individual loci have been replicated in independent cohorts, and there is considerable overlap with other lung diseases, including asthma and idiopathic pulmonary fibrosis.[18] No single gene or polymorphism would qualify as a biomarker of COPD susceptibility due to both small effect size and a lack of specificity. In the largest GWAS for COPD to date (>400,000 individuals),[19] a genetic risk score (GRS) combining 279 genetic variants associated with lung function was used to assess COPD risk. A GRS in the top decile conferred an odds ratio of 4.73 for COPD; overall, 54% of all COPD cases could be attributed to genetic architecture alone. The use of GRSs for predicting future disease risk is controversial,[20] but the complex polygenic nature of COPD makes this a promising way forward for identifying at-risk individuals.

There is some evidence that variation in airway structure may be a useful biomarker of COPD risk. In the Multi-Ethnic Study of Atherosclerosis general population cohort, airway branch variants determined by thoracic CT were present in 26% of participants, and the most common variant was associated with greater respiratory symptoms, chronic bronchitis, and a 40% increased risk of COPD.[21] In the same cohort, a GRS for COPD was associated with lung structure (luminal diameter, total small airway count, and lung density) independent of the effects of smoking.[22] Adjustment for these lung structural findings attenuated the association between the GRS and lung function, suggesting that the genetic determination of COPD risk may be explained partially by variation in lung structure. How and why anatomic variation, present from the time of lung development in utero, predisposes to COPD later in life is a matter for speculation.

Potential Diagnostic Biomarkers

Spirometry is insensitive to the narrowing and loss of small airways, which occur early in the natural history of the disease.[23,24] A significant number of people with normal spirometry report symptoms, experience exacerbation-like events, and have abnormal ventilatory mechanics during exercise—representing a form of pre-COPD.[25] Hence, there are a significant number of patients with mild or early-stage pathology who are not diagnosed by the current gold standard test. A useful diagnostic biomarker, therefore, would detect this pre-COPD, prior to the onset of spirometric abnormalities.

Physiologic tests other than spirometry may be promising diagnostic biomarkers for pre-COPD. For example, diffusing capacity for carbon monoxide (DLCO) may be abnormally low despite normal spirometry and thus represent a form of pre-COPD. In a large cohort of active smokers with normal spirometry, however, only one-quarter had reduced DLCO at baseline and, of these, only 22% went on to develop spirometrically defined COPD after approximately 4 years of follow-up,[26] meaning it may not have sufficient sensitivity to be a useful diagnostic biomarker. Similar findings have been reported for an increased residual volume to total lung capacity (RV/TLC) ratio in the presence of normal spirometry, which confers a 30% increased risk of progressing to overt COPD.[27]

Inert gas washout techniques, such as the multiple breath nitrogen washout (MBNW) test, are particularly sensitive to changes in the lung periphery.[28] MBNW measures ventilation heterogeneity (VH) arising from the uneven branching structure of the airways.[29] Up to half of current smokers with normal spirometry show increased VH on MBNW[30] which does not completely normalize after smoking cessation,[31] suggesting irreversible pathology. Recent computer modeling experiments show that increased VH on MBNW testing can be explained purely by removal of acinar units, which simulate the loss of terminal bronchioles described by Hogg and colleagues more than 50 years ago.[23] It, therefore, is highly likely that increased VH on MBNW is detecting some form of pre-COPD, but whether or not it represents a good diagnostic biomarker requires further clinicopathologic correlation.

Forced oscillometry, where low-amplitude pressure oscillations are applied to the lung via the mouth, also is sensitive to changes in the small airways.[32] Forced oscillometry measurements are abnormal in approximately half of smokers with normal spirometry,[30] but long-term evidence supporting this tool as a biomarker of pre-COPD currently is lacking.

Imaging biomarkers may prove useful for detecting changes that represent pre-COPD. Kirby and colleagues[33] performed hyperpolarized helium-3 MRI on ex-smokers with normal spirometry and no emphysema on thoracic CT. Subjects with DLCO less than 75% predicted had MRI evidence of airspace enlargement (measured by the apparent diffusion coefficient [ADC]) suggesting subtle emphysematous changes. Importantly, the increased ADC correlated with both symptom scores and 6-minute walk test distance walked. In more recent work, the same investigators found that machine learning analysis of apparently normal thoracic CT scans could detect subtle changes that differentiated between normal and abnormal DLCO subjects with 80% accuracy.[34] Further development of such findings as useful diagnostic biomarkers will require replication in larger cohorts with long-term follow-up.

Potential Prognostic Biomarkers

Lung function decline

Long-term observational data suggest that approximately half of people who develop COPD had normal FEV_1 prior to age of 40 years followed by rapid FEV_1 decline, whereas the remaining half had low (<80% predicted) FEV_1 prior to the age of 40 followed by steady/normal FEV_1 decline.[35] Furthermore, genetic signals associated with cross-sectional lung function are not necessarily predictive of longitudinal change in lung function.[36] This suggests that lung development may be just as relevant as subsequent lung function decline for the development of COPD and may explain why good biomarkers of FEV_1 decline in COPD so far have been elusive.

Several potential blood biomarkers of FEV_1 decline have been explored in longitudinal COPD cohorts. In the Evaluation of COPD Longitudinally to Identify Predictive Surrogate End-points (ECLIPSE) study, reduced serum level of the anti-inflammatory pneumoprotein club cell secretory protein 16 (CC-16) was associated independently with FEV_1 decline in participants with COPD.[11] A similar finding was reported in the Lung Health Study (LHS).[37] Reduced serum surfactant protein D (SP-D), another pneumoprotein with an important role in lung homeostasis and innate immunity, also was associated independently with FEV_1 decline in the LHS.[38] The association between these proteins and FEV_1 decline remained significant when analyzed under the mendelian randomization framework, which suggests causal roles in COPD progression.[38,39] The individual contribution of these factors to the rate of lung function decline in COPD is small. Combining biomarkers may be more advantageous: in the COPDGene Study cohort, a combination of CC-16, fibrinogen, and soluble receptor for advanced glycation end products (sRAGE), however, was the best biomarker predictor of FEV_1 decline, but it explained only an additional 6% of the variance compared with clinical factors alone.[40] By comparison, a predictive model based on clinical and physiologic factors (available as a Web-based calculator at http://resp.core.ubc.ca/ipress/FEV1Pred) explained 88% of the variance in FEV_1 decline.[41]

Exacerbations

The strongest known predictor of future exacerbations is a prior history of exacerbations,[10] and any potential biomarker of exacerbation risk would need to perform better than this simple clinical history. In order to further dissect the heterogeneity of exacerbation risk, Adibi and colleagues[42] recently developed and externally validated a tool for predicting individual exacerbation risk based on routinely available clinical information. The model predicted exacerbation frequency of greater than or equal to 2 per year with an area under the receiver operating characteristic curve of 0.81, with close agreement between the predicted and observed exacerbation rates. Importantly, the model performed well even when limited to people with a prior exacerbation history. Although it may not be considered a biomarker in the traditional sense, a clinical prediction tool based on objectively measured factors may fulfill many of the criteria of a good biomarker and may be useful particularly for determining individualized exacerbation risk or enriching clinical trials.

Several blood biomarkers of long-term exacerbation risk also have been of interest:

- Peripheral blood eosinophil count has been associated with increased exacerbation rate in some studies[43,44] and was found to have marginal additional predictive value in people experiencing frequent exacerbations in the ECLIPSE and COPDGene studies. The FDA, however, has rejected blood eosinophils as a predictive biomarker for frequent exacerbations, on the basis of heterogeneous study designs and eosinophil count thresholds.[3]
- An investigation of multiple blood biomarkers related to inflammation (inflammome) found that persistence of this inflammatory signature doubles the risk of exacerbations even after adjusting for prior exacerbation history.[45] The same study showed, however, that the inflammome is not necessarily stable over time and it is unknown whether or not exacerbation risk changes along with inflammatory status.
- Low serum level of immunoglobulin G (IgG) has been found to increase the risk of COPD exacerbations and hospitalizations by up to 40% and 92%, respectively, in a concentration-dependent manner.[46] This is a promising finding that may identify a particularly at-risk group who may benefit from a specific therapy (IgG replacement), but the nonspecific nature of IgG deficiency and the likelihood of confounding factors mean serum IgG may not turn out to be a good biomarker.

There are few studies investigating biomarkers of short-term (ie, imminent) exacerbation risk. Such studies are difficult because they require constant monitoring or sampling of patients over a long period of time. One potential biomarker, however, is the variability in physiologic indices: Zimmermann and colleagues[47] reported that the variability in forced oscillometry measurements, recorded daily through home telemonitoring, increased in the days prior to an acute exacerbation and was more sensitive than the change in symptoms. This is an intriguing use of technology to help predict exacerbations at an individual level, particularly because it may offer the chance for timely and personalized intervention.

Mortality

The causes of mortality in COPD patients vary according to disease severity.[48] Fletcher and Peto[49] acknowledged the association between low FEV_1 and mortality in their seminal work, and the addition of other clinical factors in composite scores, such as body mass index, airflow obstruction, dyspnea, and exercise capacity (BODE) index[50] increases the predictive power. The number of comorbidities also influences the likelihood of mortality in COPD.[51] It is perhaps not surprising that many of the biomarkers investigated to date do not add much additional predictive value over and above that of clinical factors. In the COPDGene study, the best-performing biomarker (SP-D) explained only an additional 2% of the variance in mortality compared with 56% for clinical factors alone.[40]

More personalized approaches that identify subpopulations at a high risk of mortality and who may benefit from a specific intervention would be more beneficial. For example, Leitao Filho and colleagues[52] studied the lung microbiome of COPD patients hospitalized for acute exacerbations and found that the presence of *Staphylococcus* sp and the absence of *Veillonella* sp in sputum conferred a markedly increased risk of death within 1 year of follow-up. Whether or not altering the microbiome can influence its association with mortality remains to be seen.

Potential Therapeutic Biomarkers

Because an entire article in this issue of *Clinics* is dedicated to the treatment of COPD, a brief discussion of some of the more interesting predictive therapeutic biomarkers is presented here.

Inhaled bronchodilators are the mainstay of maintenance therapy in COPD. Although a large proportion of COPD patients significantly increase their FEV_1 after inhaled bronchodilator, the magnitude of change in FEV_1 correlates poorly with clinical outcomes[53] and, therefore, is not considered a useful predictive therapeutic biomarker for these medications. This may reflect the insensitivity of the test rather than poor correlation between the physiology and clinical outcomes. Forced oscillometry may be more useful as a predictive therapeutic biomarker: increased respiratory system impedance is correlated with gas trapping and hyperinflation[54] and may predict a more significant deflation response to inhaled bronchodilators.[55] This physiologic change is more relevant to clinical outcomes, such as symptoms and exercise capacity.[56] This novel use of forced oscillometry for guiding bronchodilator therapy is yet to be tested, however, in a clinical trial setting.

There is great interest in peripheral blood eosinophil count as a predictive biomarker of response to inhaled corticosteroid (ICS) therapy.[57] In a meta-analysis of clinical trials of triple therapy (inhaled long-acting beta-agonists and antimuscarinics, with or without ICS), Cazzola and colleagues[58] found that the number needed to treat with ICS to prevent 1 exacerbation per year reduced from 38 to 8 when restricted to patients with blood eosinophil count greater than or equal to 300 cells/μL. A majority of clinical trials that have undergone (predominantly post hoc) subanalysis by blood eosinophil level have used a 2% cutoff to demonstrate a superior reduction in exacerbation rate with ICS therapy. There currently is no consensus, however, on what the appropriate threshold should be. This is part of the reason given by the FDA in their rejection of blood eosinophils as a predictive therapeutic biomarker.[3]

The use of the acute phase reactant C-reactive protein (CRP) to guide antibiotic therapy for COPD exacerbations recently has been explored in both inpatient[59] and community[60] settings. In these studies, patients presenting with acute exacerbations were randomized to receive antibiotics based on an elevated serum CRP level or based on usual care (ie, patient symptom–driven antibiotic prescription). In both studies, the CRP-guided treatment strategy was associated with significantly reduced antibiotic use without significant differences in clinical outcomes or treatment failures.[59,60] Although it may not predict a superior therapeutic response, CRP may be useful as a biomarker that prevents unnecessary antibiotic prescription and maximizes the benefit:harm ratio, which is consistent with the precision medicine paradigm. One of the major challenges of developing a biomarker-guided strategy, however, is clinician acceptance or beliefs. For example, a similar strategy using serum procalcitonin was investigated for antibiotic treatment of lower respiratory tract infections but did not reduce antibiotic use compared with usual care.[61] In this study, clinicians often broke with the treatment protocol and prescribed antibiotics despite a low procalcitonin level: acute COPD exacerbation was one of the most common reasons given by the physicians for ignoring the treatment protocol.

Biomarkers might be beneficial for guiding nonpharmacological therapies. The National Emphysema Treatment Trial showed that in patients undergoing lung volume reduction surgery, upper lobe–predominant emphysema on CT scan predicted a reduction in mortality compared with medical treatment in patients with poor exercise capacity.[62] Similarly, heterogeneously distributed emphysema appears to predict the success of bronchoscopic lung volume reduction.[63] Central to the success of this treatment is the presence of intact interlobar fissures, which minimize collateral ventilation between the target and adjacent lobes and allow the targeted lobe to collapse.[63,64] Assessment of fissure integrity can be performed by multiple methods, most commonly CT[65] or endoscopic methods (eg, the commonly used Chartis system).[66] An adjacent interlobar fissure that is greater than 90% complete is associated with treatment success in up to 65% of patients undergoing bronchial valve placement; fissures that are less than 90% complete confer a very low chance of treatment success.[65] Preprocedural estimation of treatment success is critical when the intervention carries significant risk, and biomarkers may play an increasing role in determining the benefit:risk ratio for each individual.

SUMMARY

There is intense interest in developing biomarkers in COPD, driven largely by the lack of progress in modifying clinical outcomes in this highly complex and heterogeneous disease. There are any number of associations between genetic, physiologic, biochemical, or radiological factors and COPD outcomes. Biomarker development is about taking these findings beyond mere association and exploring their potential roles in the context of personalized medicine. For example, a biomarker of COPD susceptibility, exacerbation risk, or mortality is of benefit only if it is used to identify a subpopulation for targeted intervention. Similarly, a predictive therapeutic biomarker is useful only if it reliably identifies patients who would gain clinically meaningful benefit or be saved from unnecessary harm. For these reasons, the authors believe the main role for COPD biomarkers in the foreseeable future will be in predicting treatment response and enriching clinical trials for high-risk patients. Biomarker research in COPD needs to move beyond discovery and instead focus on identifying and developing the most viable candidates. This undoubtedly will require ongoing collaboration and data sharing between the large, longitudinal COPD cohorts.

DISCLOSURE

There were no direct financial sponsors for the submitted work. S. Milne reports personal fees from Novartis, Boehringer Ingelheim, and Menarini and nonfinancial support from Draeger Australia, outside the submitted work. D.D. Sin reports grants from Merck; personal fees from Sanofi-Aventis, Regeneron, and Novartis; and grants and personal fees from Boehringer Ingelheim and AstraZeneca, outside the submitted work.

REFERENCES

1. United States National Institutes of Health. NIH All of Us program [online resource]. Available at: https://allofus.nih.gov/about/faq. Accessed January 23, 2020.

2. Biomarkers and surrogate endpoints: preferred definitions and conceptual framework. Clin Pharmacol Ther 2001;69(3):89–95.

3. United States Food and Drug Administration. Biomarker Qualification Submissions [online resource]. Available at: https://www.fda.gov/drugs/cder-biomarker-qualification-program/biomarker-qualification-submissions. Accessed January 17, 2020.

4. Gabay C, Kushner I. Acute-phase proteins and other systemic responses to inflammation. N Engl J Med 1999;340(6):448–54.

5. Alessandri C, Basili S, Violi F, et al. Hypercoagulability state in patients with chronic obstructive pulmonary disease. Thromb Haemost 1994;72(09):343–6.

6. Dahl M, Tybjærg-Hansen A, Vestbo J, et al. Elevated plasma fibrinogen associated with reduced pulmonary function and increased risk of chronic obstructive pulmonary disease. Am J Respir Crit Care Med 2001;164(6):1008–11.

7. Valvi D, Mannino DM, Müllerova H, et al. Fibrinogen, chronic obstructive pulmonary disease (COPD) and outcomes in two United States cohorts. Int J Chron Obstruct Pulmon Dis 2012;7:173–82.

8. Groenewegen KH, Postma DS, Hop WCJ, et al. Increased systemic inflammation is a risk factor for COPD exacerbations. Chest 2008;133(2):350–7.

9. Mannino DM, Tal-Singer R, Lomas DA, et al. Plasma fibrinogen as a biomarker for mortality and hospitalized exacerbations in people with COPD. Chronic Obstr Pulm Dis 2015;2(1):23–34.

10. Hurst JR, Vestbo J, Anzueto A, et al. Susceptibility to exacerbation in chronic obstructive pulmonary disease. N Engl J Med 2010;363(12):1128–38.

11. Vestbo J, Edwards LD, Scanlon PD, et al. Changes in forced expiratory volume in 1 second over time in COPD. N Engl J Med 2011;365(13):1184–92.

12. Miller BE, Tal-Singer R, Rennard SI, et al. Plasma fibrinogen qualification as a drug development tool in chronic obstructive pulmonary disease. Perspective of the chronic obstructive pulmonary disease biomarker qualification consortium. Am J Respir Crit Care Med 2016;193(6):607–13.

13. United States Food and Drug Administration. Executive summary for plasma fibrinogen. Available at: https://www.fda.gov/drugs/drug-development-tool-ddt-qualification-programs/plasma-biomarker-fibrinogen-reviews. Accessed January 05, 2020.

14. Tan WC, Sin DD, Bourbeau J, et al. Characteristics of COPD in never-smokers and ever-smokers in the general population: results from the CanCOLD study. Thorax 2015;70(9):822–9.

15. Park B, Koo S-M, An J, et al. Genome-wide assessment of gene-by-smoking interactions in COPD. Sci Rep 2018;8(1):9319.

16. Liao S-Y, Lin X, Christiani DC. Gene-environment interaction effects on lung function- a genome-wide association study within the Framingham heart study. Environ Health 2013;12(1):101.

17. Giacopuzzi E, Laffranchi M, Berardelli R, et al. Real-world clinical applicability of pathogenicity predictors assessed on SERPINA1 mutations in alpha-1-antitrypsin deficiency. Hum Mutat 2018;39(9):1203–13.

18. Sakornsakolpat P, Prokopenko D, Lamontagne M, et al. Genetic landscape of chronic obstructive pulmonary disease identifies heterogeneous cell-type and phenotype associations. Nat Genet 2019;51(3):494–505.

19. Shrine N, Guyatt AL, Erzurumluoglu AM, et al. New genetic signals for lung function highlight pathways and chronic obstructive pulmonary disease associations across multiple ancestries. Nat Genet 2019;51(3):481–93.

20. Lewis CM, Vassos E. Prospects for using risk scores in polygenic medicine. Genome Med 2017;9(1):96.

21. Smith BM, Traboulsi H, Austin JHM, et al. Human airway branch variation and chronic obstructive pulmonary disease. Proc Natl Acad Sci U S A 2018;115(5):E974–81.

22. Oelsner EC, Ortega VE, Smith BM, et al. A genetic risk score associated with chronic obstructive pulmonary disease susceptibility and lung structure on computed tomography. Am J Respir Crit Care Med 2019;200(6):721–31.

23. Hogg JC, Macklem PT, Thurlbeck W. Site and nature of airway obstruction in chronic obstructive lung disease. N Engl J Med 1968;278(25):1355–60.

24. Cosio M, Ghezzo H, Hogg JC, et al. The relations between structural changes in small airways and pulmonary-function tests. N Engl J Med 1978;298(23):1277–81.

25. Celli BR, Agustí A. COPD: time to improve its taxonomy? ERJ Open Res 2018;4(1):00132–2017.

26. Harvey B-G, Strulovici-Barel Y, Kaner RJ, et al. Risk of COPD with obstruction in active smokers with normal spirometry and reduced diffusion capacity. Eur Respir J 2015;46(6):1589–97.

27. Zeng S, Tham A, Bos B, et al. Lung volume indices predict morbidity in smokers with preserved spirometry. Thorax 2019;74(2):114–24.

28. Verbanck S, Schuermans D, Van Muylem A, et al. Conductive and acinar lung-zone contributions to ventilation inhomogeneity in COPD. Am J Respir Crit Care Med 1998;157(5):1573–7.

29. Crawford A, Makowska M, Paiva M, et al. Convection-and diffusion-dependent ventilation maldistribution in normal subjects. J Appl Physiol (1985) 1985; 59(3):838–46.

30. Jetmalani K, Thamrin C, Farah CS, et al. Peripheral airway dysfunction and relationship with symptoms in smokers with preserved spirometry. Respirology 2018;23(5):512–8.

31. Verbanck S, Schuermans D, Paiva M, et al. Small airway function improvement after smoking cessation in smokers without airway obstruction. Am J Respir Crit Care Med 2006;174(8):853–7.

32. Foy BH, Soares M, Bordas R, et al. Lung computational models and the role of the small airways in asthma. Am J Respir Crit Care Med 2019. https://doi.org/10.1164/rccm.201812-2322OC.

33. Kirby M, Owrangi A, Svenningsen S, et al. On the role of abnormal DLCO in ex-smokers without airflow limitation: symptoms, exercise capacity and hyperpolarised helium-3 MRI. Thorax 2013;68(8): 752–9.

34. Kirby M, McCormack DG, Parraga G. Normal thoracic CT in ex-smokers without COPD: can machine learning reveal subclinical disease? [Abstract]. Am J Respir Crit Care Med 2019;199:A5770.

35. Lange P, Celli B, Agustí A, et al. Lung-function trajectories leading to chronic obstructive pulmonary disease. N Engl J Med 2015;373(2):111–22.

36. John C, Soler Artigas M, Hui J, et al. Genetic variants affecting cross-sectional lung function in adults show little or no effect on longitudinal lung function decline. Thorax 2017;72(5):400–8.

37. Park HY, Churg A, Wright JL, et al. Club cell protein 16 and disease progression in chronic obstructive pulmonary disease. Am J Respir Crit Care Med 2013;188(12):1413–9.

38. Obeidat M, Li X, Burgess S, et al. Surfactant protein D is a causal risk factor for COPD: results of Mendelian randomisation. Eur Respir J 2017;50(5): 1700657.

39. Milne S, Li X, Cordero AIH, et al. The protective effect of club cell secretory protein (CC-16) on COPD risk and progression: a Mendelian randomisation study. bioRxiv 2019. https://doi.org/10.1101/2019.12.20.885384.

40. Zemans RL, Jacobson S, Keene J, et al. Multiple biomarkers predict disease severity, progression and mortality in COPD. Respir Res 2017;18(1):117.

41. Zafari Z, Sin DD, Postma DS, et al. Individualized prediction of lung-function decline in chronic obstructive pulmonary disease. CMAJ 2016; 188(14):1004–11.

42. Adibi A, Sin DD, Safari A, et al. The Acute COPD Exacerbation Prediction Tool (ACCEPT): development and external validation study of a personalised prediction model. bioRxiv 2019;651901. https://doi.org/10.1101/651901.

43. Yun JH, Lamb A, Chase R, et al. Blood eosinophil count thresholds and exacerbations in patients with chronic obstructive pulmonary disease. J Allergy Clin Immunol 2018;141(6):2037–47.e10.

44. Vedel-Krogh S, Nielsen SF, Lange P, et al. Blood eosinophils and exacerbations in chronic obstructive pulmonary disease. The Copenhagen General Population Study. Am J Respir Crit Care Med 2016; 193(9):965–74.

45. Agustí A, Edwards LD, Rennard SI, et al. Persistent systemic inflammation is associated with poor clinical outcomes in COPD: a novel phenotype. PLoS One 2012;7(5):e37483.

46. Leitao Filho FS, Won Ra S, Mattman A, et al. Serum IgG and risk of exacerbations and hospitalizations in chronic obstructive pulmonary disease. J Allergy Clin Immunol 2017;140(4):1164–7.e6.

47. Zimmermann S, Huvanandana J, Nguyen C, et al. Temporal variability of forced oscillometry from home telemonitoring and relationship with patient-centred outcomes and AECOPD. Eur Respir J 2019;54(suppl 63):OA477.

48. Celli BR. Predictors of mortality in COPD. Respir Med 2010;104(6):773–9.

49. Fletcher C, Peto R. The natural history of chronic airflow obstruction. Br Med J 1977;1(6077):1645–8.

50. Celli BR, Cote CG, Marin JM, et al. The body-mass index, airflow obstruction, dyspnea, and exercise capacity index in chronic obstructive pulmonary disease. N Engl J Med 2004;350(10):1005–12.

51. Sin DD, Anthonisen NR, Soriano JB, et al. Mortality in COPD: role of comorbidities. Eur Respir J 2006; 28(6):1245–57.

52. Filho FSL, Alotaibi NM, Ngan D, et al. Sputum microbiome is associated with 1-year mortality after chronic obstructive pulmonary disease hospitalizations. Am J Respir Crit Care Med 2019;199(10): 1205–13.

53. Calverley PM, Burge PS, Spencer S, et al. Bronchodilator reversibility testing in chronic obstructive pulmonary disease. Thorax 2003;58(8):659–64.

54. Milne S, Jetmalani K, Chapman DG, et al. Respiratory system reactance reflects communicating lung volume in chronic obstructive pulmonary disease. J Appl Physiol (1985) 2019;126(5):1223–31.

55. Milne S, Hammans C, Watson S, et al. Bronchodilator responses in respiratory impedance, hyperinflation and gas trapping in COPD. COPD 2018; 15(4):341–9.

56. O'Donnell DE, Casaburi R, Vincken W, et al. Effect of indacaterol on exercise endurance and lung hyperinflation in COPD. Respir Med 2011;105(7):1030–6.

57. Barnes NC, Sharma R, Lettis S, et al. Blood eosinophils as a marker of response to inhaled corticosteroids in COPD. Eur Respir J 2016;47(5):1374–82.

58. Cazzola M, Rogliani P, Calzetta L, et al. Triple therapy versus single and dual long-acting

bronchodilator therapy in COPD: a systematic review and meta-analysis. Eur Respir J 2018;52(6): 1801586.

59. Prins HJ, Duijkers R, van der Valk P, et al. CRP-guided antibiotic treatment in acute exacerbations of COPD in hospital admissions. Eur Respir J 2019;53(5):1802014.

60. Butler CC, Gillespie D, White P, et al. C-reactive protein testing to guide antibiotic prescribing for COPD exacerbations. N Engl J Med 2019;381(2):111–20.

61. Huang DT, Yealy DM, Filbin MR, et al. Procalcitonin-guided use of antibiotics for lower respiratory tract infection. N Engl J Med 2018;379(3):236–49.

62. Fishman A, Martinez F, Naunheim K, et al. A randomized trial comparing lung-volume-reduction surgery with medical therapy for severe emphysema. N Engl J Med 2003;348(21):2059–73.

63. Davey C, Zoumot Z, Jordan S, et al. Bronchoscopic lung volume reduction with endobronchial valves for patients with heterogeneous emphysema and intact interlobar fissures (the BeLieVeR-HIFi study): a randomised controlled trial. Lancet 2015; 386(9998):1066–73.

64. Koster TD, Slebos D-J. The fissure: interlobar collateral ventilation and implications for endoscopic therapy in emphysema. Int J Chron Obstruct Pulmon Dis 2016;11:765–73.

65. Schuhmann M, Raffy P, Yin Y, et al. Computed tomography predictors of response to endobronchial valve lung reduction treatment. Comparison with Chartis. Am J Respir Crit Care Med 2015;191(7):767–74.

66. Mantri S, Macaraeg C, Shetty S, et al. Technical advances: measurement of collateral flow in the lung with a dedicated endobronchial catheter system. J Bronchology Interv Pulmonol 2009;16(2):141–4.

What Is Asthma Chronic Obstructive Pulmonary Disease Overlap?

David M.G. Halpin, MB BS, MA, DPhil, FRCP, FERS

KEYWORDS

• Asthma • COPD • ACO • Diagnosis • Definition • Nosology

KEY POINTS

- Patients may be diagnosed with asthma, chronic obstructive pulmonary disease (COPD), or both diseases.
- Patients with both diseases are generally excluded from clinical trials.
- It is not known if patients with both diseases have a different prognosis or need different treatment to those with either disease alone.
- The existence of an overlap condition or syndrome has been postulated, but there is no agreement on the definition of such a condition and definitive evidence to support its existence or the need for it as a diagnosis is lacking.
- The 2020 GOLD report has abandoned the concept and no longer refers to asthma and COPD overlap (ACO), instead it emphasizes that asthma and COPD are different disorders, although they may share some common traits and clinical features.

When I use a word," Humpty Dumpty said, in rather a scornful tone, "it means just what I choose it to mean—neither more nor less.
—Lewis Carroll (Charles L. Dodgson), Through the Looking-Glass, see Claus F. Vogelmeier and Peter Alter's article, "Assessing Symptom Burden," in this issue.

Making a diagnosis has always been central to the doctor-patient relationship. Diagnoses guide patients' treatment, help set expectations about prognosis, and facilitate communication between doctors. In examining the current controversies about what is asthma chronic obstructive pulmonary disease (COPD) overlap (ACO) and whether it is a useful concept at all, it is helpful to consider how our current concepts of diseases evolved, what is meant by the term "disease," and how we identify the extent and boundaries of diseases to differentiate one from another.

DISEASES AND DIAGNOSES

Our current approach to the classification of diseases developed in the late seventeenth century when Sydenham urged physicians to organize illnesses into groups and hierarchies similar to those recently introduced by botanists to classify plants.[1] Disease names, like the names of species, gave clinicians and patients terms that facilitated communication, even though specific treatments were not available in most cases. The only way categorize diseases at that time was according to their external characteristics, as the causes and pathophysiology could not be determined, and de Sauvages suggested grouping diseases by their symptoms.[2] To be useful in classifying diseases, he said these had to be *manifest, essential, and constant*, that is, they had to be observable, not occur by accident, and always present; considerations still relevant today.

---

see Claus F. Vogelmeier and Peter Alter's article, "Assessing Symptom Burden," in this issue.
University of Exeter Medical School, College of Medicine and Health, University of Exeter, Exeter EX1 2LU, UK
E-mail address: d.halpin@nhs.net

Clin Chest Med 41 (2020) 395–403
https://doi.org/10.1016/j.ccm.2020.06.006
0272-5231/20/© 2020 Elsevier Inc. All rights reserved.

Much thought was given to how best to identify groups of symptoms and put boundaries around them to define specific diseases. This was necessary to make classification systems useful in practice and establish a set of terms that everyone associated with the same meanings. In the early eighteenth century, Drummond[3] emphasized the importance of these boundaries but cautioned on taking it too far. He offered good and bad examples of this process, beginning the debate between "lumpers" and "splitters" that continued into the twentieth century.[4] Drummond[3] wrote that no two cases of disease are "strictly parallel in every circumstance but every case should not therefore have a new name."

As pathologic and anatomic knowledge developed in the nineteenth century, new approaches to disease classification emerged and classification of disease, as promoted by Osler,[5] relied on both the clinical presentation and pathologic findings. Over the past 100 years, this approach has gradually evolved with the introduction of definitive laboratory tests, physiologic and radiological investigations, and, most recently, molecular genetics. In many fields, more and more "precise" histopathological, radiological, and molecular characterization of a disease has become possible, but in other fields, notably psychiatry, clinical features remain the most important.

Modern disease classification reflects the inexorable progression, but not necessarily triumph, of "splitting." By the end of the twentieth century, many broad disease syndromes had been split into more specific diseases, reflecting different causes, mechanisms, and responses to therapy. The continual elaboration of disease classification has led to advances in management, including more accurate prediction of prognosis, and splitting is fundamental to the concept of personalized medicine. Treatment using contemporary therapy often depends on maximal specificity in the diagnosis, as has been seen to great effect with the refinement of the classification of lung cancer and the use of targeted agents and checkpoint inhibitors.[6] However, there is a point at which splitting stops defining different diseases and moves to defining subtypes of a disease that benefit in some ways from being considered the same, whilst benefit in other ways of being considered distinct.

ASTHMA AND CHRONIC OBSTRUCTIVE PULMONARY DISEASE

How do these concepts relate to current understanding and usage of the terms asthma and COPD? The term asthma was used somewhat imprecisely from antiquity up to the middle of the past century to describe a condition of breathlessness. Its use was refined in the early nineteenth century to describe a condition associated with intermittent narrowing of the airways.[7] Emphysema was described as a postmortem finding by Bonet[8] in the late seventeenth century and the term chronic bronchitis was introduced by Badham[9] in the early nineteenth century. Emphysema was linked with chronic bronchitis by Laennec,[7] but the association with airflow obstruction was not recognized until the mid-twentieth century[10] and the term COPD was not introduced until the mid-1960s.[11]

The 1959 CIBA symposium attempted to develop definitions of asthma, chronic bronchitis, and emphysema, which included the presence of airflow obstruction and the extent of its reversibility.[12] Two umbrella terms were proposed: chronic nonspecific lung disease (CNSLD) for the whole spectrum of these diseases, and generalized obstructive lung disease for asthma and what was subsequently termed COPD. CNSLD was adopted by the Netherlands, reflecting their reluctance to divide this group of patients into those with and without asthma. Most other countries continue to divide patients into those with and without asthma, but precise criteria dividing patients into those with COPD and those with asthma were not set out originally or subsequently.[13] The terminology and definitions established at this period were provisional and expected to evolve, but although there have been many publications on these topics in the following 60 years, few modifications have been established. Yet, despite the difficulties of defining the terms of asthma and COPD, clinicians seemed to regard these terms as useful in clinical practice.[14]

In 1991, the National Asthma Education Program guidelines for the diagnosis and management of asthma produced a working definition of asthma that combined immunopathological with physiologic and clinical features.[15] Similar definitions of asthma have subsequently been proposed by the Global Initiative for Asthma (GINA)[16] and definitions of COPD proposed by Global Initiative for Chronic Obstructive Lung Disease (GOLD), including the most recent,[17] also combine pathologic and physiologic abnormalities with clinical features (**Box 1**).

THE IMPORTANCE OF DEFINITIONS

In 1959, Scadding[18] wrote, "These terminological matters are of great importance, for our choice of words inevitably influences our subsequent thought." In later work, he discussed the difficulty in defining respiratory diseases with reference to philosophic thinking on definitions.[19] In the 1940s, Popper[20] had drawn attention to two fundamentally different philosophic types of definition used in science: essentialist and nominalist. Regarding essentialist definitions he wrote:

I use the name methodological essentialism to characterise the view, held by Plato and many of his followers, that it is the task of pure knowledge or science to discover and to describe the true nature of things, i.e. their hidden reality or essence. …. And a description of the essence of a thing they all called a definition.

Essentialist definitions imply the *a priori* existence of something that can be identified and characterized by the identification of a shared and unique essence. Essentialist thinking underpins the idea that diseases are causes of illness and that diagnosis simply consists of identifying the disease that is causing the illness. In contrast, nominalists believe that diseases have no existence apart from that of patients with them. Nominalists see definitions as merely introducing a name, the defined term, as an abbreviation or convenient way of briefly stating the end point of a diagnostic process, without introducing unjustified assumptions about pathophysiology or causation.

Popper[20] criticized the essentialist view of knowledge because it implied finality and certainty. He believed we can never be sure to have reached the truth and that in the empirical sciences there are no proofs that establish once and for all the truth, or the complete characterization of a disease. To him, all definitions used in medicine were nominalist. In reality, I believe we have both. For example, streptococcal pneumonia is an essentialist definition, as the essence is a histopathological finding caused by a defined external agent, whereas asthma and COPD have nominalist definitions. Scadding[18] also believed that most respiratory diagnoses were nominalist and, for example, wrote the following:

The physician should know that in applying the diagnostic term 'asthma' he is claiming no more than that the wheezy breathlessness is due to wide variations in resistance to expiratory air-flow in the lungs. He may be able to show that the patient's bronchi are abnormally reactive to a variety of stimuli, but can only speculate about the causes of this abnormal reactivity. He will try to identify factors causing increases in resistance. In many instances, he will fail.[21]

ASTHMA CHRONIC OBSTRUCTIVE PULMONARY DISEASE OVERLAP

What then should we make of the term asthma COPD overlap (ACO)? From an essentialist's perspective, are there 3 distinct diseases, asthma, COPD, and ACO, 2 diseases that may occur in the same patient, or all subtypes of a single disease? If ACO is simply the coincident occurrence of 2 diseases, does the coexistence of the 2 conditions modify the prognosis or management sufficiently to justify a specific label or lead to distinct treatment recommendations? From a nominalist perspective, are they simply convenient labels to describe groups of patients who have certain characteristics? The GINA and GOLD definitions of asthma and COPD appear to be essentialist, but are both flawed, they are simply descriptions of the diseases and neither identifies the essence or defining characteristics that separate them from each other and other diseases. This would not matter a great deal if there was consensus among doctors when making a differential diagnosis, and this is at the root of the difficulty in addressing ACO.

As they stand, neither of the definitions of asthma and COPD is mutually exclusive and the differential diagnosis is sometimes a challenge for clinicians. Nevertheless, we persevere in trying to differentiate asthma and COPD for the very reason splitting evolved: to guide the patient's treatment, help set expectations about prognosis, and facilitate communication between doctors. However, for many years, clinicians have recognized that some patients share traits of the two conditions, and this was exemplified in the Venn diagram included in the 1995 American Thoracic Society COPD guidelines.[22]

Consider a patient in his or her late 60s who had allergic asthma when younger and became tight chested and developed airflow obstruction when exposed to cats, who has smoked all his or her adult life, and now has daily breathlessness on exertion, fixed airflow obstruction on spirometry, and emphysema on computed tomography (CT), but who still bronchoconstricts on exposure to cats. Because of the history, it is clear that the patient has both asthma and COPD concurrently.

It is more difficult to make a firm diagnosis when assessing a patient with no prior history of respiratory symptoms who presents in his or her 50s with variable breathlessness, who has a significant bronchodilator response on spirometry but the post-bronchodilator forced expiratory volume in 1 second (FEV_1)/forced vital capacity (FVC) ratio remains abnormal and has mild emphysema on CT. This patient could have asthma or COPD or ACO.

The difficulty in separating asthma and COPD arises because there are no accepted unique defining characteristics, yet in most cases a diagnosis of one or the other can be made. A major cause of the confusion that reigns is the misinterpretation of the diagnostic labels as essentialist and to unthinkingly apply criteria as disease defining. For example, bronchodilator responsiveness is seen by many as the defining physiologic characteristic of asthma, yet it can be demonstrated in many patients with COPD,[23] and markers of type 2 inflammation, thought to be common in asthma, are also found in people with COPD.[24] Similarly, fixed airflow obstruction is seen by many as the defining physiologic characteristic of COPD yet it can be found in many patients with asthma, particularly those with longstanding disease.[25–27] The reluctance to make a specific diagnosis also occurs in some cases because of laziness based on the perception that the treatment and prognosis are the same.

There is also a lack of clear and useful guidance from "experts" as to how the distinction can be made in clinical practice. A recent systematic review on the overlap syndrome provides an example of the tautology of the use of terms and the lack of precision in making the correct diagnosis. The investigators defined the overlap phenotype as any patients with COPD (defined as fixed airflow obstruction on post-bronchodilator spirometry) with at least 1 or more of the following findings[28]:

- Physician-diagnosed asthma or self-reported physician diagnosis of asthma.
- Reversibility testing ($\geq$12% and at least 200 mL change in FEV_1 from baseline).
- Peak expiratory flow (PEF) variability ($\geq$20% change in PEF).
- Airway hyperresponsiveness to methacholine or histamine.

In reality, some of these patients may have fixed airflow obstruction as part of their asthma,[29] in which case the presence of 1 or more of the 4 findings would simply confirm the diagnosis of asthma, or they may have had COPD but none of the physiologic findings prove they also have asthma. In particular, a previous physician diagnosis of asthma may simply reflect initial diagnostic uncertainty before a conclusive diagnosis of COPD was made, and up to 50% of patients with COPD have bronchodilator reversibility greater than 200 mL and greater than 12%.[23,30] Similarly problems arise in the Spanish effort to develop criteria for the diagnosis of asthma overlap in COPD without defining COPD itself.[31]

The introduction of the term asthma COPD overlap syndrome (ACOS) in 2014[32] did not help with this confusion, particularly as it has essentialist pretensions implying the existence of a distinct entity not just an overlap of 2 common conditions. The dropping of the word syndrome[33] helped undo some of the problems that had developed, but without an operational definition, the term ACO has continued to be problematic, particularly if viewed from an essentialist rather than nominalist perspective.

Much effort has been put into "defining" ACO. Many workshops have been convened, and a variety of definitions proposed by these groups as well as individual investigators (**Table 1**). In many cases, it is not possible to determine how the separate diagnoses of asthma and COPD were made or whether they are describing patients with asthma with fixed airflow obstruction or patients with COPD with a significant bronchodilator response. The GINA/GOLD document stated that one of the objectives of publishing the report was to "stimulate further study of the character and treatments for this common clinical problem"[32]; however, without an agreed definition, confusion rather than clarity has emerged.

Table 1
Examples of definitions of asthma COPD overlap

First Author, Year	Definition
Marsh et al,[47] 2008	Patients with COPD (post-BD FEV_1/FVC <0.7) and asthma (post-BD increase in FEV_1 ≥15% or peak flow variability ≥20% during 1 wk of testing or physician-diagnosed asthma in conjunction with current symptoms).
Hardin et al.[36] 2011	GOLD stage 2 or higher COPD (post-BD FEV_1/FVC <0.7 and FEV_1 <80% predicted) and a subject report of a physician diagnosis of asthma before the age of 40.
Soler-Cataluna rt al,[31] 2012	2 major criteria or 1 major and 2 minor criteria met on 2 or more occasions. The major criteria: very positive bronchodilator test (increase in FEV_1 ≥15% and ≥400 mL), eosinophilia in sputum and personal history of asthma. Minor criteria high total IgE, personal history of atopy and positive BD test (increase in FEV_1 ≥12% and ≥200 mL).
Andersen et al,[48] 2013	Hospital discharge ICD codes for treatment at some point over different treatment periods for both asthma and COPD diagnoses.
De Marco et al,[34] 2013	Self-reported doctor-diagnosed asthma and COPD.
Lim et al,[49] 2014	Age ≥40, smoking history of ≥10 pack-years, post-BD FEV_1/FVC <0.70 and a positive bronchodilator response or positive airway hyperresponsiveness. A positive bronchodilator response was defined as an increase in FEV_1 by ≥200 mL and 12% after inhalation of 200 mg of salbutamol. Airway hyperresponsiveness was defined as having a provocation concentration that caused a decrease in FEV_1 of 20% no higher than 16 mg/mL.
Fu et al,[50] 2014	Respiratory symptoms, increased airflow variability and incompletely reversible airflow obstruction: post-BD FEV_1 <80% predicted, FEV_1/FVC <0.7.
Menezes et al,[51] 2014	A combination of asthma (wheezing in the last 12 months plus post-BD increase) (or self-reported doctor diagnosis of asthma) and COPD (post-BD FEV_1/FVC <0.70).
Barrecheguren et al,[52] 2015	Age ≥40 y of age, diagnosis of COPD in medical records; smokers or ex-smokers of at least 10 pack-years; post-BD FEV_1/FVC <0.7, patient report of a previous diagnosis of asthma before the age of 40 y.
Ishiura et al,[53] 2015	Episodic respiratory symptoms, increased airflow variability (asthma; ie, ≥20% FEV_1 fall from baseline occurred after inhalation of methacholine or increase in post-BD FEV_1 ≥200 mL and 12% compared with pre-BD FEV_1), as well as incompletely reversible airway obstruction (COPD; post-BD FEV_1/FVC <70% and post-BD FEV_1 <80% of predicted).
Kiljander et al,[54] 2015	Age 18–70 y, current or ex-smoker with 10 or more pack-years, doctor-diagnosed asthma (fulfilling at least 1 of the following criteria (1): ≥12% [and 200 mL] reversibility in FEV_1 or FVC in a bronchodilation test, (2) during a 2-wk peak expiratory flow monitoring at least 3 times either a BD response of ≥15% [and 60 L/min] or a diurnal variation of ≥20%, (3) moderate-to-severe bronchial hyperresponsiveness in histamine or methacholine inhalation challenge or (4) FEV_1 had improved more than 15% during a corticosteroid treatment test) and post-BD FEV_1/FVC <0.70.

(continued on next page)

Table 1
(continued)

First Author, Year	Definition
Sin et al,[55] 2016	Presence of all 3 major criteria and at least 1 minor criterion. Major criteria: persistent airflow limitation (post-BD FEV_1/FVC <0.70 or LLN) in individuals 40 y of age or older; at least 10 pack-years of tobacco smoking, or equivalent indoor or outdoor air pollution exposure (eg, biomass); documented history of asthma before 40 y of age or BD response of >400 mL in FEV_1. Minor criteria: Documented history of atopy or allergic rhinitis; BD response of FEV_1 ≥200 mL and 12% from baseline values on 2 or more visits; peripheral blood eosinophil count of ≥300 cells/μL.
Plaza et al,[56] 2017	Age 35 y or older, smoker or ex-smoker of more than 10 pack-years, post-BD FEV_1/FVC <0.7 that persists after treatment with bronchodilators and inhaled corticosteroids (even after systemic corticosteroids in selected cases), and an objective current diagnosis of asthma based on history and/or symptoms causing clinical suspicion (family history of asthma or personal history of asthma in childhood or personal history of atopy; respiratory symptoms [wheezing, cough, chest tightness] of variable course, on occasions in the form of a dyspneic crisis also of variable intensity, or inflammation of the upper airway [rhinosinusitis with or without nasal polyposis]); and objective diagnostic confirmation (reversibility of obstruction of spirometric flows measured by spirometry or positive bronchodilator response [≥12% and ≥200 mL], or a diurnal variability of PEF ≥20%, or FeNO ≥50 ppb) or if the diagnosis of asthma cannot be demonstrated, marked positive results on a BD test (FEV_1 ≥15% and ≥400 mL) or elevated blood eosinophil count (≥300 cells/μL).
Ding et al,[57] 2017	Physician-confirmed airflow obstruction, a diagnosis of COPD (that could include emphysema and chronic bronchitis), and a physician-confirmed diagnosis of asthma, which could have occurred before, after, or simultaneously with their COPD diagnosis.
Yanagisawa et al,[58] 2018	Features of both asthma and COPD are present. COPD is likely to be present if any of the following criteria are satisfied: a smoking history or equivalent exposure to air pollution, emphysematous changes on high-resolution CT, and decreased gas exchange. Asthma is likely in the presence of the following: variable or paroxysmal clinical symptoms; a documented history of asthma before the age of 40 y; elevated FeNO; and a history of perennial allergic rhinitis, airway reactivity, elevation of peripheral blood eosinophils, or an elevated total or allergen-specific IgE level.
Krishnan et al,[59] 2019	Age >40 y, current or former smoking, post-BD airflow limitation (FEV_1/FVC <0.7), and ≥12% and ≥200 mL reversibility in post-BD FEV_1.

Abbreviations: BD, bronchodilator; COPD, chronic obstructive pulmonary disease; CT, computed tomography; FeNO, fractional exhaled nitric oxide; FEV_1, forced expiratory volume in 1 second; FVC, forced vital capacity; ICD, International Classification of Diseases; Ig, immunoglobulin; LLN, lower limit of normal; PEF, peak expiratory flow.
Data from Refs.[31,34,36,47–59]

What are the practical reasons for introducing ACO as a nominalist diagnosis? Patients with features of concurrent asthma and COPD are usually excluded from epidemiologic studies or randomized controlled trials of therapy in asthma and COPD, and it is argued, therefore, that it is not possible to say if they have a different prognosis or treatment response to those with either disease in isolation. Epidemiologic studies have tried to validate the concept of ACO as a distinct entity by demonstrating that patients meeting *their* definition of ACO have different radiological findings, and worse symptoms, quality of life, and prognosis than those with asthma or COPD alone,[34–36] but at least one study has suggested they do not.[37] However, without a universally accepted definition, it is difficult to interpret these results, as different clinicians may argue that patients considered to have ACO in these studies actually have forms of COPD or asthma, rather than overlap.

One of the principal arguments advanced for justifying the introduction of the overlap diagnosis is that it ensures that patients who need inhaled corticosteroids for their asthma are not denied them because of the diagnosis of COPD. This seems fallacious, because if both asthma and COPD are present in the same patient, both need management according to relevant guidelines.

The joint GINA and GOLD document stated that "the term asthma COPD overlap does *not* describe a single disease entity. Instead, as for asthma and COPD, it likely includes patients with several different forms of airways disease (phenotypes) caused by a range of mechanisms."[33] It further stated that "outside specialist centers, a stepwise approach to diagnosis is advised," implying that with specialist investigations or expertise, a firm diagnosis of ACO can be made, but no further clarification is given on this. It stated that "the mechanisms underlying the overlap are largely unknown, and a formal definition of asthma-COPD overlap cannot be provided."

Perversely, the American Thoracic Society/National Heart, Lung, and Blood Institute Asthma–Chronic Obstructive Pulmonary Disease Overlap Workshop participants concluded that although they recognized that the overlap occurred, it was "*not useful* (my emphasis) at this time to develop a single, universal definition of ACO for diagnosis and treatment." The group proposed that ACO should be regarded as "an interim clinical label, to identify at-risk patients on the basis of clinical features of both asthma and COPD to safely manage patients until evidence about mechanisms and targeted treatments emerges." Both this document and the 2017 GINA-GOLD document imply that ACO exists in an essentialist sense. The investigators obviously believed that with more knowledge rather than it being possible to differentiate asthma from COPD more reliably, it will be possible to identify multiple ACOs based on specific defining characteristics. Adopting similar thinking, Bateman and colleagues[38] proposed that at least four ACOs exist, with more yet to be identified.

An alternative approach that has been proposed is to move away from the diagnostic labels of asthma and COPD and to identify "treatable traits" in patients with airways disease.[39] Although it is true that there are similarities in the clinical, physiologic, and immunologic features of asthma and COPD there are also important differences in the response to therapy, even when patients are stratified by treatable traits. For example, patients with the treatable trait of higher blood eosinophil counts in both asthma and COPD respond to anti–interleukin-5 therapy, but the magnitude of the response is very much greater in patients with asthma[40–43] than with COPD,[44,45] suggesting the traits are occurring *in different diseases*. Thus, it is necessary and helpful to maintain the current diagnostic labels while continuing to characterize patients having these diseases in as detailed a way as possible to identify phenotypes and underlying endotypes using the latest molecular pathologic and genetic approaches. Although, at the same time, not falling into the trap identified by Drummond[3] nearly 250 years ago of introducing "such numbers of names to each disease, and such minute and subtle distinctions of them by which a beginner …. will be apt to imagine that each name denotes a disease very different from any other."

It is worth thinking again about the way plants and animals are classified into species. There are many different breeds of dogs, but all are the same species. Dogs and cats share many characteristics, such as having 4 legs, yet the terms dog and cat remain useful. In *On the Origin of Species*, Darwin[46] recognized that there cannot be essentialist definitions of species and said "… in determining whether a form should be ranked as a species or a variety, the opinion of naturalists having sound judgment and wide experience seems the only guide to follow." In the absence of unique defining characteristics, expert clinical opinion is also the only guide to follow when making a diagnosis.

The wheel has gone full circle. In the 2020 GOLD report, we state "We no longer refer to asthma & COPD overlap (ACO), instead we emphasize that asthma and COPD are different disorders, although they may share some common traits and clinical features (eg, eosinophilia, some degree of reversibility). Asthma and COPD may coexist in an individual patient. If a concurrent diagnosis of asthma is suspected, pharmacotherapy should primarily follow asthma guidelines, but pharmacologic and non-pharmacological approaches may also be needed for their COPD."

REFERENCES

1. Latham RG. The works of Thomas Sydenham. London: The Sydenham Society; 1848.
2. King LS. Boissier de Sauvages and 18th century nosology. Bull Hist Med 1966;40:43–51.

3. Drummond J. An essay on the improvement of medicine. In: Medical essays and observations. Edinburgh: A Society in Edinburgh; 1773. p. 453–8.

4. McKusick VA. On lumpers and splitters, or the nosology of genetic disease. Perspect Biol Med 1969;12:298–318.

5. Osler W. The principles and practice of medicine. New York: Appleton; 1892.

6. Vargas AJ, Harris CC. Biomarker development in the precision medicine era: lung cancer as a case study. Nat Rev Cancer 2016;16:525–37.

7. Laennec RTH. De l'Auscultation Médiate ou Traité du Diagnostic des Maladies des Poumons et du Coeur. Paris: Brosson & Chaudé; 1819.

8. Bonet T. Sepulchretum sive anatonia pructica ex Cadaveribus Morbo denatis, proponens Histoa's Observations omnium pené humani corporis affectuum, ipsarcomoue Causas recorditas revelans. Geneva (Switzerland): Pierre Chouet; 1679.

9. Badham C. An essay on bronchitis: with a supplement containing remarks on simple pulmonary abscess. 2nd ediiton. London: J Callow; 1814.

10. Petty TL. The history of COPD. Int J Chron Obstruct Pulmon Dis 2006;1(1):3–14.

11. Briscoe WA, Nash ES. The slow space in chronic obstructive pulmonary disease. Ann N Y Acad Sci 1965;121:706–22.

12. CIBA foundation guest symposium. Terminology, definitions and classification of chronic obstructive pulmonary emphysema and related conditions. Thorax 1959;14:286–99.

13. Standards for the diagnosis and care of patients with chronic obstructive pulmonary disease (COPD) and asthma. This official statement of the American Thoracic Society was adopted by the ATS Board of Directors, November 1986. Am Rev Respir Dis 1987;136(1):225–44.

14. Pride NB, Vermeire P, Allegra L. Diagnostic labels applied to model case histories of chronic airflow obstruction. Responses to a questionnaire in 11 North American and Western European countries. Eur Respir J 1989;2(8):702–9.

15. National Asthma Education Program. Guidelines for the diagnosis and management of asthma: expert panel report. Pub. No. 91–3042. Bethesda (MD): National Heart, Lung, and Blood Institute; 1991.

16. Global Initiative for Asthma. Global strategy for asthma management and prevention. 2019. Available at: www.ginasthma.org. Accessed January 30, 2020.

17. Global Initiative for Chronic Obstructive Lung Disease (GOLD). Global strategy for the diagnosis, management, and prevention of chronic obstructive pulmonary disease. 2020 Report. 2020. Available at: http://www.goldcopd.org/. Accessed January 30, 2020.

18. Scadding JG. Principles of definition in medicine with special reference to chronic bronchitis and emphysema. Lancet 1959;1(7068):323–5.

19. Scadding JG. Essentialism and nominalism in medicine: logic of diagnosis in disease terminology. Lancet 1996;348(9027):594–6.

20. Popper KR. The open society and its enemies. London: Routledge, Kegan Paul; 1945.

21. Scadding JG. Health and disease: what can medicine do for philosophy? J Med Ethics 1988;14(3): 118–24.

22. Standards for the diagnosis and care of patients with chronic obstructive pulmonary disease. American Thoracic Society. Am J Respir Crit Care Med 1995;152(5 Pt 2):S77–121.

23. Hanania NA, Sharafkhaneh A, Celli B, et al. Acute bronchodilator responsiveness and health outcomes in COPD patients in the UPLIFT trial. Respir Res 2011;12:6.

24. George L, Brightling CE. Eosinophilic airway inflammation: role in asthma and chronic obstructive pulmonary disease. Ther Adv Chronic Dis 2016;7(1): 34–51.

25. Brown PJ, Greville HW, Finucane KE. Asthma and irreversible airflow obstruction. Thorax 1984;39(2): 131–6.

26. Backman KS, Greenberger PA, Patterson R. Airways obstruction in patients with long-term asthma consistent with 'irreversible asthma. Chest 1997; 112(5):1234–40.

27. Vonk JM, Jongepier H, Panhuysen CI, et al. Risk factors associated with the presence of irreversible airflow limitation and reduced transfer coefficient in patients with asthma after 26 years of follow up. Thorax 2003;58(4):322–7.

28. Alshabanat A, Zafari Z, Albanyan O, et al. Asthma and COPD overlap syndrome (ACOS): a systematic review and meta analysis. PLoS One 2015;10(9): e0136065.

29. Wu W, Bleecker E, Moore W, et al. Unsupervised phenotyping of Severe Asthma Research Program participants using expanded lung data. J Allergy Clin Immunol 2014;133(5):1280–8.

30. Burge PS, Calverley PM, Jones PW, et al. Randomised, double blind, placebo controlled study of fluticasone propionate in patients with moderate to severe chronic obstructive pulmonary disease: the ISOLDE trial. BMJ 2000;320(7245):1297–303.

31. Soler-Cataluna JJ, Cosio B, Izquierdo JL, et al. Consensus document on the overlap phenotype COPD-asthma in COPD. Arch Bronconeumol 2012; 48(9):331–7.

32. Global Initiative for Asthma, Global Initiative for Obstructive Lung Disease. Diagnosis of Diseases of Chronic Airflow Limitation: Asthma, COPD and Asthma-COPD Overlap Syndrome (ACOS). 2014.

33. Global Initiative for Asthma, Global Initiative for Obstructive Lung Disease. Diagnosis and Initial Treatment of Asthma, COPD and Asthma-COPD Overlap 2017.

34. de Marco R, Pesce G, Marcon A, et al. The coexistence of asthma and chronic obstructive pulmonary disease (COPD): prevalence and risk factors in young, middle-aged and elderly people from the general population. PLoS One 2013;8(5):e62985.

35. Kauppi P, Kupiainen H, Lindqvist A, et al. Overlap syndrome of asthma and COPD predicts low quality of life. J Asthma 2011;48(3):279–85.

36. Hardin M, Silverman EK, Barr RG, et al. The clinical features of the overlap between COPD and asthma. Respir Res 2011;12(1):127.

37. Izquierdo-Alonso JL, Rodriguez-Gonzalezmoro JM, de Lucas-Ramos P, et al. Prevalence and characteristics of three clinical phenotypes of chronic obstructive pulmonary disease (COPD). Respir Med 2013;107(5):724–31.

38. Bateman ED, Reddel HK, van Zyl-Smit RN, et al. The asthma-COPD overlap syndrome: towards a revised taxonomy of chronic airways diseases? Lancet Respir Med 2015;3(9):719–28.

39. Agusti A, Bel E, Thomas M, et al. Treatable traits: toward precision medicine of chronic airway diseases. Eur Respir J 2016;47(2):410–9.

40. Bel EH, Wenzel SE, Thompson PJ, et al. Oral glucocorticoid-sparing effect of mepolizumab in eosinophilic asthma. N Engl J Med 2014;371(13):1189–97.

41. Bel EH, Ortega HG, Pavord ID. Glucocorticoids and mepolizumab in eosinophilic asthma. N Engl J Med 2014;371(25):2434.

42. FitzGerald JM, Bleecker ER, Nair P, et al. Benralizumab, an anti-interleukin-5 receptor alpha monoclonal antibody, as add-on treatment for patients with severe, uncontrolled, eosinophilic asthma (CALIMA): a randomised, double-blind, placebo-controlled phase 3 trial. Lancet 2016;388(10056):2128–41.

43. Bleecker ER, FitzGerald JM, Chanez P, et al. Efficacy and safety of benralizumab for patients with severe asthma uncontrolled with high-dosage inhaled corticosteroids and long-acting beta2-agonists (SIROCCO): a randomised, multicentre, placebo-controlled phase 3 trial. Lancet 2016;388(10056):2115–27.

44. Pavord ID, Chanez P, Criner GJ, et al. Mepolizumab for eosinophilic chronic obstructive pulmonary disease. N Engl J Med 2017;377(17):1613–29.

45. Criner GJ, Celli BR, Brightling CE, et al. Benralizumab for the prevention of COPD Exacerbations. N Engl J Med 2019;381(11):1023–34.

46. Darwin CR. On the origin of species by means of natural selection, or the preservation of favoured races in the struggle for life. London: John Murray; 1859.

47. Marsh SE, Travers J, Weatherall M, et al. Proportional classifications of COPD phenotypes. Thorax 2008;63(9):761–7.

48. Andersen H, Lampela P, Nevanlinna A, et al. High hospital burden in overlap syndrome of asthma and COPD. Clin Respir J 2013;7(4):342–6.

49. Lim HS, Choi SM, Lee J, et al. Responsiveness to inhaled corticosteroid treatment in patients with asthma-chronic obstructive pulmonary disease overlap syndrome. Ann Allergy Asthma Immunol 2014;113(6):652–7.

50. Fu JJ, Gibson PG, Simpson JL, et al. Longitudinal changes in clinical outcomes in older patients with asthma, COPD and Asthma-COPD overlap syndrome. Respiration 2014;87(1):63–74.

51. Menezes AM, Montes de Oca M, Perez-Padilla R, et al. Increased risk of exacerbation and hospitalization in subjects with an overlap phenotype: COPD-asthma. Chest 2014;145(2):297–304.

52. Barrecheguren M, Roman-Rodriguez M, Miravitlles M. Is a previous diagnosis of asthma a reliable criterion for asthma-COPD overlap syndrome in a patient with COPD? Int J Chron Obstruct Pulmon Dis 2015;10:1745–52.

53. Ishiura Y, Fujimura M, Shiba Y, et al. A comparison of the efficacy of once-daily fluticasone furoate/vilanterole with twice-daily fluticasone propionate/salmeterol in asthma-COPD overlap syndrome. Pulm Pharmacol Ther 2015;35:28–33.

54. Kiljander T, Helin T, Venho K, et al. Prevalence of asthma-COPD overlap syndrome among primary care asthmatics with a smoking history: a cross-sectional study. NPJ Prim Care Respir Med 2015;25:15047.

55. Sin DD, Miravitlles M, Mannino DM, et al. What is asthma-COPD overlap syndrome? Towards a consensus definition from a round table discussion. Eur Respir J 2016;48(3):664–73.

56. Plaza V, Alvarez F, Calle M, et al. Consensus on the asthma-COPD overlap syndrome (ACOS) between the Spanish COPD guidelines (GesEPOC) and the Spanish guidelines on the management of asthma (GEMA). Arch Bronconeumol 2017;53(8):443–9.

57. Ding B, Small M. Treatment trends in patients with asthma-COPD overlap syndrome in a COPD cohort: findings from a real-world survey. Int J Chron Obstruct Pulmon Dis 2017;12:1753–63.

58. Yanagisawa S, Ichinose M. Definition and diagnosis of asthma-COPD overlap (ACO). Allergol Int 2018;67(2):172–8.

59. Krishnan JA, Nibber A, Chisholm A, et al. Prevalence and characteristics of asthma-chronic obstructive pulmonary disease overlap in routine primary care practices. Ann Am Thorac Soc 2019;16(9):1143–50.

Multimorbidity in Patients with Chronic Obstructive Pulmonary Disease

Miguel Divo, MD, MPH*, Bartolome R. Celli, MD

KEYWORDS

• COPD comorbidities • Multimorbidity • COPD system networks

KEY POINTS

- Patients with COPD also suffer from major concurrent diseases that are more frequent in them than in patients without COPD.
- These comorbidities not only are more frequent but also appear a decade or 2 earlier in patients with the disease.
- Coronary artery disease, cardiac arrhythmias, heart failure, lung cancer, osteoporosis, gastro-esophageal reflux, interstitial lung disease, and depression, independently increase the risk of death in those patients.
- The novel use of system network analysis highlights the potential interaction of multiple diseases occurring simultaneously.
- Advances in high throughput and big data analysis provide new avenues to help understand the possible pathobiological mechanisms explaining multimorbidity co-occurrence.

INTRODUCTION

Life expectancy has increased, partly due to significant improvements in the treatment of communicable diseases. This has resulted in an epidemiologic transition from early mortality caused by transmissible diseases toward a higher prevalence of noncommunicable diseases causing deaths at an older age.[1] The challenge today is to achieve not only a longer life but also a healthier one. Given this paradigm change, we must be prepared to manage individuals with concomitant chronic diseases.

Noncommunicable chronic conditions are characterized by their slow, cumulative progression, making them clinically apparent at later stages in life, often when they can be controlled but not cured. As age advances, individuals are likely to have more than 1 co-occurring chronic condition, a phenomenon known as multimorbidity.[2] Chronic obstructive pulmonary disease (COPD), a classic model of a complex disease, may start in early life,[3] progress very slowly over time, and often is diagnosed when patients reach their sixth or seventh decade. The disease is defined by the presence of respiratory symptoms, in particular dyspnea, and is confirmed by the presence of airflow limitation that is not fully reversible using a spirometry. COPD is a syndrome rather than a single disease, with distinct phenotypes, each with its own natural course and prognosis and frequently associated with important systemic consequences, such as skeletal muscle dysfunction and impaired functional capacity.[4] Once clinically expressed, it is a disabling disease, affecting a patient's quality of life and increasing the risk of hospitalizations and death. From the Evaluation of COPD Longitudinally to Identify Predictive Surrogate Endpoints study, it has been learned that the degree of airway obstruction alone cannot identify by itself patients at risk of developing

Pulmonary and Critical Care Division, Brigham and Women's Hospital, Harvard Medical School, 75 Francis Street, Boston, MA 02460, USA
* Corresponding author.
E-mail address: mdivo@bwh.harvard.edu

Clin Chest Med 41 (2020) 405–419
https://doi.org/10.1016/j.ccm.2020.06.002

those outcomes.[5] The development of multidimensional indices like the BODE index,[6] which includes body mass index (BMI), degree of airflow obstruction, dyspnea compromise, and exercise capacity (**Table 1**), has changed the understanding, by highlighting the importance of the extrapulmonary domains in COPD that in the end influence the clinical presentation and ultimate prognosis of these patients. It also has been learned that COPD rarely presents as the only disease of a particular patient, because more than 80% of those attending clinics have 1 or more comorbidities when carefully evaluated.[7]

DYING FROM OR WITH CHRONIC OBSTRUCTIVE PULMONARY DISEASE

COPD is the third cause of death worldwide,[8] yet up to two-thirds of individuals suffering from COPD die of nonpulmonary causes, mainly cardiovascular diseases (congestive heart failure, myocardial infarction, and stroke) and lung cancer.[9,10] This means that two-thirds of COPD patients, usually those with milder degrees of COPD severity, contribute to the cardiovascular and cancer death pool. Respiratory causes of death become more prevalent in patients with more advanced disease, as measured by degree of obstruction or better yet with the BODE index.[6]

In addition, compared with the general population, comorbidities develop at an earlier age and with a higher point prevalence in patients with COPD[7,11] (**Fig. 1**).

EPIDEMIOLOGY OF CHRONIC OBSTRUCTIVE PULMONARY DISEASE–RELATED COMORBIDITIES

Most studies have centered primarily on the identification of the most frequently observed comorbidities, their prevalence in COPD patients compared with the general population without this diagnosis, and their impact on patient-centered outcomes, such as mortality, quality of life, response to pulmonary rehabilitation, and hospitalizations. A summary of selected studies is presented in **Table 2**, which compares the methods used to ascertain comorbidities in those studies, the setting where they were conducted, and the number of patients and controls included. In bold (first column), those settings with direct impact on patient-centered outcomes (listed in the fifth row) are highlighted. In this context, some general conclusions can be drawn.

The first observation is that not all comorbid diseases present in patients with COPD are associated with the same prognostic implication. As shown in **Fig. 2**, there is a group of 12 of 78 comorbidities studied in more than 1600 patients for 5 years that independently increase the risk of death in COPD patients. These diseases are important because, as shown in the **Fig. 2**, they can be screened for by health care providers with tools common to most practices, and several of them are the target of primary and secondary prevention as well as established treatment algorithms. A computed tomography (CT) scan, an electrocardiogram, a mammogram, or an echocardiogram can help detect the most prevalent of these particularly important diseases. Perhaps less prevalent, but important because of its close association to increased mortality (see **Fig. 2**), is a diagnosis of anxiety. This frequently unrecognized disease needs to be considered, because its detection and treatment can help these patients profoundly. Not only should it be able to be diagnosed but also, more importantly, patients should be referred to an appropriate health provider capable of managing this particular problem because, as can be seen in **Fig. 2**, it is associated with a poor prognosis. Keep in mind that pulmonary rehabilitation has been shown to improve depression and anxiety independent of improvements in other patient-reported outcomes.[23]

Divo and coworkers[12] developed a COPD-specific comorbidity test (COTE) index, which independently increases the predictive power of the BODE index on mortality (**Table 3**). **Fig. 3** shows that the impact of the comorbidities included in the COTE index on mortality is more pronounced in patients with BODE index lower than 4 points (less severe COPD), compared with its impact in patients with more severe disease. In other words, in patients with milder COPD, checking for the comorbidities highlighted in the comorbidome may improve the final outcome of those patients because they are more likely to be impacted by the severity of those diseases than by COPD itself. These findings are consistent with that of other studies evaluating a smaller number of comorbid conditions. One such study, that of Sin and colleagues,[10] reported that patients with milder COPD measured by airflow limitation actually have a higher chance of dying from a cardiovascular cause than from respiratory insufficiency.

COMORBIDITIES OF CLINICAL RELEVANCE IN CHRONIC OBSTRUCTIVE PULMONARY DISEASE PATIENTS

It is impossible to review all the comorbidities that patients with COPD may manifest; however, there are some organ systems and specific illnesses that

Table 1
The BODE index

	Points on BODE Index			
Variables	0	1	2	3
FEV$_1$ (% of predicted)	$\geq$65	50–64	36–49	$\leq$35
Distance walked in 6 min (m)	$\geq$350	250–349	150–249	$\leq$149
Modified Medical Research Council dyspnea scale	0–1	2	3	4
BMI	>21	$\leq$21		

deserve some attention because their detection is possible by any health care provider and should be part of the expertise of those caring for patients with COPD. Furthermore, all of them are impacted favorably by their identification and appropriate therapeutic approach.

Decreased Functional Capacity

Functional capacity relates to the ability to perform physical functions; the concept has been associated with the ability to perform aerobic work (cellular use of oxygen) and practically measured as exercise capacity. The capacity to exercise depends on the ability of the respiratory system and the cardiovascular pump to deliver oxygen to the working muscles. The assessment of functional capacity is achieved with the use of a formal cardiopulmonary exercise test with the measured peak oxygen uptake being the gold standard.[24] Simple field tests, however, such as the 6-minute walk distance and the shuttle walk test, have excellent prognostic power and wide clinical applicability.[25] The introduction of portable pedometers and accelerator-based activity monitors may help better determine the actual level of activity rather than the functional capacity or reserve of patients with COPD, but their use has not resulted in major improvements in outcomes.[26] The pulmonary physiologic factors contributing to functional limitation all are inter-related and it is difficult to separate the independent effect of each factor on overall functional capacity. Over decades, the limitation of functional capacity had been associated with worse airflow limitation; however, an increasing body of evidence shows that static and dynamic hyperinflation is more important in determining functional dyspnea than the actual degree of obstruction. The levels of arterial oxygen and carbon dioxide are important contributors to overall functional compromise in patients with COPD and, although little explored, it is possible that some of the decreased functional capacity

of patients with COPD relates to compromised cardiac function secondary to hyperinflation and increased cardiac load resulting from large swings in intrathoracic pressures.

Finally, it has also been shown that in COPD, the functional capacity is related to skeletal muscle weakness and dysfunction, which often is accompanied by loss of fat-free mass (FFM), including muscle.[27] In COPD, the loss of muscle mass (sarcopenia) occurs at a slow rate but faster than that observed during normal aging and is associated with a pathologic alteration in the structure and enzymatic component of the machinery needed for the muscles to function correctly. This muscle wasting has profound effects on morbidity, including an increased risk for hospital readmission after exacerbation as well as increased need for mechanical ventilatory support. Furthermore, muscle wasting has been identified as a significant determinant of mortality in COPD, which is independent of lung function, smoking, and BMI.[28] The exact reasons for the muscle dysfunction of COPD patients are still poorly understood, but inactivity appears to be an important factor, because muscles that are active, such as the diaphragm and adductor pollicis, usually are not weak in contrast to inactive muscles, such as quadriceps and vastus lateralis. Furthermore, the deltoid and diaphragm do not show the biopsy characteristics exhibited by the quadriceps.[29] Patients with COPD are very immobile, and this is further reduced around the time of exacerbations when patients are inactive. Whether by this inactivity, heightened inflammation, or both, the exercise capacity is decreased significantly with these events and fails to return to normal up to 1 year after the episodes.[30] Although the mechanisms classically thought to induce systemic muscle dysfunction is local or systemic inflammation, as well as increased oxidative stress, some studies have shown a lower level of inflammatory biomarkers in patients with the most intense loss of muscle in the multi-organs loss of tissue (molt)

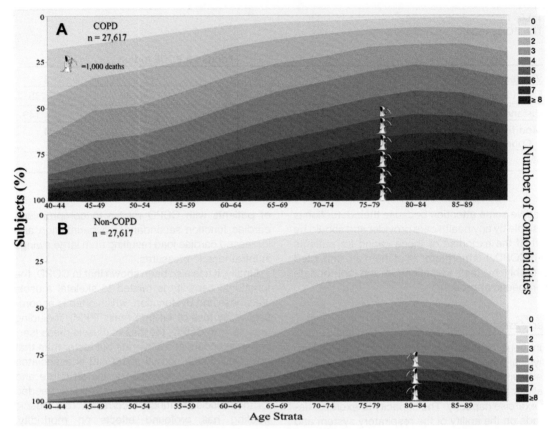

Fig. 1. Number of comorbidities per individual by age bracket and total mortality. Each band represent the number of comorbidities per patient and the width the proportion of individuals with that number of comorbidities at different age brackets (X axis). (*A*) Represent those patients carrying the diagnosis of COPD and (*B*) those without COPD. (*From* Divo MJ, Celli BR, Poblador-Plou B, et al. Chronic Obstructive Pulmonary Disease (COPD) as a disease of early aging: Evidence from the EpiChron Cohort. *PLoS ONE.* 2018;13(2):e0193143; with permission.)

phenotype. The authors suggest other mechanisms, such as inability to mount a reparative response to progressive loss of mesenchymal cells, as possible reasons for this discrepancy.

The most important reason to detect and quantify a decreased functional capacity is that pulmonary rehabilitation improves and at least partially reverses the skeletal muscle dysfunction of patients with COPD. Rehabilitation improves exercise capacity and increases the content of oxidative enzymes in the mitochondria of biopsies of the vastus lateralis muscle.[31] Attempts have been made to develop medications that can help reduce oxidative stress or alter the basic pathophysiologic mechanisms responsible for the peripheral muscle dysfunction. Unfortunately, the few trials of a group of those medications have not resulted in positive outcomes.[32]

Cardiovascular Disease

The anatomic and functional relation that exists between the lungs and the heart is such that any

dysfunction that impacts in 1 of the organs is likely to have consequences on the other. This interaction is important in patients with COPD and can be summarized in 2 types of association: first, 1 that relates pathologies that share similar risks, such as cigarette smoke and coronary artery disease (CAD) or congestive heart failure and COPD, and second, those that result in dysfunction of the heart from primary lung disease, such as secondary pulmonary hypertension and ventricular dysfunction due to increased mechanical loads.

Coronary Artery Disease and Atherosclerosis

COPD and CAD are both highly prevalent and share common risk factors, such as exposure to cigarette smoke, older age, and sedentarism. As discussed previously, patients with airflow limitation have a significantly higher risk of death from myocardial infarction and this is independent of age, gender, and smoking history.[33] The forced expiratory volume in the first second

Table 2
Summary of chronic obstructive pulmonary disease comorbidities studies describing the setting, methodology of disease ascertainment, number of subjects, prevalence, and impact on important outcomes

	Divo et al,[12] 2012	Vanfleteren et al,[13] 2013	Mapel et al,[14] 2000		Cazzola et al,[15] 2010		van Manen et al,[16] 2001		Schnell et al,[17] 2012		Putcha et al,[18] 2014	Crisafulli et al,[19] 2008	Terzano et al,[20] 2010	Almagro et al,[21] 2012	Antonelli Incalzi et al,[22] 1997
Disease ascertainment	Self-reported	Measured	Administrative database		Administrative database		Administrative database		Self-reported/measured		Administrative database	Self-reported	Self-reported/measured		
	COPD	COPD	COPD	Control	COPD	Control	COPD	Control	COPD	Control	COPD	COPD	COPD	COPD	COPD
N	1659	213	200	200	15,000	325,000	290	421	995	14,828	843	2962	288	606	288
Outcome	Mortality						QOL				QOL	Response to Rehab	Readmission	Readmission/mortality	Mortality
Setting	Outpatient	Outpatient	Acute		Outpatient		Outpatient		Outpatient		Outpatient	Outpatient	Acute	Acute	Acute
Prevalence (%)															
HTN	52	48	45	37				23*	21	60	52		38*	63	
Hyperlipidemia	44	36								48	41		9*	8	
CAD	30*	9	22	15	15	16	7					23.4*	9*	12*	21*
Obesity	29	23								40	34	40.9*		29	
DJD	29		22	20	20					55		58.6*			
Diabetes mellitus	22	54	8	7	7	19	11	7*	5	16	13	13.9*	14*	25*	21*
GERD	18														
PAD	17	53					5	6*	2				18*	17*	
Depression	17	16	17	13	13	7	5	9*	4	21	13	42.5*		15*	
CRF	17	22	2	1						16	11		26*	16*	6*
CHF	16*	14	14	3	3	8	2			12		15.1*	15*	33*	
Underweight	15														
Substance abuse	14														
Atrial fibrillation	13*														
Anxiety	12*	21								9	4			21*	18
Erectile dysfunction	12														

(continued on next page)

Table 2
(continued)

Setting	Outpatient	Acute	Outpatient	Outpatient	Outpatient	Outpatient	Outpatient	Acute	Acute	Acute	Acute	Acute
Gastric/ duodenal Ulcer	12*	32	17	7*	2				5*	10		
CVA	11		4	3*	4	9	5					
Pulmonary HTN + CP	10*								4*	11*	60*	
OSA	10								2	2		
Lung cancer	9*		2	0					2*	2		
Osteoporosis	8	31	15	11	17	9		7*	2*	16		
Hypothyroidism	7											
Breast cancer	7*											
AAA	7											
Pulmonary fibrosis	6*											
DVT	5	5										
Anemia		12	14	7	9	6	9		10.1*	10		
Cardiac arrhythmia									6*		6*	

Diseases in bold and italic font and * indicate diseases associated with a particular patient-centered outcome (see outcome row for details).

Abbreviations: AAA, abdominal aortic aneurism; CHF, congestive heart failure; CP, cor pulmonale; CRF, chronic renal failure; CVA, cerebrovascular accident; DJD, degenerative joint disease; DVT, deep vein thrombosis; GERD, gastroesophageal reflux disease; HTN, hypertension; PAD, peripheral artery disease.

Data from Refs. [12–22]

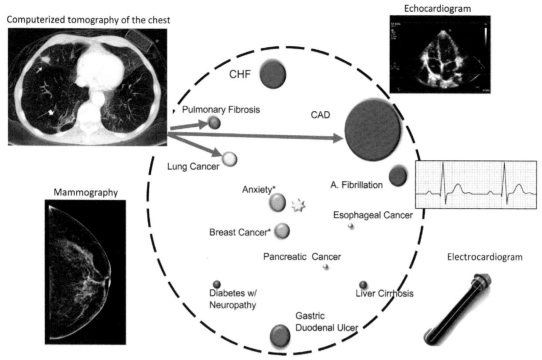

Fig. 2. The comorbidome: an orbital representation of the comorbidities that confer increased risk of 5-year mortality in patients with COPD. In the center, the yellow star represents the death; each comorbidity is represented by a circle with a diameter that is proportional to its prevalence and the distance to the center the inverse of the hazard ratio both numerically represented in **Table 3**. In addition, 5 simple tests are proposed to help diagnose some of those comorbidities. A. Fibrillation, atrial fibrillation; CHF, congestive heart failure. (*Adapted from* Divo MJ, Cote C, de Torres JP, et al. Comorbidities and risk of mortality in patients with chronic obstructive pulmonary disease. *Am J Respir Crit Care Med.* 2012;186(2):155-161; with permission.)

of expiration (FEV_1) is an independent predictor of the probability of dying from a myocardial infarction even when allowing for smoking history. The most attractive link between COPD and CAD is the presence of low-grade systemic inflammation in both diseases. Although the mechanisms responsible have not been elucidated entirely, evidence suggests that patients with COPD should be screened for the presence of concomitant atherosclerosis and, just as importantly, patients evaluated for the presence of atherosclerotic heart disease should be investigated for the concomitant presence of airflow limitation.

Heart Failure

Much less evidence exists for an association between COPD and left ventricular congestive failure of the classic type, that characterized by the presence of cardiomegaly and a poor ejection fraction in an echocardiogram.[34] There is some evidence that, if anything, the cardiac size is decreased, at least in patients with emphysema, and that the

actual volume of intrathoracic blood also is decreased in patients with hyperinflation.[35] Similarly, a majority of patients with milder COPD have normal right heart function at rest. Although there is a modest but statistically significant relationship between FEV_1 and pulmonary artery pressure, the presence of true pulmonary hypertension is rare in patients with COPD. Their existence suggests, however, that there may be an independent phenotype of patients with COPD who manifest pulmonary hypertension with COPD rather than as a result of it. The prevalence of true cor pulmonale with its clinical expression of the blue-bloated patient seems to be decreasing. The exact reason for this is not clear but could be related to the early supplementation of oxygen in patients with hypoxemia. Several studies relating the CT determined ratio of the pulmonary artery diameter to the aortic arch diameter to outcomes. If that ratio is higher than 1, there is an increased risk not only of exacerbations[36] but also of death over time, independent of other COPD-related prognostic factors.[37] If pulmonary hypertension is present, long-term

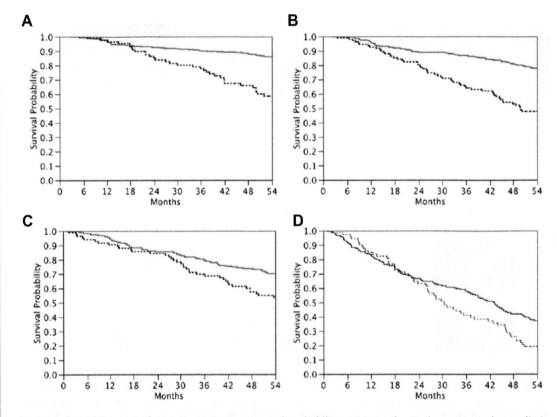

Fig. 3. Kaplan-Meier survival curves representing survival probability at 54 months. To demonstrate the predictive contribution of the COTE to the BODE index, the survival curves were represented for each BODE score quartile (see **Table 1**). (*A*) BODE quartile 1 (scores 0, 1, and 2). (*B*) BODE quartile 2 (scores 3 and 4). (*C*) BODE quartile 3 (scores 5 and 6). (*D*) BODE quartile 5 (scores 7, 8, 9, and 10). In each panel, patients were categorized as COTE score of 0 to 3 (*solid line*) or those greater than or equal to 4 points (*dotted line*). (*From* Divo MJ, Cote C, de Torres JP, et al. Comorbidities and risk of mortality in patients with chronic obstructive pulmonary disease. *Am J Respir Crit Care Med.* 2012;186(2):155-161; with permission.)

oxygen therapy is the most effective treatment because its administration slows down the progression of pulmonary arterial hypertension (PAH). Systemic and selective vasodilators, so useful in primary PAH, are not recommended routinely for the treatment of PAH in COPD because there no evidence of clinical benefit observed in several well controlled trials.

Finally, physical constraint of heart function as a consequence of static and dynamic hyperinflation has come to be regarded an important factor limiting heart function in patients with COPD. As the disease progresses, the most important factor limiting exercise is the ceiling imposed by ventilatory limitation.[38] During exercise, patients develop relatively high intrathoracic pressures due to impedance to increased ventilatory demands as a consequence of dynamic hyperinflation with large swings of the intrathoracic pressures during inspiration. Right heart catheterization shows that patients with severe COPD who hyperinflate either during exercise or by voluntary hyperventilation develop high intrathoracic pressures resulting in increased pulmonary and capillary wedge pressures, suggestive of left ventricular dysfunction.[39] These studies suggest that the function of the heart is mechanically constrained by the dynamic hyperinflation that is associated with increased ventilatory demand in patients with COPD, particularly during exercise and episodes of exacerbations. Treatment with bronchodilators, oxygen, pulmonary rehabilitation, and even lung volume reduction procedures reduces hyperinflation by prolonging expiratory time. This results in a delay in the development of hyperinflation and critical dyspnea during situations of increased ventilatory demand.

Lung Cancer

Lung cancer is a common cause of death in COPD patients[40] and patients with COPD, in particular those with emphysema, are 3 times to 4 times

Table 3
The COPD comorbity test (COTE) index

Comorbidity	Points	Prevalence (%)	Hazard Ratio
Lung, esophageal, pancreatic, and breast[a] cancers	6	9.1, 0.4, 0.4, and 7, respectively	2.02–6.18
Anxiety[a]	6	13.8	13.8
All other cancers	2		
Liver cirrhosis	2	2.5	1.68
Atrial fibrillation/flutter	2	13	1.56
Diabetes with neuropathy	2	4	1.54
Pulmonary fibrosis	2	6.1	1.51
Congestive heart failure	1	15.7	1.33
Gastric/duodenal ulcers	1	11.5	1.32
CAD	1	30.2	1.27

[a] Comorbidity with significant impact in women.

more likely to develop lung cancer than smokers with normal lung function.[41] This may be independent of the effect of cigarettes smoke, because it has been diagnosed more frequently in subjects with spirometric airflow limitation who had never smoked than in those with normal spirometry. The increased prevalence of lung cancer in COPD patients probably is linked to the increased inflammation and oxidative stress of cigarette smoke. Whatever the reason for the association between airflow limitation, emphysema, and lung cancer, what is clear is that lung cancer early detection is effective in reducing lung cancer mortality. This brings the discussion back to the value of CT scanning in patients with COPD. In cancer screening studies, there was a 20% reduction in mortality in those subjects undergoing yearly CT screening over 3 years, compared with subjects using routine chest x-ray evaluation.[42] These findings have been confirmed in other randomized trials exploring the value of lung cancer screening in high-risk patients, thus providing a supportive argument to consider a chest CT in most patients with COPD attending clinics.

Depression and Anxiety

Anxiety and depression are frequent in COPD patients and these diseases often are undiagnosed and untreated in clinical practice.[43] Depressive symptoms that are clinically relevant are estimated to occur in between 10% and 80% of all patients. On the other hand, in clinically stable outpatients with COPD, the prevalence of major depression (that requires medical intervention) ranges between 19% and 42%.[44] Smoking is more frequent in patients with anxiety and depression, so the presence of continued smoking in spite of medical advice and treatment should warn the clinician to a diagnosis of depression or anxiety. The effect of aging, smoking, and hypoxemia on brain function also is likely to contribute to its genesis. Whatever the cause, untreated depression increases length of hospital stay and frequency of hospital admissions and leads to impaired quality of life and premature death.[18,45,46] The benefit of antidepressants in the treatment of depression in COPD has been inconclusive in several small clinical trials, although these have often been poorly designed and there is a need for larger properly controlled trials in the future. In a recent study, the improvement in depression and anxiety after rehabilitation was unrelated to the improvement in dyspnea, suggesting that, if present, depression itself should be targeted for therapy independent of the treatment offered for the other better-known manifestations of COPD.[23] Psychotherapy added to pulmonary rehabilitation significantly reduces depression in COPD patients. Cognitive behavioral therapy also improves the quality of life in COPD patients with depression.

Osteoporosis

Several studies have shown a very high prevalence of osteoporosis and low bone mineral density (BMD) in patients with COPD, even with milder stages of disease.[47] The prevalence is as high as 40% in men and even higher in women. Vertebral compression fractures are relatively common among COPD patients and the resultant increased kyphosis may further reduce pulmonary function. COPD patients have several risk factors for osteoporosis, including advanced age, poor mobility, smoking, poor nutrition, low BMI, and high doses of inhaled corticosteroids as well as courses of oral steroids. Low BMD is correlated with reduced FFM in COPD patients. It follows that BMD should be measured, either by dual-energy x-ray absorptiometry or CT, particularly in patients with a low FFM. Regardless of gender, patients with COPD attending clinics should be treated with a bisphosphonate, as recommended clinically.[48]

Obstructive Sleep Apnea

Epidemiologic studies have shown that approximately 20% of patients with obstructive sleep apnea (OSA) also have COPD, whereas approximately 10% of patients with COPD have OSA independent of disease severity. OSA patients also share several of the comorbidities of COPD, such as endothelial dysfunction, cardiac failure, diabetes, and metabolic syndrome.[49] There is recent evidence that OSA patients have local upper airway inflammation as well as systemic inflammation and oxidative stress. Although there is no evidence of increased incidence of OSA in patients with COPD, the presence of OSA in such a patient is associated with oxygen desaturation and a worse outcome than with either disease alone. Treatment with continuous positive airway pressure in those patients with COPD who also have OSA improves survival.[50]

Anemia

Contrary to common teaching, recent studies have shown that there is a high prevalence of anemia in COPD patients, ranging between 15% and 30%, particularly in patients with severe disease, whereas polycythemia (erythrocytosis) is relatively rare (6%).[51]

The level of hemoglobin is associated strongly and independently with increased functional dyspnea and decreased exercise capacity and, therefore, is an important contributor to functional capacity as well as poor quality of life and even mortality.[52] The anemia usually is of the normochromic normocytic type characteristic for diseases of chronic inflammation and appears to be due to resistance to the effects of erythropoietin, the concentration of which is elevated in these patients. Although there has been no trial evaluating specific therapy for this anemia, correction of all potential causes of anemia must be evaluated and addressed.

A NOVEL APPROACH TO CHRONIC OBSTRUCTIVE PULMONARY DISEASE COMORBIDITIES

The greatest challenge remains on how to approach and treat multiple comorbidities.

Following individual practice guidelines for each condition in a typical COPD patient will result in an overwhelming task, including not only multiple laboratory tests of significant cost but also the prescription of multiple medications for the different diseases, with great potential to develop adverse interactions.[53] To address this challenge, several reviews have been published to guide clinicians in the management of COPD comorbidities. These reviews are characterized by recommendations made on single comorbidities and using a dichotomic approach; for example, COPD and congestive heart failure or COPD and osteoporosis.[54–56] Although it is a step in the right direction, this approach fails to consider that a majority of COPD patients have more than 2 comorbidities and that addressing the most prevalent ones may not necessarily address those that have an impact on important outcomes. As discussed previously and shown graphically in **Fig. 2**, a plan can be drafted to concentrate on those diseases that have a direct impact on mortality. The authors propose the use of simple diagnostic tests, available to most health care practitioners, that can diagnose and grade the severity of those important and frequent comorbidities and that with current approaches may have their natural course modified.

ADDRESSING THE COMPLEXITY OF MULTIMORBIDITY

Multimorbidity is more than just experiencing the additive effect of having more than 1 disease, it actually implies a complex synergistic interaction between diseases. Unfortunately it has been learned that, despite having effective treatments to improve airflow limitation and to reduce the number of COPD exacerbations, bronchodilators have limited impact on mortality.[57,58] This observation is in part due to the fact that, as discussed previously, up to two-thirds of individuals suffering from COPD die of nonpulmonary causes.[9,10] These observations support the need to understand how co-occurring diseases interact with each other and their effect on outcomes. Those synergistic interactions amongst concurrent diseases can be illustrated by a bicycle team racing in the Tour de France. The Tour is not a 100-m sprint, where pure speed is key to crossing the finish line first; instead, it is a strategy game. In the Tour, there are several stages, with a constant synergistic interaction among the cyclists in the form of competitions or coalitions. Those interactions could be simultaneous or sequential throughout the race, allowing a cyclist to interact differently in time.[59] At the end, the winner is the one who benefits the most from those alliances, team effort, and own cycling capacity. The life course study of chronic diseases has emerged as a branch of public health and epidemiology that has as its goal, "learning the tour of life." This emerging field aims to study the temporal relationship, from gestation to adult life (Tour stages) and the synergistic interactions (alliances or competitions) between exposures, with the development of chronic diseases and their effect on health.[60]

The temporal relationships and the different courses diseases can take over time are highlighted by several recent observation. For example, it has been learned that the development of airway obstruction can follow different trajectories starting at early age and that clinically significant COPD can occur in close to half of subjects without accelerated lung function decline.[61] Another example of differential course of diseases evaluating the occurrence of multimorbidity is a Danish study that reviewed an electronic health registry that included 6.2 million individuals followed over time. The investigators used this longitudinal database and evaluated the temporal disease trajectories of several diseases over a period of 15 years. They found that COPD anteceded several other diagnoses and was a key driver of other comorbidities. The same study also pointed out that behavioral diseases anteceded COPD itself, which suggests that COPD is a consequence of personal misbehavior, which in theory could be altered to prevent that dreaded consequence.[62]

Evidence on the synergistic interactions between diseases can be found in other related fields; for example, it has been shown that the FEV_1 is an independent predictor of the probability of dying from a myocardial infarction even when adjusting for smoking history.[33] As for lung cancer, patients with COPD are 3 times to 4 times more likely to develop lung cancer than smokers with normal lung function,[63] more specifically, those COPD patients with milder obstruction and a lower BMI and diffusing capacity of the lungs for carbon monoxide (DLCO)[64] are at even higher risk than patients with more severe airflow limitation. Finding synergistic interactions requires a multivariate integrative approach rather than a reductionist one by providing a more complete view of the interactive role of many diseases coexisting in an individual.

THE USE OF NOVEL TOOLS TO ANALYZE COMPLEX INTERACTIONS

With that in mind, the authors' group used a multidimensional network analysis and explored the associations between 79 different comorbidities and phenotypic characteristics in a cohort of more than 2000 individuals. That study found that comorbidities are interlinked beyond simple coincidence, and diseases aggregate in clusters with meaningful syndromic associations supporting the existence of a unified intermediate mechanism targeting different organs. **Fig. 4** illustrates an example of interlinked comorbidities and phenotypic features in 1 of the 6 clusters in that study. It consists of younger COPD patients (less than 55 years old), with BMI lower than 21 kg/m² and low DLCO, who manifest a predominantly psychiatric and behavioral cluster of illnesses that are associated to other comorbidities linked to high-risk behaviors.[65] This finding, although observed in this cross-sectional study, coincides with the observational longitudinal study by Jensen and colleagues,[62] discussed previously, where behavioral diseases clustered and actually preceded the ulterior development of COPD.

Studying comorbidities and COPD phenotypes using this integrative network or other clustering techniques, rather than studying each component separately, helps better understand the underlying relationships among diseases. The sum is more meaningful than its individual parts. Examples of such studies are listed in the references section for the interested reader.[13,65–69]

The biggest limitation of these clustering studies is their cross-sectional nature and the way comorbidities are ascertained. Despite this shortcoming, if those clusters are analyzed, relations between co-occurring diseases can be inferred based on knowledge of the natural history of some disease. For example, the cluster in **Fig. 4** shows the links among hepatitis-cirrhosis and liver cancer, which appear to follow the known natural history of that complex of diseases. Cluster analysis can provide new insight in possible interactions between comorbidities previously undetected with univariate analysis and could help generate testable hypothesis of disease associations.

Beginning in the nineteenth century, the classification of diseases and their diagnoses was made from observational correlations between pathologic analysis and clinical syndromes. With time, the use of laboratory and radiological markers has helped make this process less invasive and more objective, increasing the confidence of assessments. This classic diagnostic strategy, however, lacks sensitivity to identify preclinical disease and also lacks the specificity to unequivocally define a disease.[70] One such example is the lack of precise categorizations in clinical guidelines in terms of defining different COPD phenotypes, such as the recently described MOLT

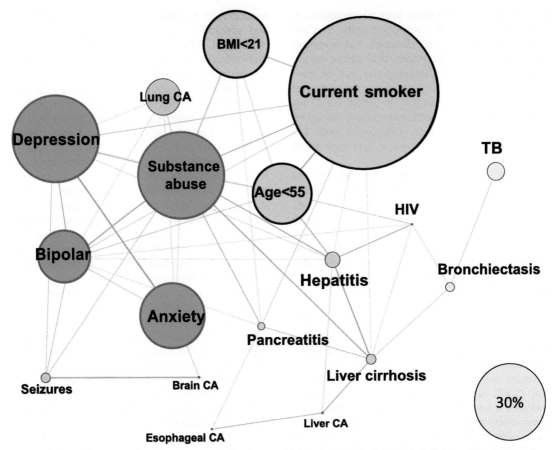

Fig. 4. This graph represents a cluster or module of comorbidities and clinical characteristics resulting from a clustering algorithm applied to the COPD comorbidities network. The module contains correlated comorbidities and clinical characteristics tightly connected. The size of the nodes represents the prevalence, and the links represent statistically significant correlations between connected nodes. CA, cancer; HIV, human immunodefficiency virus; TB, tuberculosis. (*Adapted from* Divo MJ, Casanova C, Marin JM, et al. COPD comorbidities network. *Eur Respir J.* 2015;46(3):640-650; with permission.)

phenotype.[71] This phenotype expands on the old characterization of the classic pink puffer phenotype, described more than 60 years ago,[72] with the application of newer diagnostic tools that were nonexistent then, now allowing a better description of this subgroup of COPD patients.

One added problem affecting the field of comorbidities in COPD is the lack of a clear taxonomy. For example, the terms, *extrapulmonary manifestations* and *comorbidities*, are still interchanged when referring to sarcopenia, osteoporosis, anemia, or cachexia. Although this seems an issue of semantics, recognizing the extrapulmonary manifestation of the disease would allow clinicians to follow COPD patients in a more integrative way, like endocrinologists follow their diabetic patients for retinopathy or nephropathy. A suggested approach is described in a review by Loscalzo and colleagues,[70] where the proposed response to environmental exposures (temperature,

radiation, hydration, oxygen tension, micronutrients and macronutrients, infective agents and parasitism, and toxins) the gene expression can ultimately modify. In contrasts to the classic genetic concepts, whose actions are uniquely affected by the primary genetic mutation that determine a particular disease trait, other modifiable genes, whose actions reflect generic responses to the stress evoked by environmental exposures, may lead to imbalanced response in different pathobiological pathways. These responses include inflammation, thrombosis and hemorrhage, fibrosis, the immune response, proliferation, and apoptosis/necrosis,[70] mechanisms that may interact to simultaneously have an impact on different organ systems, leading to different phenotypical and clinical manifestations. For the clinician, this is recognized as different diseases because a clinical approach has been developed that partitions diseases according to the organs affected. In this new paradigm, those diseases would be grouped according to the pathobiological mechanism responsible for its development, thereby changing the way diseases and their treatment are thought of.

SUMMARY

The vision of COPD, as a relatively simple disease affecting only the airways and lung parenchyma, has changed over the past 2 decades to include important systemic consequences. Above and beyond that, novel studies have provided evidence of the occurrence of multiple morbidities in patients with COPD that not only have a higher prevalence in those patients but also, equally important, begin at an earlier age. In particular, diseases of the heart, lung cancer, osteoporosis, anxiety, and depression are extremely frequent in those patients and some of them are independent predictors of mortality these patients. In patients with mild obstruction, cardiovascular diseases and lung cancer are more frequent causes of death than any respiratory cause. Importantly, most of these comorbidities can be detected with tools currently available to most clinicians and a majority have treatments capable of improving them. Novel approaches, using big data and system biology that allow exploration of multiple variables simultaneously, are increasing understanding of the potentially common pathobiological mechanisms that those diseases may share. Exploration of the hypothesis generated by those findings may lead to novel therapies directed at those pathobiological processes rather than to the treatment of single organ affliction. In the meantime, health care providers caring for COPD patients should be aware of the multiple diseases that they can be suffering from and address them properly with the many tools currently available.

DISCLOSURE

The authors have no relevant financial interest related to the material in the article.

REFERENCE

1. Affairs DOEAS, Population. United Nations, Department of Economic and Social Affairs, Population Division (2013). World Population Prospects: the 2012 Revision, Highlights and Advance Tables. Working Paper No. ESA/P/WP.228.; 2013.

2. Barnett K, Mercer SW, Norbury M, et al. Epidemiology of multimorbidity and implications for health care, research, and medical education: a cross-sectional study. Lancet 2012;380(9836):37–43.

3. Martinez FD. Early-life origins of chronic obstructive pulmonary disease. N Engl J Med 2016;375(9): 871–8.

4. Celli BR. COPD: time to improve its taxonomy? ERJ Open Res 2018;4(1):1–8.

5. Agustí A, Calverley PMA, Celli B, et al. Characterisation of COPD heterogeneity in the ECLIPSE cohort. Respir Res 2010;11(1):122.

6. Celli BR, Cote CG, Marin JM, et al. The body-mass index, airflow obstruction, dyspnea, and exercise capacity index in chronic obstructive pulmonary disease. N Engl J Med 2004;350(10):1005–12.

7. Divo MJ, Celli BR, Poblador-Plou B, et al. Chronic Obstructive Pulmonary Disease (COPD) as a disease of early aging: evidence from the epichron cohort. PLoS One 2018;13(2):e0193143.

8. Naghavi M, Abajobir AA, Abbafati C, et al. Global, regional, and national age-sex specific mortality for 264 causes of death, 1980â€"2016: a systematic analysis for the Global Burden of Disease Study 2016. Lancet 2017;390(10100):1151–210.

9. McGarvey LP, John M, Anderson JA, et al. Ascertainment of cause-specific mortality in COPD: operations of the TORCH clinical Endpoint Committee. Thorax 2007;62(5):411–5.

10. Sin DD, Anthonisen NR, Soriano JB, et al. Mortality in COPD: role of comorbidities. Eur Respir J 2006; 28(6):1245–57.

11. Agustí A, Noell G, Brugada J, et al. Lung function in early adulthood and health in later life: a transgenerational cohort analysis. Lancet Respir Med 2017;5(12):935–45.

12. Divo MJ, Cote C, de Torres JP, et al. Comorbidities and risk of mortality in patients with chronic obstructive pulmonary disease. Am J Respir Crit Care Med 2012;186(2):155–61.

13. Vanfleteren LEGW, Spruit MA, Groenen M, et al. Clusters of comorbidities based on validated objective measurements and systemic inflammation in patients with chronic obstructive pulmonary disease. Am J Respir Crit Care Med 2013;187(7):728–35.

14. Mapel DW, Hurley JS, Frost FJ, et al. Health care utilization in chronic obstructive pulmonary disease. A case-control study in a health maintenance organization. Arch Intern Med 2000;160(17):2653–8.

15. Cazzola M, Bettoncelli G, Sessa E, et al. Prevalence of comorbidities in patients with chronic obstructive pulmonary disease. Respiration 2010; 80(2):112–9.

16. van Manen JG, Bindels PJ, IJzermans CJ, et al. Prevalence of comorbidity in patients with a chronic airway obstruction and controls over the age of 40. J Clin Epidemiol 2001;54(3):287–93.

17. Schnell K, Weiss CO, Lee T, et al. The prevalence of clinically-relevant comorbid conditions in patients

with physician-diagnosed COPD: a cross-sectional study using data from NHANES 1999-2008. BMC Pulm Med 2012;12(1):26.

18. Putcha N, Han MK, Martinez CH, et al. Comorbidities of COPD have a major impact on clinical outcomes, particularly in African Americans. Chronic Obstr Pulm Dis 2014;1(1):105–14.

19. Crisafulli E, Costi S, Luppi F, et al. Role of comorbidities in a cohort of patients with COPD undergoing pulmonary rehabilitation. Thorax 2008;63(6):487–92.

20. Terzano C, Conti V, Di Stefano F, et al. Comorbidity, hospitalization, and mortality in COPD: results from a longitudinal study. Lung 2010;188(4):321–9.

21. Almagro P, Cabrera FJ, Diez J, et al. Comorbidities and short-term prognosis in patients hospitalized for acute exacerbation of COPD: the EPOC en Servicios de medicina interna (ESMI) study. Chest 2012; 142(5):1126–33.

22. Antonelli Incalzi R, Fuso L, De Rosa M, et al. Comorbidity contributes to predict mortality of patients with chronic obstructive pulmonary disease. Eur Respir J 1997;10(12):2794–800.

23. Paz-Díaz H, Montes de Oca M, López JM, et al. Pulmonary rehabilitation improves depression, anxiety, dyspnea and health status in patients with COPD. Am J Phys Med Rehabil 2007;86(1):30–6.

24. Puente-Maestu L, Palange P, Casaburi R, et al. Use of exercise testing in the evaluation of interventional efficacy: an official ERS statement. Eur Respir J 2016;47:429–60.

25. Celli B, Tetzlaff K, Criner G, et al. The 6-minute-walk distance test as a chronic obstructive pulmonary disease stratification tool. Insights from the COPD biomarker qualification Consortium. Am J Respir Crit Care Med 2016;194(12):1483–93.

26. Armstrong M, Winnard A, Chynkiamis N, et al. Use of pedometers as a tool to promote daily physical activity levels in patients with COPD: a systematic review and meta-analysis. Eur Respir Rev 2019; 28(154):190039.

27. Montes de Oca M, Torres SH, Gonzalez Y, et al. Peripheral muscle composition and health status in patients with COPD. Respir Med 2006;100(10):1800–6.

28. Swallow EB, Reyes D, Hopkinson NS, et al. Quadriceps strength predicts mortality in patients with moderate to severe chronic obstructive pulmonary disease. Thorax 2007;62(2):115–20.

29. Gea JG, Pasto M, Carmona MA, et al. Metabolic characteristics of the deltoid muscle in patients with chronic obstructive pulmonary disease. Eur Respir J 2001;17(5):939–45.

30. Cote CG, Dordelly LJ, Celli BR. Impact of COPD exacerbations on patient-centered outcomes. Chest 2015;131(3):696–704.

31. Bui K-L, Nyberg A, Rabinovich R, et al. The relevance of limb muscle dysfunction in chronic obstructive pulmonary disease: a review for clinicians. Clin Chest Med 2019;40(2):367–83.

32. Abdulai RM, Jensen TJ, Patel NR, et al. Deterioration of limb muscle function during acute exacerbation of chronic obstructive pulmonary disease. Am J Respir Crit Care Med 2018;197(4):433–49.

33. Sin DD, Wu L, Man SFP. The relationship between reduced lung function and cardiovascular mortality: a population-based study and a systematic review of the literature. Chest 2005;127(6):1952–9.

34. Padeletti M, Jelic S, LeJemtel TH. Coexistent chronic obstructive pulmonary disease and heart failure in the elderly. Int J Cardiol 2008;125(2):209–15.

35. Barr RG, Bluemke DA, Ahmed FS, et al. Percent emphysema, airflow obstruction, and impaired left ventricular filling. N Engl J Med 2010;362(3):217–27.

36. Wells JM, Washko GR, Han MK, et al. Pulmonary arterial enlargement and acute exacerbations of COPD. N Engl J Med 2012;367(10):913–21.

37. de Torres JP, Ezponda A, Alcaide AB, et al. Pulmonary arterial enlargement predicts long-term survival in COPD patients. PLoS One 2018;13(4). e0195640–13.

38. O'Donnell DE, Elbehairy AF, Webb KA, et al, Canadian Respiratory Research Network. The link between reduced inspiratory capacity and exercise intolerance in chronic obstructive pulmonary disease. Ann Am Thorac Soc 2017;14(Supplement_1): S30–9.

39. Butler J, Schrijen F, Henriquez A, et al. Cause of the raised wedge pressure on exercise in chronic obstructive pulmonary disease. Am Rev Respir Dis 1988;138(2):350–4.

40. Turner MC, Chen Y, Krewski D, et al. Chronic obstructive pulmonary disease is associated with lung cancer mortality in a prospective study of never smokers. Am J Respir Crit Care Med 2007;176(3):285–90.

41. de Torres JP, Bastarrika G, Wisnivesky JP, et al. Assessing the relationship between lung cancer risk and emphysema detected on low-dose CT of the chest. Chest 2007;132(6):1932–8.

42. de Koning HJ, van der Aalst CM, de Jong PA, et al. Reduced lung-cancer mortality with volume CT screening in a randomized trial. N Engl J Med 2020;382(6):503–13.

43. Yohannes AM, Kaplan A, Hanania NA. Anxiety and depression in chronic obstructive pulmonary disease: recognition and management. Cleve Clin J Med 2018;85(2 Suppl 1):S11–8.

44. Hill K, Geist R, Goldstein RS, et al. Anxiety and depression in end-stage COPD. Eur Respir J 2008; 31(3):667–77.

45. Cully JA, Graham DP, Stanley MA, et al. Quality of life in patients with chronic obstructive pulmonary disease and comorbid anxiety or depression. Psychosomatics 2006;47(4):312–9.

46. Ng T-P, Niti M, Tan W-C, et al. Depressive symptoms and chronic obstructive pulmonary disease: effect on mortality, hospital readmission, symptom burden, functional status, and quality of life. Arch Intern Med 2006;167(1):60–7.

47. Jørgensen NR, Schwarz P. Osteoporosis in chronic obstructive pulmonary disease patients. Curr Opin Pulm Med 2008;14(2):122–7.

48. Ebeling PR. Clinical practice. Osteoporosis in men. N Engl J Med 2008;358(14):1474–82.

49. Fabbri LM, Luppi F, Beghe B, et al. Complex chronic comorbidities of COPD. Eur Respir J 2008;31(1): 204–12.

50. Marin JM, Soriano JB, Carrizo SJ, et al. Outcomes in patients with chronic obstructive pulmonary disease and obstructive sleep apnea: the overlap syndrome. Am J Respir Crit Care Med 2010;182(3):325–31.

51. John M, Lange A, Hoernig S, et al. Prevalence of anemia in chronic obstructive pulmonary disease: comparison to other chronic diseases. Int J Cardiol 2006;111(3):365–70.

52. Cote C, Zilberberg MD, Mody SH, et al. Haemoglobin level and its clinical impact in a cohort of patients with COPD. Eur Respir J 2007;29(5):923–9.

53. Boyd CM, Darer J, Boult C, et al. Clinical practice guidelines and quality of care for older patients with multiple comorbid diseases: implications for pay for performance. JAMA 2005;294(6):716–24.

54. Vanfleteren LEGW, Spruit MA, Wouters EFM, et al. Management of chronic obstructive pulmonary disease beyond the lungs. Lancet Respir Med 2016; 4(11):911–24.

55. Vanfleteren L, Spruit MA, Franssen F. Tailoring the approach to multimorbidity in adults with respiratory disease: the NICE guideline. Eur Respir J 2017; 49(2):1601696.

56. Fabbri LM, Boyd C, Boschetto P, et al. How to integrate multiple comorbidities in guideline development: article 10 in integrating and coordinating efforts in COPD guideline development. an official ATS/ERS Workshop Report. Proc Am Thorac Soc 2012;9(5):274–81.

57. Calverley PMA, Anderson JA, Celli B, et al. Salmeterol and fluticasone propionate and survival in chronic obstructive pulmonary disease. N Engl J Med 2007;356(8):775–89.

58. Vestbo J, Anderson JA, Brook RD, et al. Fluticasone furoate and vilanterol and survival in chronic obstructive pulmonary disease with heightened cardiovascular risk (SUMMIT): a double-blind randomized controlled trial. Lancet 2016;387(10030): 1817–26.

59. Mignot J. Strategic behavior in road cycling competitions. The Economics of Professional Road Cycling https://doi.org/10.1007/978-3-319-22312-4.

60. Ben-Shlomo Y, Kuh D. A life course approach to chronic disease epidemiology: conceptual models, empirical challenges and interdisciplinary perspectives. Int J Epidemiol 2002;31(2):285–93.

61. Lange P, Celli B, Agusti A, et al. Lung-function trajectories leading to chronic obstructive pulmonary disease. N Engl J Med 2015;373(2):111–22.

62. Jensen AB, Moseley PL, Oprea TI, et al. Temporal disease trajectories condensed from population-wide registry data covering 6.2 million patients. Nat Commun 2014;5(1):1769.

63. Wasswa-Kintu S, Gan WQ, Man SFP, et al. Relationship between reduced forced expiratory volume in one second and the risk of lung cancer: a systematic review and meta-analysis. Thorax 2005;60(7): 570–5.

64. de-Torres JP, Marin JM, Casanova C, et al. Identification of COPD patients at high risk for lung cancer mortality using the COPD-LUCSS-DLCO. Chest 2016;149(4):936–42.

65. Divo MJ, Casanova C, Marin JM, et al. COPD comorbidities network. Eur Respir J 2015;46(3):640–50.

66. Rennard SI, Locantore N, Delafont B, et al. Identification of five chronic obstructive pulmonary disease subgroups with different prognoses in the ECLIPSE cohort using cluster analysis. Ann Am Thorac Soc 2015;12(3):303–12.

67. Burgel PR, Paillasseur JL, Caillaud D, et al. Clinical COPD phenotypes: a novel approach using principal component and cluster analyses. Eur Respir J 2010;36(3):531–9.

68. Burgel P-R, Paillasseur J-L, Janssens W, et al. A simple algorithm for the identification of clinical COPD phenotypes. Eur Respir J 2017;50(5): 1701034.

69. Garcia-Aymerich J, Gómez FP, Benet M, et al. Identification and prospective validation of clinically relevant chronic obstructive pulmonary disease (COPD) subtypes. Thorax 2011;66(5):430–7.

70. Loscalzo J, Kohane I, Barabási A-L. Human disease classification in the postgenomic era: a complex systems approach to human pathobiology. Mol Syst Biol 2007;3:124.

71. Celli BR, Locantore N, Tal-Singer R, et al. Emphysema and extrapulmonary tissue loss in COPD: a multi-organ loss of tissue phenotype. Eur Respir J 2018;51(2):1702146.

72. Dornhorst AC. Respiratory insufficiency. Lancet 1955;268(6876):1185–7.

Section III : Exacerbations

Definition, Causes, Pathogenesis, and Consequences of Chronic Obstructive Pulmonary Disease Exacerbations

Andrew I. Ritchie, MBChB, Jadwiga A. Wedzicha, PhD*

KEYWORDS

• Chronic obstructive pulmonary disease • Exacerbations • Pathogenesis

KEY POINTS

- Acute exacerbations of chronic obstructive pulmonary disease (AECOPD) are episodes of symptom worsening which have significant adverse consequences for patients.
- Highly heterogeneous events associated with increased airway and systemic inflammation and physiological changes.
- They are triggered predominantly by respiratory viruses and bacteria, which infect the lower airway and increase airway inflammation.
- A proportion of patients appear to be more susceptible to exacerbations, with poorer quality of life and more aggressive disease progression.
- Prevention and mitigation of exacerbations are therefore key goals of COPD management.

INTRODUCTION

Acute exacerbations of chronic obstructive pulmonary disease (AECOPDs) are episodes of symptom worsening[1] that have significant adverse consequences for patients.[2] The important causes of exacerbations include airway bacteria, viruses, and pollution; however, the interplay of these triggers must also be considered. It is recognized that defects in immunity and host defense lead to more frequent AECOPDs. Greater frequency of exacerbations is associated with accelerated lung function decline,[3] quality-of-life impairment,[4] and increased mortality.[5] Furthermore, as the incidence of chronic obstructive pulmonary disease (COPD) increases, exacerbations place a greater burden on health care systems, accounting for more than 10 million unscheduled attendances per year in the United States.[6] The direct costs of COPD treatment in the United States are greater than $32 billion per year,[7,8] with exacerbations estimated to account for 50% to 75% of these health care costs.[9] Exacerbations are also important outcome measures in COPD, with acute treatment targeting accelerated recovery, whereas long-term maintenance therapy is designed to prevent and reduce their frequency and severity.

Although half of the patients treated in the community recover to their baseline symptoms by

Dr. Wedzicha reports grants from GSK, grants from Johnson and Johnson, other from Novartis, other from Boehringer Ingelheim, other from Astra Zeneca, other from GSK, grants from GSK, grants from Astra Zeneca, grants from Boehringer Ingelheim, grants from Novartis, outside the submitted work; Dr Ritchie reports no disclosures.
National Heart and Lung Institute, Guy Scadding Building, Imperial College London, Dovehouse Street, London SW3 6JY, United Kingdom
* Corresponding author.
E-mail address: j.wedzicha@imperial.ac.uk

Clin Chest Med 41 (2020) 421–438
https://doi.org/10.1016/j.ccm.2020.06.007

7 days, a study of the time course found that, despite treatment, 14% had still not fully recovered by 5 weeks. Moreover, in a small proportion of exacerbations, symptoms never returned to the baseline level.[10] Consequently, a substantial number of COPD exacerbations can be prolonged, which culminates in greater morbidity associated with such an event. A key audit examining hospital admissions showed that more than one-quarter of patients experience another event during the following 8 weeks.[11] In a cohort of patients with moderate to severe COPD followed up after exacerbation, 22% had a recurrent event within 50 days of the first (index) exacerbation. Such events are therefore complex, and an initial exacerbation seems to increase the susceptibility to a subsequent exacerbation.[12] These recurrent events are associated with substantially increased mortality[13] and this has driven financial incentives for health care services aiming to avoiding hospital readmission.[14,15]

Exacerbations Definition

AECOPDs are transient periods of increased symptoms of dyspnea, sputum purulence, and sputum volume, but they may also encompass minor symptoms of nasal blockage/discharge, wheeze, sore throat, cough, fever, chest tightness or discomfort, fatigue/reduced energy, sleep disturbance, or limited physical activity.[16] COPD exacerbations are associated with several features, including increased airway inflammation, mucus hypersecretion, and gas trapping. There is a degree of controversy over the precise definition of exacerbation events. The 2017 Global Initiative for Chronic Obstructive Lung Disease (GOLD) document AECOPD definition slightly differs from this as "an acute worsening of respiratory symptoms that results in additional therapy." This definition requires the patient to seek or use treatment and is an example of a health care use (HCU) exacerbation in which the patient or clinician decides whether treatment is warranted. The disadvantage with only considering this definition is that it risks not accounting for important events in certain key scenarios; for example, those of lesser severity that do not trigger increased treatment use, where respiratory deterioration with an alternative cause is misdiagnosed, or events in resource-poor areas with a lack of access to treatment or clinicians.

The alternative to an HCU definition is to measure the increase in symptoms and to classify an exacerbation when this change crosses a threshold (regardless of whether the patient receives treatment). This approach has been widely accepted in research, using several validated patient-reported outcome (PRO) tools such as symptom/treatment diary cards and questionnaire tools such as the EXACT (Exacerbations of Chronic Obstructive Pulmonary Disease Tool) and CAT (The COPD Assessment Test). When implemented, it was discovered that a large number of events are unreported and untreated.[4] Studies using symptom-based definitions typically report an incidence of exacerbations that is approximately twice as high as with HCU definitions. One reason for this is that the method captures additional milder events that the HCU definition does not.[17] Although unreported exacerbations are milder than reported events, they do not seem to be inconsequential. However, the science of measuring symptoms is challenging, both in the collection of (daily) data and in their analysis. Analysis challenges include defining the threshold for exacerbation, ceiling effects, and how and when to reset the baseline symptom level in the event of incomplete exacerbation recovery.[18] Two of the most extensively validated PROs in exacerbation studies are the EXACT[17] and CAT,[19] which seem to be valuable in the assessment of exacerbation frequency, duration, and severity and have been qualified as an exploratory end point by both the US Food and Drug Administration (FDA) and the European Medicines Agency (EMA).[20] A particular strength of the EXACT is its ability to detect unreported events, and, in the ATTAIN (Aclidinium to Treat Airway Obstruction in COPD Patients),[21] comparing a long-acting muscarinic antagonist with placebo, unreported (untreated) symptom (EXACT)-defined events had the same medium-term health consequences as reported (treated) HCU exacerbations. Moreover, the trial intervention reduced the rate of both symptom (EXACT)-defined and HCU events. However, a challenge with interpreting PROs such as the EXACT tool is the discordance between HCU exacerbations and symptom (EXACT)-defined events, with discrepancies found in both observational studies[17] and clinical trials.[21]

A major challenge is the heterogeneous nature of the clinical presentation, and alternative causes for acute deterioration, such as heart failure, pneumothorax, pulmonary emboli, or anxiety, must be considered. Traditionally, infective exacerbations are thought to be driven by infection of the airway lumen (bronchi/bronchioles), whereas pneumonia represents alveolar infection. However, it is likely that these distinct processes overlap. A chest radiograph is not routinely performed during a COPD exacerbation,[1] and consolidation may be missed if it is early in the infective process, or through the insensitivity of the test.

Exacerbation Severity

The latest GOLD guidelines define exacerbation severity by the treatment that is required.[1]

- Mild: treatment with short-acting bronchodilators only
- Moderate: treated with short-acting bronchodilators plus antibiotics and/or oral corticosteroids
- Severe: requires either hospitalization or a visit to the emergency department and may also be associated with respiratory failure.

Exacerbation Cause

Exacerbations are airway inflammatory events that are triggered by infection in most cases. Respiratory viral infections are the predominant cause, although bacterial infections and environmental factors such as air pollution and ambient temperature trigger or worsen these events.[22,23] Although early studies focused on bacteria as the primary cause of exacerbations, the development of highly specific molecular diagnostic techniques has highlighted the importance of viruses as key triggers for exacerbations.[24–26] The primary role of different exacerbation triggers and important aspects of their interplay, including viral-bacterial

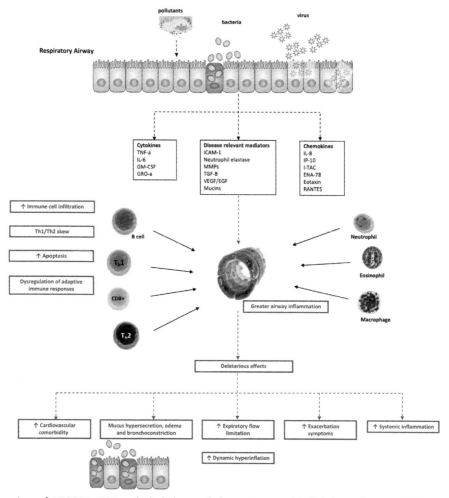

Fig. 1. Overview of AECOPD. EGF, endothelial growth factor; ENA, epithelial-derived neutrophil-activating peptide; ICAM-1, intercellular adhesion molecule 1; IL, interleukin; IP, interferon γ–induced protein; I-TAC, interferon-inducible T-cell alpha chemoattractant; GM-CSF, granulocyte-macrophage colony–stimulating factor; GRO, growth-regulated oncogene; MMP, matrix metalloproteinase; RANTES, regulated upon activation, normal T Cell expressed and presumably secreted; TGF, transforming growth factor; Th, T helper; TNF, tumor necrosis factor; VEGF, vascular endothelial growth factor.

coinfection, deficient host response to bacteria, and the lung microbiome in exacerbation are described here (**Fig. 1**). It has long been observed that the frequency of AECOPD doubles in winter months,[27,28] with more than 50% of exacerbations preceded by coryzal symptoms (**Table 1**).[10,29,30]

Viruses

Earlier studies using culture-based methods underestimated the prevalence of respiratory viruses during COPD exacerbations. However, with the advent of polymerase chain reaction (PCR) methods, the detection of viruses in COPD exacerbations increased to 22% to 64%.[30–52] The wide variations in virus detection are likely to be the consequence of whether patients were sampled at true onset of symptoms or sampling was delayed. Additional factors could include variation in the range of viruses tested for, sensitivity of the assays, the study period (eg, winter vs yearlong, variation in virus epidemics; eg, respiratory syncytial virus [RSV]), population (eg, community vs inpatient, uptake of the influenza vaccine), and sampling method (eg, nasopharyngeal swabs, sputum). In studies where patients reported exacerbation symptoms at onset, there is a greater prevalence of viral infection, because viral load is higher at exacerbation onset[53,54] and may therefore be undetectable by the time patients present to hospital.[29,30,34,41,50,55]

Rhinoviruses are the most prevalent in most of these studies, accounting for up to 60% of all exacerbations.[53] Influenza viruses and RSVs are also commonly detected, being identified in up to 36%[52] and 28%[55] of AECOPDs respectively. Parainfluenza viruses, human metapneumoviruses, coronaviruses, and adenoviruses are detected, but less frequently. Importantly, viral AECOPDs are associated with more severe symptoms, greater airflow limitation, and delayed recovery compared with exacerbations where no virus is detected.[47,56] The greater incidence of rhinovirus in induced sputum, as opposed to nasal aspirates at exacerbation,[57] further supports the theory that naturally occurring rhinovirus drive most exacerbations. Although these studies have shown an association between respiratory virus infection and exacerbations, they do not prove causation because PCR detects viral nucleic acid but it cannot prove the presence of live, replicating virus. Consequently, secondary causes cannot be excluded. However, in 2011, Mallia and colleagues[54] provided novel evidence of a causal relationship between respiratory virus infection and exacerbations in patients with COPD through their experimental rhinovirus infection in patients with mild COPD. In their human model, they showed clearly that respiratory viruses produce symptoms that are typical of an exacerbation, confirming that respiratory viruses can infect the lower airway and contribute to inflammatory changes.[54]

Chronic viral infection is another key aspect to examine when considering the role played by viruses such as RSV. Although RSV infection has been seen at exacerbation,[55] whether it alone drives the event is not entirely clear, because this virus is found incidentally within the airways of patients with COPD at stable state where it is associated with increased airway inflammation.[58] Latent expression of adenoviral E1A protein in alveolar epithelial cells can potentiate the effects of lung

Table 1
Noteworthy studies showing the winter/summer seasonality incidence of acute exacerbations of chronic obstructive pulmonary disease

Study Name	Study Findings
TORCH[27]	80% winter/summer excess (9% of patients exacerbating in December-February compared with 5% in June to August) in the northern hemisphere and a 71% excess (12% vs 7% of patients) in the southern hemisphere
POET[28]	7.63 vs 3.63 exacerbations (per 100 patient months)
Donaldson et al,[140] 2012	1052 exacerbations in winter vs 652 in summer. Winter exacerbations lasted longer and were more severe: 8.4% of exacerbations resulted in patients who were hospitalized, compared with 4.6% of exacerbations in the warm seasons
TIOSPIR[141]	6646 exacerbations in winter compared with 3198 in summer

Abbreviations: TORCH, TOwards a Revolution in COPD Health; POET, prevention of exacerbations with Tiotropium; TIOSPR; The Tiotropium Safety and Performance in Respimat.
Data from Refs.[27,28,140,141]

inflammation induced by cigarette smoke.[59] It is therefore plausible that chronic viral infection could contribute to disease severity in COPD, and further work is required to understand how viruses detected in the stable state relate to exacerbations.

Impaired Antiviral Immunity in Chronic Obstructive Pulmonary Disease

It is not fully understood why patients develop an exacerbation following respiratory virus infection but never smokers do not often go on to develop significant lower respiratory symptoms. Furthermore, there is a subgroup of COPD that seems to be more susceptible to infection, irrespective of disease severity (the frequent-exacerbator phenotype).[60] COPD is associated with substantial changes in innate immunity that are likely to be relevant in the pathogenesis of exacerbations. Tobacco smoking impairs mucociliary clearance,[61] and the rhinovirus binding receptor intercellular adhesion molecule 1 (ICAM-1) is upregulated by bronchial epithelial cells in COPD.[62] Alveolar macrophages, which are numerous and form a first line of defense in the respiratory tract, are defective in COPD, with impairments in their ability to phagocytose bacteria[63,64] and clear dead and dying cells[65] compared with alveolar macrophages from healthy smoking and nonsmoking controls.

In the human experimental rhinovirus infection model, Mallia and colleagues[54] found nasal lavage viral load was significantly higher in patients with COPD following rhinovirus infection compared with age-matched healthy controls. Because all subjects were inoculated with the same virus dose, this suggests impairment in the immune response that controls viral replication in COPD. This finding supports the work by Hurst and colleagues,[29] who earlier showed that exacerbation frequency was related to cold acquisition rather than the propensity to develop an exacerbation following a cold.

The most abundant cells in the airway are bronchial epithelial cells (BECs) and alveolar macrophages. Interferon (IFN) deficiency has been observed in these important cells and, therefore, proposed as a potential mechanism of increased susceptibility to rhinovirus infection. Respiratory viruses such as human rhinovirus (HRV) replicate within the respiratory epithelium triggering the production of type I (FN-α, IFN-β) and type III IFNs (IFN-λ), which limit viral replication, protein synthesis, and protein trafficking (**Table 2**).[66] However, IFN deficiency remains controversial in COPD. Mallia and colleagues[54] found that

bronchoalveolar lavage (BAL) cells of subjects with COPD had a deficient IFN-β response to ex vivo infection with HRV-16, but did not identify any deficiency in BEC responses. In contrast, Hsu and colleagues[67] recently showed impaired IFN responses to influenza virus in BECs from COPD. These findings are supported by a study that showed a decrease in expression of IFN stimulated genes in the induced sputum of COPD participants compared with healthy controls.[68] However, Schneider and colleagues[69] and Baines and colleagues[70] showed increased IFN-λ responses to HRV-39 and HRV-1B infection of COPD BECs respectively compared with healthy controls.[69] Further studies of IFN induction in response to viral infection in epithelial and BAL cells in COPD are clearly needed because this is a potential therapeutic target.

Viral infection in COPD also leads to the production of disease-relevant proinflammatory cytokines such as interleukin (IL)-8 (CXCL8), IL-6, chemokine ligand 5 (CCL5/RANTES), tumor necrosis factor alpha (TNF-α), and IFN-γ–induced protein (IP-10/CXCL10) via the nuclear factor κB pathway leading to the recruitment of neutrophils, macrophages, natural killer cells, T cells, and dendritic cells at the site of infection enhancing viral clearance. Importantly, the magnitude of this response is greater in patients with COPD compared with healthy controls[37,38,71] and may explain how increased airway inflammation contributes to lower airway symptoms in COPD exacerbations.

In general, exacerbations become both more frequent and more severe as the severity of the underlying COPD increases,[72,73] although the reason some patients with COPD experience more frequent exacerbations than others remains unclear. The Evaluation of COPD Longitudinally to Identify Predictive Surrogate Endpoints (ECLIPSE) cohort study identified a distinct frequent-exacerbator phenotype. This group, irrespective of disease severity, was more susceptible to exacerbations and could be identified by a previous history of 2 or more exacerbations in a preceding year.[60] There is some indirect evidence that an increased susceptibility to virus infection may be a characteristic of frequent exacerbators. In studies of naturally acquired virus-induced COPD exacerbations, virus infection was detected more commonly in exacerbation-prone patients.[30,53] Alveolar macrophages taken from such patients (defined as having had an exacerbation during a 1-year period) and exposed to bacteria or toll-like receptor ligands ex vivo showed impaired induction of CXCL8/IL-8 and TNF-α, compared with macrophages from patients who were

Table 2
Inflammatory changes in viral infections in chronic obstructive pulmonary disease exacerbations

Mediator	Naturally Occurring Infection[1]	Experimental Infection in Humans
Chemokines		
CXCL10/IP-10	↑ Serum + sputum[38]	↑ BAL[106]
CXCL8/IL-8	↔ Serum[36,142] + sputum[37,57]	↑ Sputum ↔ BAL[54,106] ↑ Nasal lavage[143]
CCL5/RANTES	↑ Sputum[38] ↔ Serum[36]	—
CCL2/MCP1	↑ Sputum[38] ↔ Serum[36]	—
CXCL11	↑ Serum + sputum[38]	—
Inflammatory Cells		
Neutrophils	↔ Sputum[37]	↑ BAL, sputum, blood[54,106]
Lymphocytes	—	↑ BAL[54,144]
Eosinophils	↑ Sputum[47]	—
Cytokines		
IL-6	↑ Sputum[57,71] ↔ Serum[36,142]	↑ BAL ↔ Sputum[54] ↑ Nasal lavage[143]
TNF-α	↔ Serum[36] or sputum[37]	↔ BAL, sputum[54] ↑ Sputum[106]
IL-1β	↔ Serum[36]	↑ Sputum[106]
IL-10	↑ Serum[36]	—
IL-13	↔ Serum[36]	—
Type II IFN (γ)	↑ Serum[38] ↔ Serum[36]	—
Selected Others		
Neutrophil elastase	—	↑ Sputum ↔ BAL[54,92,106]
MMP-9	—	↑ Sputum[106]
Antimicrobial peptides (secretory leukoprotease inhibitor, elafin)	—	↓ Sputum[92]
Markers of oxidative stress (8-hydroxy-2′-deoxyguanosine, 3-nitrotyrosine)	—	↑ Sputum[106]

Abbreviations: BAL, bronchoalveolar lavage; IL, interleukin; MMP, matrix metalloproteinase; TNF, tumor necrosis factor.
Data from Refs.[36–38,47,54,57,71,92,106,142–144]

exacerbation free for a year.[73] Nevertheless, the description of frequent exacerbators remains essentially clinical and further studies are warranted to elucidate differences in the immune responses and conclusively provide an underlying mechanism to explain this phenotype.

Bacteria

Bacteria are also extremely important in the pathogenesis of COPD exacerbations. Studies using traditional sputum culturing techniques have isolated bacteria in 40% to 60% of exacerbations of COPD.[25,74] The most frequently identified species are nontypeable *Haemophilus influenzae*, *Moraxella catarrhalis*, *Streptococcus pneumoniae*, and *Pseudomonas aeruginosa*.[44,47,75] Atypical bacteria are infrequently isolated, with *Mycoplasma pneumoniae* and *Chlamydophila pneumoniae* implicated in only 4% to 5% of episodes.[74] Studies have also shown that bacterial colonization is common in COPD and is associated with greater airway inflammation and increased risk of exacerbation.[12,56,75] However, it remains unclear from these studies whether exacerbations occur because of the acquisition of new bacterial strains or an outgrowth of preexisting bacteria.[26]

The Microbiome Changes During Chronic Obstructive Pulmonary Disease Exacerbations

In up to 50% of AECOPDs showing the hallmarks of a bacterial cause, the causative pathogens are not recovered from respiratory samples by traditional culture methods. The application of microbiome techniques, which are culture independent, is giving rise to a new understanding

of the interaction between the host and the millions of microorganisms that are present on bodily surfaces. Studies identifying bacteria based on 16S ribosomal RNA gene sequences have shown that the lungs of healthy people and patients with COPD are colonized by rich, complex bacterial communities.[76–78] Recently, researchers have begun to highlight the shifts in microbial communities during COPD exacerbations (**Table 3**).

One of the first longitudinal studies, by Huang and colleagues,[79] found that the sputum microbiome did not show any significant changes in the key characteristics of community richness, evenness, and diversity. However, substantial taxonomic composition variation was seen during exacerbations, with an increase in Proteobacteria

Table 3
Summary of studies examining microbiome changes at chronic obstructive pulmonary disease exacerbation

Study	Subjects and Samples	Lung Sample/Site	Key Finding
Huang et al,[76] 2010	8 intubated patients with COPD 8 tracheal aspirates	Tracheal aspirates	Individuals have distinct airway bacterial communities Intubation duration ↓ α diversity
Huang et al,[79] 2014	12 subjects with COPD	Sputum	↑Proteobacteria at exacerbation onset In recovery: ↓Proteobacteria with antibiotic treatment ↑Proteobacteria, Bacteroidetes, and Firmicutes with oral corticosteroids
Millares et al,[158] 2014	16 subjects with COPD 5 Pseudomonas colonized, 11 uncolonized	Paired baseline and exacerbation sputum samples	No significant difference in microbiome at exacerbation between Pseudomonas colonized and uncolonized
Molyneux et al,[82] 2014	14 patients with COPD 17 Healthy subjects	RV Interventional study; sputum preinfection, 5, 15, and 52 d postinfection	Rhinovirus infection led to an outgrowth of preexisting Haemophilus and Neisseria at day 15
Wang et al,[84] 2016 BEAT-COPD	87 patients with COPD 476 sputum samples	Sputum at baseline, exacerbation onset, recovery	Distinct bacterial and eosinophilic exacerbation microbiome Biomarkers relate to diversity
Mayhew et al,[81] 2018 AERIS cohort	101 patients with COPD	Sputum	↑Proteobacteria with ↑ disease severity ↑Haemophilus with bronchiectasis ↑Dysbiosis in frequent exacerbations
Wang et al,[80] 2018 COPD-MAP	281 patients with COPD	Sputum	Distinct microbiome for eosinophilic and bacterial exacerbations Similar taxa at baseline and exacerbation

but a decrease in Actinobacteria, Clostridia, and Bacteroidia. Furthermore, when levels of important pathogens such as *H influenzae* increase at AECOPD, closely related bacterial taxa were also enriched, whereas the phylogenetically distant taxa declined.[79] The larger COPD-MAP and AERIS longitudinal studies found no significant change in Shannon diversity or core taxa abundancies at exacerbation, However, both studies suggested that exacerbations result from dysbiosis caused by changes in preexisting bacteria in the lung rather than complete removal or appearance of a novel species.[80,81] Overall, these findings suggest that, although the bacteria cultured at exacerbation undoubtedly drive events, enrichment of taxa closely related to a dominant pathogen could also contribute to pathogenesis. Therefore, exacerbations can be considered polymicrobial infections.

A study of the microbiome following experimental rhinovirus infection also showed an outgrowth in *Haemophilus* and *Neisseria* that were present in lower numbers before rhinovirus infection.[82] These changes were correlated with increased neutrophil concentration and neutrophil elastase levels, and were not observed in the healthy control group.[82] These findings support the hypothesis that the bacteria identified at exacerbation are not newly acquired but are caused by an outgrowth of preexisting bacteria that have experienced newly favored conditions.[82]

Both the BEAT-COPD cohort and COPD-MAP cohorts identified distinct microbiome compositions between bacterial and eosinophilic exacerbations, suggesting that these are stable exacerbation phenotypes. The AERIS study found that individuals with concomitant bronchiectasis had a greater abundance of *Haemophilus*. It suggested that frequent exacerbators may have greater dysbiosis compared with infrequent exacerbators, thus providing a potential mechanism by which AECOPDs arise.

Treatment Effects on the Lung Microbiome

Events treated by antibiotics alone led to a reduction in the relative abundance of Proteobacteria, whereas treatment with corticosteroids alone led to an enrichment of multiple taxa, including members of Bacteroidetes, Firmicutes, and Proteobacteria.[83,84] This finding was supported by an earlier study of tracheal aspirates from intubated patients in whom the investigators observed that bacterial communities became less diverse as the duration of intubation and antibiotic administration increased, suggesting that microbial communities are influenced by therapeutic interventions.[76]

When both steroids and antibiotics were used to treat an exacerbation, a mixed effect on the airway microbiome was seen.[79]

Host Response to Bacteria and Bacterial Susceptibility

A current hypothesis is that bacteria enter the lower respiratory tract by microaspiration during sleep or inhalation.[85] In healthy lungs, pathogens either fill an ecological niche or are eradicated with minimal inflammation by the innate immune response. However, in patients with COPD, a combination of defective innate immunity including impaired mucociliary clearance and variation in antigenic structure among strains allow these bacteria to persist and proliferate.[85]

A complex host-pathogen interaction in the lower airway determines this outcome. In a mouse model, *H influenzae* strains associated with COPD exacerbations induced greater airway neutrophil recruitment compared with colonization-associated strains.[86] Exacerbation-associated *M catarrhalis* strains interact differently with primary human airway epithelial cells, showing greater adherence and eliciting more IL-8.[87] Sputum immunoglobulin (Ig)A levels, representing the mucosal host response to the infecting strain, were greater with colonization, whereas the systemic serum IgG host response was larger during exacerbations.[88] It is thought that a robust mucosal immune response diminishes bacterial interaction with the airway epithalamium, resulting in less airway inflammation, thus favoring colonization.

Recent studies focusing on the immune response to bacterial infection have shown the development of specific antibodies to important species, including *H influenzae*, *M catarrhalis*, *S pneumoniae*, and *P aeruginosa* following exacerbations. Some of these show bactericidal and opsonophagocytic function, thereby aiding bacterial clearance.[88–90] However, the multitude of strains may result in recurrent exacerbations with the same species and also creates a challenge for effective vaccine development.

Viral-Bacterial Coinfection

Coinfection with bacteria and viruses is common, occurring in 6% to 27% of exacerbations.[44,47,91] The dynamics of viral and bacterial infection have been examined by Hutchinson and colleagues,[32] who collected respiratory samples from patients with COPD at exacerbation onset, and also 5 to 7 days later: 36% of patients who had a virus detected at exacerbation onset went on to have a bacterial infection. George and colleagues[53] reported that, when HRV was detected at exacerbation onset, 60% of patients developed a bacterial infection at 14 days. Mallia and colleagues[92] found comparable results in experimental rhinovirus infection in COPD, with 60% of patients with COPD showing bacterial infection in their sputum at day 15 compared with only 10% in healthy volunteers. Those who developed a bacterial infection had prolonged respiratory symptoms and delayed recovery compared with those in whom bacteria were not detected.[92]

Exacerbations with coinfection with viruses and bacteria are associated with greater airflow limitation, increased airway inflammation, and delayed exacerbation recovery.[47,56] However, mechanisms underpinning how HRV infection leads to a secondary bacterial infection have not been fully elucidated. Possible mechanisms include viral impairment of macrophage response to bacteria[93–95] leading to a reduction in neutrophil recruitment and bacterial clearance[96] or, alternatively, an upregulation of adhesion molecules in the bronchial epithelium.[97] However, further work is needed to understand the complex pathogen-host interactions to direct further therapeutics.

Airway Inflammation and Cells of Interest

COPD is characterized by aberrant airway inflammation.[1] A further increase in airway inflammation is seen in most exacerbations, but this process is not uniform and inflammation is related to exacerbation cause. Frequent exacerbators also show greater inflammation, and exacerbation nonrecovery is associated with persistent inflammation and a shorter time to the next exacerbation.[12]

Eosinophils

Traditionally, airway eosinophilia and T-helper cell type 2 (Th2) inflammation has been considered associated with allergic airway disorders such as asthma, and airway neutrophilia with COPD. However recent studies have reported that 20% to 40% of patients with COPD show sputum eosinophilia in the stable state.[98–100] The SPIROMICS (SubPopulations and InteRmediate Outcome Measures In COPD Study) cohort has found that sputum eosinophilia at stable state is associated with more severe disease and increased exacerbation frequency.[101] Interventional studies additionally suggest that high blood eosinophilia level at stable state might predict a better treatment response to inhaled corticosteroid use and could therefore be used to guide therapy.[102,103]

Acute exacerbations may be associated with further enhancement of eosinophilic airway inflammation, with up to 30% of COPD exacerbations being associated with sputum eosinophilia.[38,99] Although there is biological plausibility for viral infection leading to sputum eosinophilia,[104] studies of exacerbations to date have been conflicting.[38,47,105] As a result, despite the considerable interest in the role of sputum and blood eosinophilia at stable state as biomarkers for disease outcome and steroid responsiveness, further work is needed to evaluate the significance of increased Th2 inflammation during COPD exacerbations.

Neutrophils

COPD exacerbations associated with bacterial pathogens show significantly more airway neutrophilic inflammation compared with nonbacterial episodes.[88] Furthermore, the exacerbation severity and degree of airway bacterial concentration are related to the degree of neutrophilic inflammation.[88,89] Important mediators of this airway neutrophilia in bacterial exacerbations include IL-8, leukotriene B4, and TNF-α.[44,90] Studies examining bacterial exacerbations have identified an IL-1β signature comprising TNF-α, granulocyte colony–stimulating factor (Growth-regulated oncogene-α), IL-6, cluster of differentiation (CD) 40 ligand, and macrophage inflammatory protein 1 (MIP-1).[92] IL-17A has been associated specifically with *H influenzae* exacerbations.[54] Neutrophil degranulation and necrosis can cause significant damage related to the release of neutrophil elastase and matrix metalloproteinases.[69] Clinical resolution of the symptoms of exacerbation is associated with a consistent decrease in mediators of neutrophilic airway inflammation, whereas nonresolving exacerbations show a sustained level of exaggerated airway inflammation.[88] Studies from experimental infections also indicate that viral infection induces airway neutrophilic inflammation and innate inflammatory mediators such as IL-1β, granulocyte colony–stimulating factor (GM-CSF), CXCL8/IL-8, and TNF-α.[54,106,107]

Macrophages

Alveolar macrophages play a key role in the host defense against invasive pathogens by removing bacteria from the lung by phagocytosis, mediating inflammatory responses. There is increasing evidence of macrophage dysfunction in COPD.[108] Alveolar macrophages and monocyte-derived macrophages show impaired phagocytosis of *H influenzae*, *S pneumoniae*, and *Escherichia coli* compared with healthy controls.[63,64,109] Bewley and colleagues[110] also found that phagocytosis of *H influenzae* was impaired in subjects with COPD with a history of exacerbations. Alveolar macrophages of exacerbation-prone subjects with COPD also showed impaired production of inflammatory cytokines CXCL8 and TNF-α in response to *H influenzae* compared with non–exacerbation-prone subjects with COPD, implicating macrophage dysfunction as a potential mechanism responsible for increased exacerbation frequency in COPD.[64]

Macrophages from patients with COPD stimulated ex vivo with respiratory virus produce less IFN compared with healthy subjects.[54] However, in vitro studies have not necessarily supported this, with similar[70] and even increased[69] IFN released by cells taken from patients with COPD. In a murine model of COPD, IFN-α and IFN-β responses as a result of virus infection were reported as deficient in 1 study and viral clearance was impaired[111]; conversely, another study reported reduced IFN-λ (but not in IFN-β) and no difference in virus load. Therefore, it remains unclear whether production of IFN in response to virus infection is impaired in patients with COPD.

Biomarkers of Acute Exacerbations of Chronic Obstructive Pulmonary Disease

A reliable and objective biomarker of an AECOPD would be invaluable to aid in reliable diagnosis and guide appropriate treatment. The patient samples most investigated are serum or plasma, although sputum, urine, or exhaled breath may also contain useful biomarkers. Several studies have shown that the levels of a variety of immunoinflammatory cells and molecules are increased during exacerbations in respiratory samples, including exhaled breath, sputum, bronchoalveolar lavage, and bronchial biopsy (**Table 4**).

Biomarkers of Viral Exacerbations

A viral exacerbation is suggested with a history of coryzal symptoms and can subsequently be confirmed by PCR from a respiratory sample. However, a reliable biomarker would be invaluable for guiding therapy and antibiotic stewardship (see **Tables 2** and **4**). To date, serum CXCL10 (IP-10) seems the most promising,[112] with Bafadhel and colleagues[38] reporting a cutoff of 56 pg/mL to distinguish viral from nonviral exacerbations, giving a specificity of 65% and sensitivity of 75%. Quint and colleagues[142] reported an area under the curve for serum IP-10 alone of 0.78 (95% confidence interval, 0.65–091) for detecting a human rhinovirus infection at exacerbation. Other biomarkers have

been investigated, with levels of IL-6, monocyte chemoattractant protein-1 (MCP-1), and TNF-α all being increased in viral-associated AECOPD compared with viral-negative subjects and controls.[113] Procalcitonin has also been used to try to detect viral-associated AECOPD, but the evidence so far is equivocal.[114]

Biomarkers of Bacterial Exacerbations

Bafadhel and colleagues[38] suggested that a useful biomarker for determining bacterial-associated AECOPD was sputum IL-1β, with a cutoff of 125 pg/mL having a specificity of 80% and sensitivity of 90%. The serum biomarker best suited for distinguishing a bacterial cause in this study was C-reactive protein (CRP) at a cutoff of 10 mg/L, having a specificity of 70% and sensitivity of 60%.[38] Dal Negro and colleagues[115] also found that high sputum TNF-α level was associated with *Pseudomonas*-related exacerbations, and, in those subjects without high TNF-α level, high levels of IL-8 and IL-1β in the sputum distinguished bacterial from viral and noninfective exacerbations. An electronic nose used in the detection of cardinal volatile organic compounds has recently been used in a pilot study to distinguish bacterial from viral AECOPD,[116] although development and proof of concept are needed before this technology can play a role in outpatient diagnostics.

A Danish study investigating biomarkers indicative of frequent exacerbators discovered that simultaneously increased fibrinogen, CRP, and white blood cell counts indicated an increased risk of frequent exacerbation.[117] Increased plasma fibrinogen level in patients at risk of frequent exacerbation has also been replicated in further studies.[118,119] The FDA has gone on to qualify fibrinogen as an end point of exacerbations and mortality. High levels of serum surfactant protein D have been shown to predict exacerbations when at their highest levels.[120] However, the most comprehensive study to date, which included 2000 patients and examined 90 markers, in 2 separate cohorts (Spiromics and COPDGene), found no biomarker showed a significant relationship to exacerbation frequency in either cohort (after adjustment for recognized confounders: age, gender, percentage predicted forced expiratory volume in 1 second [FEV1], smoking and health status [quality of life], and self-report of gastroesophageal reflux).[121]

Consequences of Exacerbations

Lung function decline

Several studies have now shown that COPD exacerbations affect disease progression. Donaldson

Table 4
Common biomarkers examined in acute exacerbations of chronic obstructive pulmonary disease

Biomarker	Study Findings
CRP	• Most widely used biomarker when investigating and monitoring respiratory infections • CRP level is increased consistently in AECOPD in multiple studies compared with recovery[145] • In 86 patients during AECOPD, the CRP levels did not distinguish viral from bacterial causes[48] • In 118 patients studied for 1 y, a slightly higher level of CRP in bacterial compared with viral AECOPD or cases in which no pathogen was identified (58.3 mg/L, IQR 21–28.2, vs 37.3 mg/L, IQR 18.6–79.1)[48] • AECOPD associated with *H influenzae* or *S pneumoniae* incurred the highest CRP levels[146]
PCT	• Levels of PCT ≥0.25 ng/mL have been shown to indicate an AE-COPD requiring hospital admission for ≥7 d[147] • A meta-analysis investigating procalcitonin-based protocols in guiding antibiotic usage during an AECOPD found that they were clinically effective and safe[148] • However, concerns regarding these conclusions remain because of the inclusion of suboptimal studies into the meta-analysis
BNP	• 60 patients with COPD (17 exacerbations) found BNP level was significantly increased with an AECOPD (79.9 ± 16.2 pg/mL at exacerbation vs 41.2 ± 8.7 pg/mL at stable state)[149] • Higher BNP levels indicate a more severe exacerbation and a longer hospital stay[150,151]
Plasma fibrinogen	• Fibrinogen increases during COPD exacerbation (0.36 g/L SD = 0.74), and then returns to the patient's baseline over a period of 2 to 6 wk[119,152] • This process is associated with a concurrent increase in IL-6 • A large meta-analysis of more than 154,000 participants indicated that a 1-g/L increase in plasma fibrinogen resulted in a 3.7-fold increase in COPD-specific mortality[119]
IL-6	• IL-6 has been shown to be a better predictor of mortality than both CRP and plasma fibrinogen[153]
Urine metabolomics	• Few biomarkers isolated from the urine are clinically useful in AECOPD • One study that shows promise for the future has indicated that certain metabolomics can be used to differentiate COPD from asthma with a >90% accuracy[154]
Sputum eosinophilia	• Sputum eosinophil levels have been found to negatively correlate with bacterial load at exacerbation[155] • Serum peripheral blood eosinophil count at a cutoff of 2% is likely to be the best measure of sputum eosinophilia, with Bafadhel et al[38] reporting a specificity of 60%, sensitivity of 90%
Exhaled nitric oxide	• Several studies of AECOPD show an increase, with 1 showing an increase of 1.9 ppb (−0.4 to 4.0 ppb) at exacerbation[156,157]

Abbreviations: BNP, brain natriuretic peptide; CRP, C-reactive protein; IQR, interquartile range; PCT, procalcitonin; SD, standard deviation.
  Data from Refs.[38,48,119,145–157]

and colleagues[3] showed that patients with a history of frequent exacerbations show accelerated decline, at around 25%, whereas Kanner and colleagues[122] also showed that episodes of respiratory infections affect FEV1 decline. However, some of the earlier studies did not show a relationship between exacerbations and FEV1 decline.[123–125] A review by Silverman[126] suggested that this heterogeneity could be caused by the general/unselected or chronic bronchitis/

emphysema populations studied in the early, negative studies in contrast with the COPD patient populations studied in the later, positive studies. A recent COPDGene study showed that the effect of exacerbations on decline was greatest in patients with mild (GOLD stage 1) COPD, with each event associated with an additional 23 mL/y decline.[127] On occasion, lung function following an exacerbation does not fully recover, and then a group of patients who experience frequent exacerbations (because they have more events) are likely to have a faster lung function decline than patients who have zero or few exacerbations.[128]

Mortality

According to the latest Global Burden of Disease study estimates for 2015, COPD accounted worldwide for 3.2 million deaths.[129] Exacerbations are the predominant cause of mortality, and Soler-Cataluña and colleagues[5] showed that AECOPDs requiring hospitalization are independently associated with mortality (after adjusting for confounding variables such as age, FEV1, body mass index, and Charlson comorbidity index), and that the mortality risk increases with exacerbation frequency. A Canadian mortality study showed that rates after the first hospitalized COPD exacerbation were 50% at 3·6 years and 75% at 7·7 years.[130] The mortality risk peaks sharply in the first 7 days after hospitalization and gradually declines over the subsequent 3 months. With every new hospitalized exacerbation, the risk of death increased, and the interval between hospitalizations decreased over time. For AECOPDs requiring hospitalization, patients with older age, higher arterial $Paco_2$, prolonged oral corticosteroid use, or admission to intensive care unit are more likely to die.[131] In a large analysis of a UK primary care population, Rothnie and colleagues[132] show a clear association between both the increasing frequency and the severity of AECOPDs and mortality.

Quality of life

The relationship between COPD exacerbations and health-related quality of life was first reported by Seemungal and colleagues,[4] who found that patients with frequent exacerbations (>3 per year) had a 14.8-unit higher total St George's Respiratory Questionnaire (SGRQ) score, indicating poorer quality of life, than patients with infrequent exacerbations (≤2 per year). Patients with COPD with frequent exacerbations (>3 per year) also have a faster deterioration in SGRQ scores over time (almost 2 units per year).[133] Quality of life also worsens acutely at exacerbation compared with preexacerbation levels using several difference indices. These studies include worse activity and affect SGRQ, CCQ (clinical COPD Questionnaire), EQ-5D (European Quality of Life – 5 Dimensions questionnaire), MRC (Medical Research Council) dyspnea, ADL (Activities of Daily Living), CAT (The COPD Assessment Test), and EXACT (Exacerbations of Chronic Obstructive Pulmonary Disease Tool) scores.[17,19,134] Exacerbations also worsen patients' mental health with an increase in anxiety and depression[135] and feelings of fatigue.[136] Hospital admission and readmission for acute exacerbations have a particularly negative impact on quality-of-life scores.[4,137]

Physical activity

Acutely at exacerbation, patients spend less time outside of their homes, and patients who experience frequent exacerbation have a faster decline in time spent outdoors compared with infrequent exacerbators.[138] Peripheral muscle weakness also deteriorates during an AECOPD.[139] Patients who maintain physical activity at a low level reduce the risk of hospital admission for COPD by 28% (P = .033) compared with little or no physical activity[136]

SUMMARY

AECOPDs are episodes of symptom worsening that have significant adverse consequences for patients. Exacerbations are highly heterogeneous events associated with increased airway and systemic inflammation and physiologic changes. The frequency of exacerbations is associated with accelerated lung function decline, quality of life impairment, and increased mortality. They are triggered predominantly by respiratory viruses and bacteria, which infect the lower airway and increase airway inflammation. A proportion of patients seem to be more susceptible to exacerbations, with poorer quality of life and more aggressive disease progression than those who have infrequent exacerbations. Exacerbations also contribute significantly to health care expenditure. Prevention and mitigation of exacerbations are therefore key goals of COPD management.

REFERENCES

1. Vogelmeier CF, Criner GJ, Martinez FJ, et al. Global strategy for the diagnosis, management, and prevention of chronic obstructive lung disease 2017 report. GOLD executive summary. Am J Respir Crit Care Med 2017;195(5):557–82.

2. Wedzicha JA, Seemungal TA. COPD exacerbations: defining their cause and prevention. Lancet 2007;370(9589):786–96.

3. Donaldson GC, Seemungal TA, Bhowmik A, et al. Relationship between exacerbation frequency and lung function decline in chronic obstructive pulmonary disease. Thorax 2002;57(10):847–52.

4. Seemungal TA, Donaldson GC, Paul EA, et al. Effect of exacerbation on quality of life in patients with chronic obstructive pulmonary disease. Am J Respir Crit Care Med 1998;157(5 Pt 1):1418–22.

5. Soler-Cataluña JJ, Martinez-Garcia MA, Roman Sanchez P, et al. Severe acute exacerbations and mortality in patients with chronic obstructive pulmonary disease. Thorax 2005;60(11):925–31.

6. Mannino DM, Braman S. The epidemiology and economics of chronic obstructive pulmonary disease. Proc Am Thorac Soc 2007;4(7):502–6.

7. Guarascio AJ, Ray SM, Finch CK, et al. The clinical and economic burden of chronic obstructive pulmonary disease in the USA. Clinicoecon Outcomes Res 2013;5:235–45.

8. Toy EL, Gallagher KF, Stanley EL, et al. The economic impact of exacerbations of chronic obstructive pulmonary disease and exacerbation definition: a review. COPD 2010;7(3):214–28.

9. Celli BR, MacNee W. Standards for the diagnosis and treatment of patients with COPD: a summary of the ATS/ERS position paper. Eur Respir J 2004;23(6):932–46.

10. Seemungal TA, Donaldson GC, Bhowmik A, et al. Time course and recovery of exacerbations in patients with chronic obstructive pulmonary disease. Am J Respir Crit Care Med 2000;161(5):1608–13.

11. Hurst JR, Donaldson GC, Quint JK, et al. Temporal clustering of exacerbations in chronic obstructive pulmonary disease. Am J Respir Crit Care Med 2009;179(5):369–74.

12. Perera WR, Hurst JR, Wilkinson TMA, et al. Inflammatory changes, recovery and recurrence at COPD exacerbation. Eur Respir J 2007;29(3):527–34.

13. Roberts CM, Lowe D, Bucknall CE, et al. Clinical audit indicators of outcome following admission to hospital with acute exacerbation of chronic obstructive pulmonary disease. Thorax 2002;57(2):137–41.

14. Stolz D, Christ-Crain M, Bingisser R, et al. Antibiotic treatment of exacerbations of COPD: a randomized, controlled trial comparing procalcitonin-guidance with standard therapy. Chest 2007;131(1):9–19.

15. Shah T, Churpek MM, Coca Perraillon M, et al. Understanding why patients with COPD get readmitted: a large national study to delineate the Medicare population for the readmissions penalty expansion. Chest 2015;147(5):1219–26.

16. Anthonisen NR, Manfreda J, Warren CPW, et al. Antibiotic therapy in exacerbations of chronic obstructive pulmonary disease. Ann Intern Med 1987;106(2):196.

17. Mackay AJ, Donaldson GC, Patel AR, et al. Detection and severity grading of COPD exacerbations using the exacerbations of chronic pulmonary disease tool (EXACT). Eur Respir J 2014;43(3):735–44.

18. Burgel P, Contoli M, López-Campos JL, editors. Acute exacerbations of pulmonary diseases. European Respiratory Society; 2017.

19. Mackay AJ, Donaldson GC, Patel AR, et al. Usefulness of the chronic obstructive pulmonary disease assessment test to evaluate severity of COPD exacerbations. Am J Respir Crit Care Med 2012;185(11):1218–24.

20. Mackay AJ, Kostikas K, Murray L, et al. Patient-reported outcomes for the detection, quantification, and evaluation of chronic obstructive pulmonary disease exacerbations. Am J Respir Crit Care Med 2018;198(6):730–8.

21. Jones PW, Lamarca R, Chuecos F, et al. Characterisation and impact of reported and unreported exacerbations: results from ATTAIN. Eur Respir J 2014;44(5):1156–65.

22. Li J, Sun S, Tang R, et al. Major air pollutants and risk of COPD exacerbations: a systematic review and meta-analysis. Int J Chron Obstruct Pulmon Dis 2016;11:3079–91.

23. Woodhead M, Blasi F, Ewig S, et al. Guidelines for the management of adult lower respiratory tract infections–full version. Clin Microbiol Infect 2011;17(Suppl 6):E1–59.

24. Ritchie AI, Farne HA, Singanayagam A, et al. Pathogenesis of viral infection in exacerbations of airway disease. Ann Am Thorac Soc 2015;12(Suppl 2):S115–32.

25. Tager I, Speizer FE. Role of infection in chronic bronchitis. N Engl J Med 1975;292(11):563–71.

26. Sethi S, Evans N, Grant BJ, et al. New strains of bacteria and exacerbations of chronic obstructive pulmonary disease. N Engl J Med 2002;347(7):465–71.

27. Jenkins CR, Celli B, Anderson JA, et al. Seasonality and determinants of moderate and severe COPD exacerbations in the TORCH study. Eur Respir J 2012;39(1):38–45.

28. Rabe KF, Fabbri LM, Vogelmeier C, et al. Seasonal distribution of COPD exacerbations in the prevention of exacerbations with Tiotropium in COPD trial. Chest 2013;143(3):711–9.

29. Hurst JR, Donaldson GC, Wilkinson TM, et al. Epidemiological relationships between the common cold and exacerbation frequency in COPD. Eur Respir J 2005;26(5):846–52.

30. Seemungal T, Harper-Owen R, Bhowmik A, et al. Respiratory viruses, symptoms, and inflammatory markers in acute exacerbations and stable chronic obstructive pulmonary disease. Am J Respir Crit Care Med 2001;164(9):1618–23.

31. Ko FW, Ip M, Chan PK, et al. Viral etiology of acute exacerbations of COPD in Hong Kong. Chest 2007; 132(3):900–8.

32. Hutchinson AF, Ghimire AK, Thompson MA, et al. A community-based, time-matched, case-control study of respiratory viruses and exacerbations of COPD. Respir Med 2007;101(12):2472–81.

33. Daubin C, Parienti JJ, Vabret A, et al. Procalcitonin levels in acute exacerbation of COPD admitted in ICU: a prospective cohort study. BMC Infect Dis 2008;8:145.

34. Camargo CA Jr, Ginde AA, Clark S, et al. Viral pathogens in acute exacerbations of chronic obstructive pulmonary disease. Intern Emerg Med 2008; 3(4):355–9.

35. Bozinovski S, Hutchinson A, Thompson M, et al. Serum amyloid a is a biomarker of acute exacerbations of chronic obstructive pulmonary disease. Am J Respir Crit Care Med 2008;177(3):269–78.

36. Almansa R, Sanchez-Garcia M, Herrero A, et al. Host response cytokine signatures in viral and nonviral acute exacerbations of chronic obstructive pulmonary disease. J Interferon Cytokine Res 2011;31(5):409–13.

37. Pant S, Walters EH, Griffiths A, et al. Airway inflammation and anti-protease defences rapidly improve during treatment of an acute exacerbation of COPD. Respirology 2009;14(4):495–503.

38. Bafadhel M, McKenna S, Terry S, et al. Acute exacerbations of chronic obstructive pulmonary disease: identification of biologic clusters and their biomarkers. Am J Respir Crit Care Med 2011; 184(6):662–71.

39. Singh M, Lee SH, Porter P, et al. Human rhinovirus proteinase 2A induces TH1 and TH2 immunity in patients with chronic obstructive pulmonary disease. J Allergy Clin Immunol 2010;125(6): 1369–78.e2.

40. De Serres G, Lampron N, La Forge J, et al. Importance of viral and bacterial infections in chronic obstructive pulmonary disease exacerbations. J Clin Virol 2009;46(2):129–33.

41. McManus TE, Marley AM, Baxter N, et al. Respiratory viral infection in exacerbations of COPD. Respir Med 2008;102(11):1575–80.

42. Beckham JD, Cadena A, Lin J, et al. Respiratory viral infections in patients with chronic, obstructive pulmonary disease. J Infect 2005;50(4):322–30.

43. Cameron RJ, de Wit D, Welsh TN, et al. Virus infection in exacerbations of chronic obstructive pulmonary disease requiring ventilation. Intensive Care Med 2006;32(7):1022–9.

44. Perotin JM, Dury S, Renois F, et al. Detection of multiple viral and bacterial infections in acute exacerbation of chronic obstructive pulmonary disease: a pilot prospective study. J Med Virol 2013;85(5): 866–73.

45. Bandi V, Jakubowycz M, Kinyon C, et al. Infectious exacerbations of chronic obstructive pulmonary disease associated with respiratory viruses and non-typeable Haemophilus influenzae. FEMS Immunol Med Microbiol 2003;37(1):69–75.

46. Qiu Y, Zhu J, Bandi V, et al. Biopsy neutrophilia, neutrophil chemokine and receptor gene expression in severe exacerbations of chronic obstructive pulmonary disease. Am J Respir Crit Care Med 2003;168(8):968–75.

47. Papi A, Bellettato CM, Braccioni F, et al. Infections and airway inflammation in chronic obstructive pulmonary disease severe exacerbations. Am J Respir Crit Care Med 2006;173(10):1114–21.

48. Kherad O, Kaiser L, Bridevaux PO, et al. Upper-respiratory viral infection, biomarkers, and COPD exacerbations. Chest 2010;138(4):896–904.

49. Dimopoulos G, Lerikou M, Tsiodras S, et al. Viral epidemiology of acute exacerbations of chronic obstructive pulmonary disease. Pulm Pharmacol Ther 2012;25(1):12–8.

50. Rohde G, Wiethege A, Borg I, et al. Respiratory viruses in exacerbations of chronic obstructive pulmonary disease requiring hospitalisation: a case-control study. Thorax 2003;58(1):37–42.

51. Minosse C, Selleri M, Zaniratti MS, et al. Frequency of detection of respiratory viruses in the lower respiratory tract of hospitalized adults. J Clin Virol 2008;42(2):215–20.

52. Tan WC, Xiang X, Qiu D, et al. Epidemiology of respiratory viruses in patients hospitalized with near-fatal asthma, acute exacerbations of asthma, or chronic obstructive pulmonary disease. Am J Med 2003;115(4):272–7.

53. George SN, Garcha DS, Mackay AJ, et al. Human rhinovirus infection during naturally occurring COPD exacerbations. Eur Respir J 2014;44(1): 87–96.

54. Mallia P, Message SD, Gielen V, et al. Experimental rhinovirus infection as a human model of chronic obstructive pulmonary disease exacerbation. Am J Respir Crit Care Med 2011;183(6):734–42.

55. Falsey AR, Formica MA, Hennessey PA, et al. Detection of respiratory syncytial virus in adults with chronic obstructive pulmonary disease. Am J Respir Crit Care Med 2006;173(6):639–43.

56. Wilkinson TM, Hurst JR, Perera WR, et al. Effect of interactions between lower airway bacterial and rhinoviral infection in exacerbations of COPD. Chest 2006;129(2):317–24.

57. Seemungal TA, Harper-Owen R, Bhowmik A, et al. Detection of rhinovirus in induced sputum at

exacerbation of chronic obstructive pulmonary disease. Eur Respir J 2000;16(4):677–83.

58. Wilkinson TMA, Donaldson GC, Johnston SL, et al. Respiratory syncytial virus, airway inflammation, and FEV1 decline in patients with chronic obstructive pulmonary disease. Am J Respir Crit Care Med 2006;173(8):871–6.

59. Retamales I, Elliott WM, Meshi B, et al. Amplification of inflammation in emphysema and its association with latent adenoviral infection. Am J Respir Crit Care Med 2001;164(3):469–73.

60. Hurst JR, Vestbo J, Anzueto A, et al. Susceptibility to exacerbation in chronic obstructive pulmonary disease. N Engl J Med 2010;363(12):1128–38.

61. Leopold PL, O'Mahony MJ, Lian XJ, et al. Smoking is associated with shortened airway cilia. PLoS One 2009;4(12):e8157.

62. Di Stefano A, Maestrelli P, Roggeri A, et al. Upregulation of adhesion molecules in the bronchial mucosa of subjects with chronic obstructive bronchitis. Am J Respir Crit Care Med 1994;149(3 Pt 1):803–10.

63. Taylor AE, Finney-Hayward TK, Quint JK, et al. Defective macrophage phagocytosis of bacteria in COPD. Eur Respir J 2010;35(5):1039–47.

64. Berenson CS, Kruzel RL, Eberhardt E, et al. Phagocytic dysfunction of human alveolar macrophages and severity of chronic obstructive pulmonary disease. J Infect Dis 2013;208(12):2036–45.

65. Hodge S, Hodge G, Scicchitano R, et al. Alveolar macrophages from subjects with chronic obstructive pulmonary disease are deficient in their ability to phagocytose apoptotic airway epithelial cells. Immunol Cell Biol 2003;81(4):289–96.

66. Vareille M, Kieninger E, Edwards MR, et al. The airway epithelium: soldier in the fight against respiratory viruses. Clin Microbiol Rev 2011;24(1):210–29.

67. Hsu ACY, Parsons K, Moheimani F, et al. Impaired antiviral stress granule and IFN-β enhanceosome formation enhances susceptibility to influenza infection in chronic obstructive pulmonary disease epithelium. Am J Respir Cell Mol Biol 2016;55(1):117–27.

68. Hilzendeger C, da Silva J, Henket M, et al. Reduced sputum expression of interferon-stimulated genes in severe COPD. Int J Chron Obstruct Pulmon Dis 2016;11:1485–94.

69. Schneider D, Ganesan S, Comstock AT, et al. Increased cytokine response of rhinovirus-infected airway epithelial cells in chronic obstructive pulmonary disease. Am J Respir Crit Care Med 2010;182(3):332–40.

70. Baines KJ, Hsu ACY, Tooze M, et al. Novel immune genes associated with excessive inflammatory and antiviral responses to rhinovirus in COPD. Respir Res 2013;14(1):15.

71. Rohde G, Borg I, Wiethege A, et al. Inflammatory response in acute viral exacerbations of COPD. Infection 2008;36(5):427–33.

72. Burge S, Wedzicha JA. COPD exacerbations: definitions and classifications. Eur Respir J Suppl 2003;41:46s–53s.

73. Berenson CS, Kruzel RL, Eberhardt E, et al. Impaired innate immune alveolar macrophage response and the predilection for COPD exacerbations. Thorax 2014;69(9):811–8.

74. Sethi S, Murphy TF. Infection in the pathogenesis and course of chronic obstructive pulmonary disease. N Engl J Med 2008;359(22):2355–65.

75. Hurst JR, Wilkinson TM, Perera WR, et al. Relationships among bacteria, upper airway, lower airway, and systemic inflammation in COPD. Chest 2005;127(4):1219–26.

76. Huang YJ, Kim E, Cox MJ, et al. A persistent and diverse airway microbiota present during chronic obstructive pulmonary disease exacerbations. OMICS 2010;14(1):9–59.

77. Erb-Downward JR, Thompson DL, Han MK, et al. Analysis of the lung microbiome in the "healthy" smoker and in COPD. PLoS One 2011;6(2):e16384.

78. Cabrera-Rubio RI, Garcia-Núñez M, Set L, et al. Microbiome diversity in the bronchial tracts of patients with chronic obstructive pulmonary disease. J Clin Microbiol 2012;50(11):3562–8.

79. Huang YJ, Sethi S, Murphy T, et al. Airway microbiome dynamics in exacerbations of chronic obstructive pulmonary disease. J Clin Microbiol 2014;52(8):2813–23.

80. Wang Z, Singh R, Miller BE, et al. Sputum microbiome temporal variability and dysbiosis in chronic obstructive pulmonary disease exacerbations: an analysis of the COPDMAP study. Thorax 2018;73(4):331–8.

81. Mayhew D, Devos N, Lambert C, et al. Longitudinal profiling of the lung microbiome in the AERIS study demonstrates repeatability of bacterial and eosinophilic COPD exacerbations. Thorax 2018;73(5):422–30.

82. Molyneaux PL, Mallia P, Cox MJ, et al. Outgrowth of the bacterial airway microbiome after rhinovirus exacerbation of chronic obstructive pulmonary disease. Am J Respir Crit Care Med 2013;188(10):1224–31.

83. Chronic obstructive pulmonary disease | Topic | NICE.

84. Wang Z, Bafadhel M, Haldar K, et al. Lung microbiome dynamics in COPD exacerbations. Eur Respir J 2016;47(4):1082–92.

85. Dickson RP, Erb-Downward JR, Huffnagle GB. The role of the bacterial microbiome in lung disease. Expert Rev Respir Med 2013;7(3):245–57.

86. Chin CL, Manzel LJ, Lehman EE, et al. Haemophilus influenzae from patients with chronic

obstructive pulmonary disease exacerbation induce more inflammation than colonizers. Am J Respir Crit Care Med 2005;172(1):85–91.

87. Parameswaran GI, Wrona CT, Murphy TF, et al. Moraxella catarrhalis acquisition, airway inflammation and protease-antiprotease balance in chronic obstructive pulmonary disease. BMC Infect Dis 2009;9:178.

88. Murphy TF, Brauer AL, Grant BJB, et al. *Moraxella catarrhalis* in chronic obstructive pulmonary disease. Am J Respir Crit Care Med 2005;172(2): 195–9.

89. Bogaert D, van der Valk P, Ramdin R, et al. Host-pathogen interaction during pneumococcal infection in patients with chronic obstructive pulmonary disease. Infect Immun 2004;72(2): 818–23.

90. Sethi S, Wrona C, Grant BJB, et al. Strain-specific immune response to *Haemophilus influenzae* in chronic obstructive pulmonary disease. Am J Respir Crit Care Med 2004;169(4):448–53.

91. Hurst JR, Perera WR, Wilkinson TMA, et al. Systemic and upper and lower airway inflammation at exacerbation of chronic obstructive pulmonary disease. Am J Respir Crit Care Med 2006;173(1): 71–8.

92. Mallia P, Footitt J, Sotero R, et al. Rhinovirus infection induces degradation of antimicrobial peptides and secondary bacterial infection in chronic obstructive pulmonary disease. Am J Respir Crit Care Med 2012;186(11):1117–24.

93. Oliver BG, Lim S, Wark P, et al. Rhinovirus exposure impairs immune responses to bacterial products in human alveolar macrophages. Thorax 2008;63(6): 519–25.

94. Cooper GE, Pounce ZC, Wallington JC, et al. Viral inhibition of bacterial phagocytosis by human macrophages: redundant role of CD36. PLoS One 2016;11(10):e0163889.

95. Finney LJ, Belchamber KBR, Fenwick PS, et al. Human rhinovirus impairs the innate immune response to bacteria in alveolar macrophages in chronic obstructive pulmonary disease. Am J Respir Crit Care Med 2019;199(12):1496–507.

96. Unger BL, Faris AN, Ganesan S, et al. Rhinovirus attenuates non-typeable Hemophilus influenzae-stimulated IL-8 responses via TLR2-dependent degradation of IRAK-1. PLoS Pathog 2012;8(10): e1002969.

97. Wang JH, Kwon HJ, Jang YJ. Rhinovirus enhances various bacterial adhesions to nasal epithelial cells simultaneously. Laryngoscope 2009;119(7): 1406–11.

98. Leigh R, Pizzichini MMM, Morris MM, et al. Stable COPD: predicting benefit from high-dose inhaled corticosteroid treatment. Eur Respir J 2006;27(5): 964–71.

99. Eltboli O, Bafadhel M, Hollins F, et al. COPD exacerbation severity and frequency is associated with impaired macrophage efferocytosis of eosinophils. BMC Pulm Med 2014;14(1):112.

100. Brightling CE, Monteiro W, Ward R, et al. Sputum eosinophilia and short-term response to prednisolone in chronic obstructive pulmonary disease: a randomised controlled trial. Lancet 2000; 356(9240):1480–5.

101. Hastie AT, Martinez FJ, Curtis JL, et al. Association of sputum and blood eosinophil concentrations with clinical measures of COPD severity: an analysis of the SPIROMICS cohort. Lancet Respir Med 2017;5(12):956–67.

102. Pascoe S, Locantore N, Dransfield MT, et al. Blood eosinophil counts, exacerbations, and response to the addition of inhaled fluticasone furoate to vilanterol in patients with chronic obstructive pulmonary disease: a secondary analysis of data from two parallel randomised controlled trials. Lancet Respir Med 2015;3(6):435–42.

103. Pavord ID, Lettis S, Locantore N, et al. Blood eosinophils and inhaled corticosteroid/long-acting β-2 agonist efficacy in COPD. Thorax 2016;71(2): 118–25.

104. Edwards MR, Strong K, Cameron A, et al. Viral infections in allergy and immunology: how allergic inflammation influences viral infections and illness. J Allergy Clin Immunol 2017;140(4): 909–20.

105. Saetta M, Di Stefano A, Maestrelli P, et al. Airway eosinophilia in chronic bronchitis during exacerbations. Am J Respir Crit Care Med 1994;150(6): 1646–52.

106. Footitt J, Mallia P, Durham AL, et al. Oxidative and nitrosative stress and histone deacetylase-2 activity in exacerbations of chronic obstructive pulmonary disease. Chest 2016;149(1):62–73.

107. Mallia P, Message SD, Contoli M, et al. Neutrophil adhesion molecules in experimental rhinovirus infection in COPD. Respir Res 2013;14(1):72.

108. Hiemstra PS. Altered macrophage function in chronic obstructive pulmonary disease. Ann Am Thorac Soc 2013;10(Suppl):S180–5.

109. Berenson CS, Wrona CT, Grove LJ, et al. Impaired alveolar macrophage response to Haemophilus antigens in chronic obstructive lung disease. Am J Respir Crit Care Med 2006;174(1):31–40.

110. Bewley MA, Belchamber KBR, Chana KK, et al. Differential effects of p38, MAPK, PI3K or rho kinase inhibitors on bacterial phagocytosis and efferocytosis by macrophages in COPD. PLoS One 2016; 11(9):e0163139.

111. Sajjan U, Ganesan S, Comstock AT, et al. Elastase-and LPS-exposed mice display altered responses to rhinovirus infection. Am J Physiol Lung Cell Mol Physiol 2009;297(5):L931–44.

112. Yin T, Zhu Z, Mei Z, et al. Analysis of viral infection and biomarkers in patients with acute exacerbation of chronic obstructive pulmonary disease. Clin Respir J 2018;12(3):1228–39.

113. Zheng J, Shi Y, Xiong L, et al. The expression of IL-6, TNF-α, and MCP-1 in respiratory viral infection in acute exacerbations of chronic obstructive pulmonary disease. J Immunol Res 2017;2017:8539294.

114. Pantzaris N-D, Spilioti D-X, Psaromyalou A, et al. The use of serum procalcitonin as a diagnostic and prognostic biomarker in chronic obstructive pulmonary disease exacerbations: a literature review update. J Clin Med Res 2018;10(7):545–51.

115. Dal Negro RW, Micheletto C, Tognella S, et al. A two-stage logistic model based on the measurement of pro-inflammatory cytokines in bronchial secretions for assessing bacterial, viral, and non-infectious origin of COPD exacerbations. COPD 2005;2(1):7–16.

116. van Geffen WH, Bruins M, Kerstjens HAM. Diagnosing viral and bacterial respiratory infections in acute COPD exacerbations by an electronic nose: a pilot study. J Breath Res 2016;10(3):036001.

117. Pais R. Biomarkers for predicting COPD exacerbations. Thorax 2014;69(8):767.

118. Faner R, Agusti A. Fibrinogen and COPD: now what? Chronic Obstr Pulm Dis 2015;2(1):1–3.

119. Duvoix A, Dickens J, Haq I, et al. Blood fibrinogen as a biomarker of chronic obstructive pulmonary disease. Thorax 2013;68(7):670–6.

120. Leung JM, Sin DD. Biomarkers in airway diseases. Can Respir J 2013;20(3):180–2.

121. Keene JD, Jacobson S, Kechris K, et al. Biomarkers predictive of exacerbations in the SPIROMICS and COPDGene cohorts. Am J Respir Crit Care Med 2017;195(4):473–81.

122. Kanner RE, Anthonisen NR, Connett JE. Lower respiratory illnesses promote FEV1 decline in current smokers but not ex-smokers with mild chronic obstructive pulmonary disease. Am J Respir Crit Care Med 2001;164(3):358–64.

123. Casanova C, de Torres JP, Aguirre-Jaime A, et al. The progression of chronic obstructive pulmonary disease is heterogeneous: the experience of the BODE cohort. Am J Respir Crit Care Med 2011;184(9):1015–21.

124. Celli BR, Thomas NE, Anderson JA, et al. Effect of pharmacotherapy on rate of decline of lung function in chronic obstructive pulmonary disease: results from the TORCH study. Am J Respir Crit Care Med 2008;178(4):332–8.

125. Howard P. A long-term follow-up of respiratory symptoms and ventilatory function in a group of working men. Br J Ind Med 1970;27(4):326–33.

126. Silverman EK. Exacerbations in chronic obstructive pulmonary disease: do they contribute to disease progression? Proc Am Thorac Soc 2007;4(8):586–90.

127. Dransfield MT, Kunisaki KM, Strand MJ, et al. Acute exacerbations and lung function loss in smokers with and without COPD. Am J Respir Crit Care Med 2016;195(3). rccm.201605-2016201014OC.

128. Donaldson GC, Law M, Kowlessar B, et al. Impact of prolonged exacerbation recovery in chronic obstructive pulmonary disease. Am J Respir Crit Care Med 2015;192(8):943–50.

129. Gbd Chronic Respiratory Disease Collaborators JB, Abajobir AA, Abate KH, et al. Global, regional, and national deaths, prevalence, disability-adjusted life years, and years lived with disability for chronic obstructive pulmonary disease and asthma, 1990-2015: a systematic analysis for the Global Burden of Disease Study 2015. Lancet Respir Med 2017;5(9):691–706.

130. Suissa S, Dell'Aniello S, Ernst P. Long-term natural history of chronic obstructive pulmonary disease: severe exacerbations and mortality. Thorax 2012;67(11):957–63.

131. Groenewegen KH, Schols AMWJ, Wouters EFM. Mortality and mortality-related factors after hospitalization for acute exacerbation of COPD. Chest 2003;124(2):459–67.

132. Rothnie KJ, Müllerová H, Smeeth L, et al. Natural history of chronic obstructive pulmonary disease exacerbations in a general practice–based population with chronic obstructive pulmonary disease. Am J Respir Crit Care Med 2018;198(4):464–71.

133. Miravitlles M, Ferrer M, Pont A, et al. Effect of exacerbations on quality of life in patients with chronic obstructive pulmonary disease: a 2 year follow up study. Thorax 2004;59(5):387–95.

134. Bourbeau J, Ford G, Zackon H, et al. Impact on patients' health status following early identification of a COPD exacerbation. Eur Respir J 2007;30(5):907.

135. Laurin C, Moullec G, Bacon SL, et al. Impact of anxiety and depression on chronic obstructive pulmonary disease exacerbation risk. Am J Respir Crit Care Med 2012;185(9):918–23.

136. Garcia-Aymerich J, Farrero E, Felez MA, et al. Risk factors of readmission to hospital for a COPD exacerbation: a prospective study. Thorax 2003;58(2):100–5.

137. Baghai-Ravary R, Quint JK, Goldring JJ, et al. Determinants and impact of fatigue in patients with chronic obstructive pulmonary disease. Respir Med 2009;103(2):216–23.

138. Donaldson GC, Wilkinson TMA, Hurst JR, et al. Exacerbations and time spent outdoors in chronic obstructive pulmonary disease. Am J Respir Crit Care Med 2005;171(5):446–52.

139. Spruit MA, Gosselink R, Troosters T, et al. Muscle force during an acute exacerbation in hospitalised

patients with COPD and its relationship with CXCL8 and IGF-I. Thorax 2003;58(9):752–6.

140. Donaldson GC, Goldring JJ, Wedzicha JA. Influence of season on exacerbation characteristics in patients with COPD. Chest 2012;141(1): 94–100.

141. Wise RA, Calverley PM, Carter K, et al. Seasonal variations in exacerbations and deaths in patients with COPD during the TIOSPIR((R)) trial. Int J Chron Obstruct Pulmon Dis 2018;13:605–16.

142. Quint JK, Donaldson GC, Goldring JJ, et al. Serum IP-10 as a biomarker of human rhinovirus infection at exacerbation of COPD. Chest 2010;137(4): 812–22.

143. Mallia P, Message SD, Kebadze T, et al. An experimental model of rhinovirus induced chronic obstructive pulmonary disease exacerbations: a pilot study. Respir Res 2006;7:116.

144. Mallia P, Message SD, Contoli M, et al. Lymphocyte subsets in experimental rhinovirus infection in chronic obstructive pulmonary disease. Respir Med 2014;108(1):78–85.

145. Chen Y-WR, Leung JM, Sin DD. A systematic review of diagnostic biomarkers of COPD exacerbation. PLoS One 2016;11(7):e0158843.

146. Gallego M, Pomares X, Capilla S, et al. C-reactive protein in outpatients with acute exacerbation of COPD: its relationship with microbial etiology and severity. Int J Chron Obstruct Pulmon Dis 2016; 11:2633–40.

147. Kawamatawong T, Apiwattanaporn A, Siricharoonwong W. Serum inflammatory biomarkers and clinical outcomes of COPD exacerbation caused by different pathogens. Int J Chron Obstruct Pulmon Dis 2017;12:1625–30.

148. Mathioudakis AG, Chatzimavridou-Grigoriadou V, Corlateanu A, et al. Procalcitonin to guide antibiotic administration in COPD exacerbations: a meta-analysis. Eur Respir Rev 2017;26(143): 160073.

149. Inoue Y, Kawayama T, Iwanaga T, et al. High plasma brain natriuretic peptide levels in stable COPD without pulmonary hypertension or cor pulmonale. Intern Med 2009;48(7):503–12.

150. European Respiratory Society SS, Calistru PI. European respiratory journal, vol. 42. ERS Journals; 2013.

151. Adrish M, Nannaka VB, Cano EJ, et al. Significance of NT-pro-BNP in acute exacerbation of COPD patients without underlying left ventricular dysfunction. Int J Chron Obstruct Pulmon Dis 2017;12: 1183–9.

152. Wedzicha JA, Seemungal TA, MacCallum PK, et al. Acute exacerbations of chronic obstructive pulmonary disease are accompanied by elevations of plasma fibrinogen and serum IL-6 levels. Thromb Haemost 2000;84(2):210–5.

153. Celli BR, Locantore N, Yates J, et al. Inflammatory biomarkers improve clinical prediction of mortality in chronic obstructive pulmonary disease. Am J Respir Crit Care Med 2012; 185(10):1065–72.

154. Adamko DJ, Nair P, Mayers I, et al. Metabolomic profiling of asthma and chronic obstructive pulmonary disease: a pilot study differentiating diseases. J Allergy Clin Immunol 2015;136(3): 571–80.e3.

155. Kolsum U, Donaldson GC, Singh R, et al. Blood and sputum eosinophils in COPD; relationship with bacterial load. Respir Res 2017;18(1):88.

156. Malerba M, Radaeli A, Olivini A, et al. Exhaled nitric oxide as a biomarker in COPD and related comorbidities. Biomed Res Int 2014;2014:271918.

157. Bhowmik A, Seemungal TAR, Donaldson GC, et al. Effects of exacerbations and seasonality on exhaled nitric oxide in COPD. Eur Respir J 2005; 26(6):1009–15.

158. Millares L, Ferrari R, Galleg M, et al. Bronchial microbiome of severe COPD patients colonised by Pseudomonas aeruginosa. Eur J Clin Microbiol Infect Dis 2014;33(7):1101–11.

Treatment of Acute Exacerbations in Chronic Obstructive Pulmonary Disease

Rajesh Kunadharaju, MD[a], Sanjay Sethi, MD[a,b,*]

KEYWORDS

- Chronic obstructive pulmonary disease • Exacerbation • Antibiotics • Corticosteroids

KEY POINTS

- Exacerbations in patients with chronic obstructive pulmonary disease are events that worsen quality of life, impact on lung function decline, and increase the risk of subsequent events and death.
- The diagnosis rests on a clinical diagnosis based on the presence of worsening dyspnea and cough and phlegm.
- Its clinical presentation ranges from a mild illness only requiring additional rescue inhaler use to acute respiratory failure requiring ventilatory support.
- Irrespective of the site of treatment, the treatment modalities are the same, with the universal intensification of bronchodilator therapy and selective application of systemic corticosteroids and antibiotics.

INTRODUCTION

An acute exacerbation of chronic obstructive pulmonary disease (AECOPD) is a flare of chronic respiratory symptoms, including worsening shortness of breath, cough, and sputum production requiring an increase in need of rescue medications or/and supplementation of additional treatment.[1] It has a heterogeneous presentation and is one of the most common reasons for hospitalization, with an in-hospital mortality rate of 3.9%.[2] Its severity spectrum ranges from a mild illness only requiring additional rescue inhaler use to acute respiratory failure requiring ventilatory support. The treatment of exacerbations depends on the severity, which itself is a complex sum of the severity of the acute event, the underlying chronic disease, and associated patient comorbidities.

DIAGNOSIS

A careful history and physical examination remain the basis of the diagnosis of an AECOPD. Despite years of study, there is no specific diagnostic test or biomarker that is the sine qua non for exacerbations. It is a diagnosis of exclusion. Most laboratory and radiological evaluation in a patient with suspected AECOPD is to exclude other cardiopulmonary causes and determine the contribution of comorbidities. Therefore, use of evaluation methods are not prescriptive and formulaic, but should be guided by the clinical assessment.

The diagnosis of an AECOPD requires the presence of underlying COPD (**Fig. 1**). Similar respiratory symptoms in an individual without COPD should be designated as acute bronchitis, a clinical entity with substantially different etiology, prognosis, and treatment. This is easy in patients

[a] Division of Pulmonary/Critical Care and Sleep Medicine, Department of Medicine, Jacobs School of Medicine and Biomedical Sciences, University at Buffalo, SUNY, Buffalo, NY, USA; [b] Clinical and Translational Research Center, Room 6045A, 875 Ellicott Street, Buffalo, NY 14203, USA
* Corresponding author. Clinical and Translational Research Center, Room 6045A, 875 Ellicott Street, Buffalo, NY 14203.
E-mail address: ssethi@buffalo.edu

Clin Chest Med 41 (2020) 439–451
https://doi.org/10.1016/j.ccm.2020.06.008

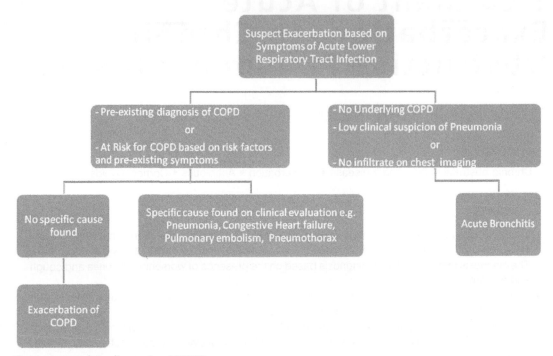

Fig. 1. Approach to diagnosing AECOPD.

with established COPD diagnosis and previous spirometry demonstrating airflow obstruction. However, not infrequently the first presentation of COPD is an acute exacerbation episode. In fact, an average delay of 2 years between the first acute episode and the establishment of a COPD diagnosis has been described.[3] An assessment for COPD risk factors is indicated in every adult patient with a lower respiratory tract infection. If present, consideration for treatment as an exacerbation and an evaluation for undiagnosed COPD in the convalescent phase are indicated.

Once the presence of COPD is established or suspected, the health care practitioner needs to consider other entities in the differential diagnosis. These include common ones such as pneumonia and congestive heart failure and less common ones such as pneumothorax, pulmonary embolism, pleural effusion, lung carcinoma, and rib fractures.[1,4,5] Recently added to the list is vaping-associated lung injury.[6] The extent of evaluation is dictated by the severity of the exacerbation and the site of treatment (**Table 1**). In mild-moderate exacerbations that are being evaluated in the office, ascertaining absence of hypoxemia with pulse oximetry is the only essential test, if the clinical assessment does not support an alternative diagnosis. In patients who are severe enough to require emergency department evaluation, a more extensive evaluation is indicated to ensure appropriate management and prevent

poor outcomes. A small autopsy study showed that in patients who died within 24 hours of admission for a COPD exacerbation, the primary causes of death were heart failure, pneumonia, pulmonary thromboembolism, and COPD in 37%, 28%, 21%, and 14% of patients, respectively.[5]

Usually the testing described in **Table 1** is sufficient to rule out alternative diagnoses. On occasion, depending on clinical circumstances and the result of these evaluations, further tests might be indicated. For example, an atypical presentation with sudden onset of dyspnea with or without an elevated D-dimer, would lead to a computed tomography (CT) pulmonary angiogram to evaluate for pulmonary embolism. The presence of atelectasis or mass lesion on the chest radiograph would require a CT scan for further characterization.

DETERMINATION OF ETIOLOGY

Around 30% to 50% of AECOPD cases are associated with a bacterial infection.[7] However, sputum Gram stain and culture are not recommended in the management of most exacerbations. Studies using molecular diagnostics have shown that sputum cultures have limited sensitivity.[8] The presence of a respiratory pathogen on culture does not distinguish between chronic colonization and acute infection, therefore having limited specificity.[9] The usual turn-around time of sputum

Table 1
Diagnostic evaluation of patients with suspected chronic obstructive pulmonary disease exacerbation

Clinical Setting	Test	Potential Diagnosis
Physician's office	Pulse oximetry	Hypoxemia
Emergency department	Complete blood count	Anemia, leukocytosis
	Comprehensive metabolic panel	Electrolyte abnormalities, liver failure, kidney failure
	Brain natriuretic peptide	Heart failure
	Cardiac enzymes	Heart failure, myocardial infarction
	D Dimer	Pulmonary embolism
	Arterial blood gas measurement	Hypoxemia, hypercapnia, and respiratory acidosis
	Electrocardiography	Myocardial infarction, arrhythmias
	Chest radiography	Pneumonia, congestive heart failure, pneumothorax, pleural effusion, rib fractures
	Point of care ultrasound – if available	Heart failure, pneumothorax, pleural effusion, pericardial effusion, venous thromboembolism

Data from Global Initiative for Chronic Obstructive Pulmonary Disease. Global Strategy for the Diagnosis, Management, and Prevention of COPD: 2020 Report. Available at: https://goldcopd.org/wp-content/uploads/2019/11/GOLD-2020-REPORT-ver1.0wms.pdf.

culture results of 48 to 72 hours also limits their utility, as clinical decisions regarding treatment of an AECOPD require point-of-care results.

There are situations where a sputum culture could be useful. These include patients who fail to respond to initial empiric antibiotic therapy, patients with risk factors for *Pseudomonas aeruginosa* or other antibiotic-resistant bacteria, and patients requiring hospitalization. Even in these scenarios, the limited accuracy of this test should be kept in mind when interpreting the results, with the clinical picture taking precedence. For instance, in a hospitalized patient responding well to current antibiotics despite the sputum culture yielding a resistant pathogen, a change of antibiotics is unnecessary.[10]

Around 30% to 50% of AECOPD cases are associated with a viral infection.[7] Viral cultures are now rarely performed. During the influenza season, a rapid diagnostic test for influenza is useful if acute onset of fever, myalgias, and coryza are seen with exacerbation symptoms. More extensive respiratory viral diagnostic panels have limited utility in the absence of specific antiviral treatment. Detection of a virus does not mean absence of a concurrent bacterial infection; as such, coinfection is seen in about 25% of exacerbations.[11]

Biomarkers for bacterial infection like procalcitonin and C-reactive protein (CRP) have been evaluated in AECOPD to guide antibiotic therapy. Although these biomarkers perform well with parenchymal and systemic infections such as pneumonia and sepsis, they have been unreliable in AECOPD.[12,13] A likely explanation is that bacterial exacerbations are mucosal infections, and therefore not enough of a stimulus to induce robust hepatic production of these acute phase reactants. Studies with these biomarkers in AECOPD have not correlated them with careful sputum microbiology and have not used the speed of resolution as an endpoint. They have not shown their utility beyond the reliable, simple and no-cost clinical symptom biomarkers of bacterial infection in exacerbations.

Clinical symptom biomarkers of bacterial infection are useful and accurate in AECOPD. These include the presence of purulent sputum, especially when the purulence emerged or increased with the onset of the exacerbation. Also useful are the Anthonisen criteria, where the probability of bacterial etiology in type 1 and 2 exacerbations is substantial and reliable enough to recommend antibiotic use (**Box 1**).[14] Sputum purulence can be assessed readily by questioning the patient or visual examination of a sputum sample if available. Another option is the use of a standardized color chart that has a sensitivity of 94.4% and specificity of 77.0% for a positive sputum culture and provides greater reproducibility.[15]

DETERMINATION OF THE SEVERITY OF AN EXACERBATION

The symptomatic criteria proposed by Anthonisen have been sometimes thought of as a measure of exacerbation severity (see **Box 1**). However, they are more useful as an indication of etiology rather than as a measure of severity. For example, a patient could have a single symptom of increased dyspnea of such severity that it requires hospitalization but still have a type 3 exacerbation, which clearly is not a mild exacerbation.

Ideally, measures of severity of exacerbations should reflect the extent of acute pathophysiology (eg, the severity of lung dysfunction or the degree of mucosal inflammation). An exacerbation is an amplification of chronic disease. Therefore, a single measurement at the time of an acute exacerbation will not inform of the severity of the acute change, unless one takes the patient's stable baseline state into account. For instance, a measured peak expiratory flow rate (PEFR) of 60 L/min at the time of an exacerbation could represent a small acute change in an individual whose baseline PEFR is 80 L/min or a large acute change in an individual with a baseline PEFR of 240 L/min. Although both will require the same level of care, the second individual has a more severe exacerbation based on pathophysiological impact.

The most used severity classification of AECOPD is based on the requirement for health care resources or the required level of care[1] (**Box 2**). However, this classification does not help in deciding how to manage an exacerbation. Other limitations of such an approach to defining severity include the inability to assess acute change and the variability in the application of health care interventions among practitioners and systems. However, such a severity classification is useful in clinical trials and is also used in determining future preventative care for exacerbations in an individual patient. More work needs to be done to develop a uniform, reproducible, and clinically relevant severity classification system for COPD exacerbations.

SITE OF TREATMENT

Although more than 80% of patients with exacerbations are managed as outpatients,[16,17] patients with respiratory distress or at risk of such distress should be hospitalized to provide access to higher levels of care[1] (**Box 3**). Mortality risk in AECOPD increases with the development of respiratory acidosis, change in mental status, presence of significant comorbidities, and the need for ventilatory support. The emergency department plays an essential role in the triage and initial management of severe COPD exacerbations. A well-developed algorithm to standardize diagnosis, evaluation, treatment, and triage decisions in the emergency department can improve the care of COPD exacerbations.

OUTPATIENT MANAGEMENT OF CHRONIC OBSTRUCTIVE PULMONARY DISEASE EXACERBATION

Outpatient management of AECOPD includes the intensification of bronchodilator therapy and

---

Box 1
Anthonisen classification of AECOPD based on clinical findings

Major Criteria:

- Increased breathlessness,
- Increased sputum volume
- New or increased sputum purulence

Minor criteria:

- Fever without other cause
- Increased wheezing or cough
- 20% increase in respiratory or heart rate compared with baseline
- Upper respiratory tract infection in the previous 5 days

Types of exacerbation:

- Type 1 exacerbations – All of major criteria.
- Type 2 exacerbations - Any 2 major criteria
- Type 3 exacerbations - consist of any 1 of major criteria along with at least 1 of the minor criteria

Data from Anthonisen NR, Manfreda J, Warren CP, et al. Antibiotic therapy in exacerbations of chronic obstructive pulmonary disease. Ann Intern Med 1987;106(2):196-204.

Box 2
GOLD severity classification based on resource requirements

- Mild exacerbation – treated with rescue inhalers that is, short-acting bronchodilators
- Moderate exacerbation – treated with rescue inhalers, antibiotics and/or oral corticosteroids
- Severe exacerbation – Requires Emergency Room visit or hospitalization including an Intensive care unit admission

Data from Global Initiative for Chronic Obstructive Pulmonary Disease. Global Strategy for the Diagnosis, Management, and Prevention of COPD: 2020 Report. Available at: https://goldcopd.org/wp-content/uploads/2019/11/GOLD-2020-REPORT-ver1.0wms.pdf.

decisions about the use of oral glucocorticoids and oral antibiotics.

Bronchodilator Therapy

Airway caliber is reduced in exacerbations by a combination of increased luminal mucus, mucosal edema, and inflammation and bronchospasm. Therefore, bronchodilators, primarily by the inhaled route, are universally indicated in AECOPD management. The goal of bronchodilator therapy is to reduce dyspnea and improve exercise tolerance, and it may help with mucus clearance by improving the effectiveness of cough.

Inhaled short-acting β-adrenergic agonists (SABAs) are the mainstay of therapy because of their rapid onset of action and efficacy. Albuterol and levalbuterol are the most used formulations delivered by a multidose inhaler (MDI) with or without a spacer device or via a nebulizer. In the outpatient setting, the usual instructions are to use the MDI every 3 to 4 hours as needed (maximum 6 times/d) or the nebulizer every 5 to 6 hours as needed (maximum 4 times/d). If such frequency of use is not adequate to alleviate dyspnea, that usually indicates the need for further in-person evaluation. Although a nebulizer is easier to use in the acute setting, it should be noted that there is no significant efficacy difference between properly administered MDI and nebulizer treatments.[18] Common adverse effects are headache, nausea, palpitations, tremor, and vomiting.

Inhaled short-acting muscarinic antagonists (SAMAs) can provide additional bronchodilation in combination with inhaled SABAs. Ipratropium is the most used formulation by MDI or nebulizer every 4 to 6 hours. Common adverse effects are dry mouth, tremor, and urinary retention.[19]

Systemic Corticosteroids

Oral corticosteroids are commonly prescribed in outpatients with AECOPD despite scant data. Most trials of systemic corticosteroids in AECOPD have been in hospitalized or emergency department patients, who are likely more severe than office-based patients. A short course of systemic corticosteroids is thought to be benign; however, studies in asthma demonstrate that intermittent steroid courses are associated with worse long-term health outcomes.[20] Emerging data also show that higher levels of blood and sputum eosinophils are a biomarker for steroid response, and conversely, when eosinophils are not elevated, clinical failure may be increased in AECOPD with systemic corticosteroids.[21,22] Microbiome studies have demonstrated that a short course of oral corticosteroids used to treat AECOPD can cause an increased abundance of airway microbial species that lasts for several weeks.[23] All these data points do not support universal prescription of systemic corticosteroids in AECOPD, and suggest that such a practice could do more harm than good in some patients.

How does one choose when to use systemic corticosteroids in AECOPD? No clear guidelines exist, but the criteria the authors use are outlined in **Box 4**. When indicated, the usual dose is oral prednisone 40 mg every day for five days.[1] Whether extended courses up to 14 days are useful has never been systematically examined in outpatients, although they are not better than short courses in hospitalized patients. Having said that, if there appears to be an incomplete or short-lived response after 5 days, a longer course could be tried if other reasons for nonresponse are ruled out clinically. Adverse effects include hyperglycemia, heartburn, infection, gastrointestinal bleeding, psychomotor disturbance, and steroid myopathy, although most of these (except hyperglycemia) are usually seen after prolonged use.[1,24]

Antibiotics

The primary role of antibiotics in AECOPD is to hasten the host response-dependent resolution process and prevent complications. The weight of evidence, from meta-analyses, placebo-controlled trials, and database studies, supports improved outcomes with antibiotics in all but mild single-symptom exacerbations. The evidence from placebo-controlled randomized trials was recently summarized in a 2018 meta-analysis that included 19 randomized trials in 2663 patients.[25] Unlike corticosteroid trials, several of these antibiotic trials have been done in the outpatient setting. Among outpatients, a significant risk reduction (risk ratio 0.69, 95% confidence interval (CI) 0.53 to 0.90) for treatment failure within 4 weeks was shown in 9 trials with 1332 participants. Common adverse effects are diarrhea and the concern of the promotion of antibiotic resistance.[26]

As about half the exacerbations are bacterial, the first decision is who to treat. That is based on looking for evidence for bacterial infection, as discussed above. A lack of bronchitic symptoms and

prominent wheezing may indicate less probability of antibiotic benefit. Once it is determined who to treat, the next important question is the choice of specific antibiotics. Unlike corticosteroids, there is significant variation in antimicrobial activity, pharmacokinetic/pharmacodynamic properties, and adverse event profiles among antibiotics, making use of the same antibiotic in all exacerbations inappropriate. Rational antibiotic choice for AECOPD requires a risk stratification approach (**Fig. 2**). In AECOPD, one can define 2 categories of risk[26]: the risk for a poor clinical outcome (ie, treatment failure, early relapse, hospitalization, death) or the risk of antimicrobial resistance. Individuals who carry these risks need early, broad-spectrum aggressive antibiotic therapy to optimize outcomes.

The risk factors for poor outcomes in AECOPD have been reproducibly identified in several observational studies and secondary analyses of randomized controlled trials. It is a simple matter to determine these risk factors and then stratify an AECOPD patient as complicated or uncomplicated. Absence of all the risk factors defines an uncomplicated patient, whereas a complicated patient will have 1 or more of these risk factors (see **Fig. 2**).[27–30] As these risk factors have been independently associated with poor outcome in exacerbations, it is likely they are additive. Complicated patients are more likely to be hospitalized or die because of an exacerbation, making the failure of initial antibiotic treatment expensive and severely detrimental in these patients.

The risk for infection by an antimicrobial-resistant pathogen includes the risk for infection with intrinsically drug-resistant pathogens (eg, *P aeruginosa*) and the risk of infection with antibiotic-resistant strains of pathogens that are generally antibiotic susceptible (eg, *Streptococcus pneumoniae*). Because *P aeruginosa* is associated with severe COPD, patients at risk for this pathogen are a subgroup of complicated patients with additional risk factors (**Fig. 3**). Presence of risk for *P aeruginosa* requires the selection of antibiotics that are active against this pathogen. The risk for antibiotic-resistant strains of the common pathogens is best predicted by recent antibiotic use for any reason, with recent usually defined as the past 3 months.[31] Selection of resistant pathogens because of recent use is often specific to that antibiotic class. Therefore, this risk is easily handled by using an antimicrobial from a different class.

Antibiotic choices for uncomplicated patients include a macrolide, a cephalosporin, or trimethoprim/sulfamethoxazole. Amoxicillin is inadequate because of the substantial incidence of β-

---

Box 4
Proposed indications for systemic steroid use in acute exacerbation of chronic obstructive pulmonary disease

- Prominent wheezing
- Severe underlying COPD where treatment failure could result in hospitalization
- Blood eosinophils that are elevated or high normal (at baseline or at exacerbation)
- Absent or minimal bronchitic symptoms (cough and sputum) of exacerbation
- Previous exacerbations have required corticosteroid treatment for resolution

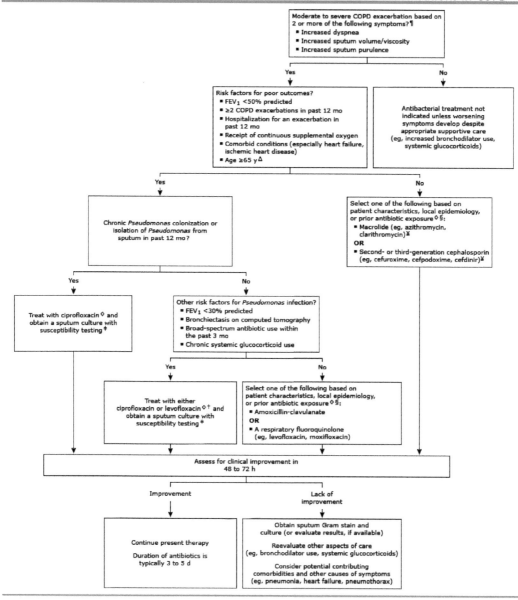

Fig. 2. The authors' approach to antibiotic treatment of AECOPD in outpatients. * Antiviral therapy for influenza is also indicated for exacerbations triggered by influenza infection ¶ Suspicion for other cardiopulmonary disorders (heart failure, pneumothorax) and more severe infections (eg, pneumonia) should be absent for the diagnosis of an acute COPD exacerbation. Δ Age alone is not a strict risk factor but should be considered as additive to other risk factors. ◊ Selection among antibiotic choices is based on local microbial sensitivity patterns, patient comorbidities, prior infecting organisms, potential adverse events and drug interactions, and also provider and patient preferences. In particularly, modifications to this regimen may be needed for patients with a history of drug-resistant Pseudomonas based on severity of illness, degree of suspicion for Pseudomonas, and prior susceptibility profiles of pseudomonal isolates. § If recent antibiotic exposure (eg, within the past 3 months), select an antibiotic from a different class than the most recent agent used. ¥ Trimethoprim-sulfamethoxazole is a reasonable alternative when macrolides and cephalosporins cannot be used due to allergy, potential adverse effects, or availability. ‡ Because fluoroquinolone resistance is prevalent among Pseudomonas aeruginosa strains, we obtain a sputum Gram stain and culture with susceptibility testing for these patients to help guide subsequent management decisions. For most other outpatients, obtaining a sputum culture is not needed unless the patient fails to respond to empiric treatment. † Levofloxacin has lesser activity against Pseudomonas than ciprofloxacin but has greater activity against S. pneumoniae and M. catarrhalis is thus a reasonable alternative to ciprofloxacin for patients who are at increased risk of Pseudomonas infection but lack microbiologic evidence of Pseudomonas infection or colonization. *Adapted with permission from*: Sethi S, Murphy TF. Management of infection in exacerbations of chronic obstructive pulmonary disease. In: UpToDate, Post TW (Ed), UpToDate, Waltham, MA. (Accessed on [Date].) Copyright © 2020 UpToDate, Inc. For more information visit HYPERLINK "http://www.uptodate.com" www.uptodate.com.

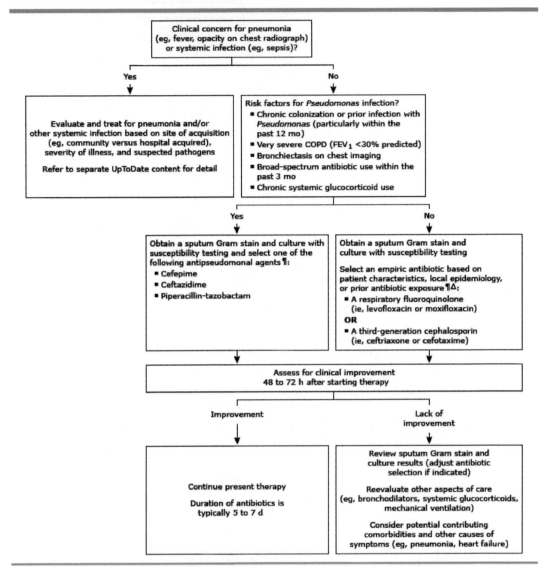

Fig. 3. The authors' approach to antibiotic treatment of AECOPD in the hospitalized patient. * Antiviral therapy for influenza is also indicated for exacerbations triggered by influenza infection. ¶ Selection among antibiotic choices is based on local microbial sensitivity patterns, patient comorbidities, prior infecting organisms, potential adverse events and drug interactions, and also provider and patient preferences. Modifications to these regimens may be needed for patients with suspicion for specific pathogens and/or history of drug-resistant organisms (eg, drug-resistant *Pseudomonas*). Δ If recent antibiotic exposure (eg, within the past 3 months), select an antibiotic from a different class than the most recent agent used. *Adapted with permission from*: Sethi S, Murphy TF. Management of infection in exacerbations of chronic obstructive pulmonary disease. In: UpToDate, Post TW (Ed), UpToDate, Waltham, MA. (Accessed on [Date].) Copyright © 2020 UpToDate, Inc. For more information visit HYPERLINK "http://www.uptodate.com" www.uptodate.com.

lactamase production among common pathogens involved in AECOPD.[32] The authors also avoid tetracyclines, because recent studies with doxycycline have shown limited bacteriologic and clinical efficacy.[33,34] Complicated patients can be treated with amoxicillin/clavulanate or a respiratory fluoroquinolone. Ciprofloxacin is recommended in the subgroup at risk for *P aeruginosa*, with the caveat that emerging resistance to this antibiotic has compromised its efficacy.[35] Therefore, it is prudent to obtain a sputum culture if possible before starting antibiotic treatment whenever this pathogen is suspected, to allow for subsequent adjustment of antibiotics.

Adjunctive Care

Exacerbations are an opportune time to discuss and encourage smoking cessation in current smokers. An assessment of proper inhaler technique and education is another important intervention. The data showing benefit with mucolytics, expectorants, and cough suppressants in AECOPD are scant and of poor quality. The use of these agents beyond the provision of adequate hydration is best individualized.

Failure to Respond to Initial Treatment

Clinical improvement in an AECOPD after commencing treatment should be expected within 48 to 72 hours, although complete resolution takes several more days. Absence of improvement or deterioration should lead to a prompt reassessment in person. This should include a careful clinical evaluation to exclude conditions described in the differential diagnosis, and to assess the worsening of comorbidities that have symptoms that overlap with AECOPD. A classic example is the decompensation of chronic congestive heart failure following an exacerbation induced by increased stress, hypoxemia, and steroid-related fluid retention. Additional diagnostic tests could be useful, as indicated in **Table 1**. If bacterial infection indicators have developed or persisted, a sputum Gram stain and culture should be considered to identify resistant pathogens. If alternative diagnoses and comorbid conditions are excluded as a cause of treatment nonresponse, switching to an alternative antibiotic and/or the addition of systemic corticosteroids should be considered.

HOSPITAL MANAGEMENT OF CHRONIC OBSTRUCTIVE PULMONARY DISEASE EXACERBATION

Patients who progress despite outpatient management or have indications for hospitalization are managed on the medical floor or intensive care unit (ICU) based on the severity of the presentation. The basic tenets of therapy of the exacerbation with bronchodilators, antibiotics, and corticosteroids do not change with hospitalization. However, hospitalization does allow for the provision of these treatments in a more intensive manner and by alternative routes. In addition, frequent assessment for signs of respiratory distress and changes in mental and hemodynamic status is possible in the inpatient setting, as well as the provision of supplemental oxygen and ventilatory support.

CARE ON THE GENERAL MEDICAL FLOOR

Management of AECOPD on the general medical floor involves reversing airflow limitation with inhaled short-acting bronchodilators and systemic glucocorticoids, treating infection, addressing comorbid conditions, ensuring adequate oxygenation, and close monitoring.

Bronchodilator Therapy

The principles of bronchodilator treatment for AECOPD in the hospital setting are similar to outpatients. Most commonly, SABA and SAMA agents are administered together. The nebulized route is often preferred initially because of ease and reliability. As the patient improves, the frequency of short-acting bronchodilators can be reduced and switched over to MDI. Long-acting bronchodilators are not appropriate during an exacerbation and usually can be resumed or initiated on discharge.

Corticosteroids

The benefit of systemic corticosteroids for AECOPD is supported by randomized controlled trials in the hospitalized setting. Systematic reviews and meta-analyses of these trials have shown that systemic corticosteroids improve lung function, reduce treatment failure and relapse, and shorten the length of hospital stay. However, they do not reduce mortality, and the most common adverse effect is hyperglycemia.[36]

Unless specific contraindications exist, systemic corticosteroids should be prescribed in all hospitalized exacerbations. Although this has been common practice for the last several decades, there has been a substantial change in steroid dose and duration in recent years. After the SCCOPE (Systemic Corticosteroids in Chronic Obstructive Pulmonary Disease Exacerbations) trial published in 1999 established the benefit of steroids in hospitalized AECOPD, the study dose, methylprednisolone 125 mg four times daily for 3 days, followed by oral steroid taper for a total of 14 days became the standard dose and duration.[37] Although subsequent trials suggested that lower doses and shorter durations of systemic corticosteroids are sufficient, it was only after the recent REDUCE trial published in 2013 that the current dose of prednisone 40 mg for 5 days became the standard of care.[38] Observational studies have shown the previous dosing regimens to be associated with more adverse effects such as hyperglycemia and infections. There appears to be no significant difference in clinical outcomes between the parenteral and oral route.[36] Most clinicians prefer to give the first 1 to 2 doses parenterally to avoid any undetected impaired absorption, and then switch to the oral route.

Although often practiced, the use of a longer course of steroids (eg, 14 days with tapering) in patients who appear to be slowly responding or failed a prior short course is not supported by current evidence and needs to be studied.

Antibiotics

Antibiotics are of proven benefit in hospitalized exacerbations of COPD. In the 2018 meta-analysis of placebo-controlled randomized trials, 5 trials in 803 hospitalized patients showed reduced treatment failure with a relative risk of 0.76 (95% confidence interval [CI] 0.58–1.00) favoring antibiotic use.[25] Two large database studies from the United States also strongly support the benefit of antibiotics in hospitalized AECOPD, demonstrating less treatment failure in antibiotic-treated patients (odds ratio [OR], 0.87; 95% CI, 0.82–0.92),[39] as well as reductions in in-hospital mortality (relative risk [RR], 0.60; 95% CI, 0.50–0.73) and 30-day readmission for COPD (RR, 0.87; 95% CI, 0.79–0.96).[40]

Whether all hospitalized patients should be treated with antibiotics is unclear, with 1 study suggesting that it is safe to withhold antibiotics in patients who are milder and do not have any clinical signs of bacterial infection. However, the accuracy of the criteria of bacterial infection has not been adequately tested in hospitalized patients. In the authors' experience, often hospitalized AECOPD patients, when asked about the color of sputum, state they can feel chest congestion but are unable to expectorate sputum because of severely limited expiratory flow. Unless specific contraindications are present, the authors treat all hospitalized patients with an antibiotic.

Almost all patients hospitalized primarily for the exacerbation will fall into the complicated group. Furthermore, the Pseudomonas subgroup is likely larger among patients requiring hospitalization compared with complicated outpatients, and its isolation has been associated with increased mortality.[41–44] A careful assessment for risk factors for Pseudomonas infection is important in hospitalized patients, including a review of previous sputum microbiology. Antibiotic choices for hospitalized patients without risk factors for P aeruginosa include a respiratory fluoroquinolone or a third-generation cephalosporin (see Fig. 3). Among hospitalized patients at risk for P aeruginosa, antibiotic choices include cefepime, ceftazidime, piperacillin/tazobactam, or ciprofloxacin. Intravenous therapy for the first 1 to 2 days is preferred, and the total duration of 5 to 7 days is adequate.

Antiviral Agents

Antiviral therapy is recommended in patients who are either outpatients or hospitalized for an AECOPD with clinical and laboratory evidence of influenza infection. Oseltamivir is the most commonly used antiviral medication, with baloxavir a newly available alternative choice.[45]

Oxygen Supplementation

In AECOPD patients presenting with hypoxia, supplemental oxygen is a critical component of treatment with a target arterial oxygen tension of 60 to 70 mm Hg or an oxygen saturation of 88% to 92%.[46,47] Supplemental oxygen use in severe COPD carries the risk of worsening hypercapnia due to combinations of blunting of ventilatory drive, the Haldane effect in the red blood cell, and worsening ventilation-perfusion mismatch. Therefore, the paradigm of oxygen supplementation in AECOPD should be start low, go slow, with careful titration. The use of titrated oxygen treatment in hospitalized AECOPD is associated with lower mortality rates and a lower likelihood of hypercapnia or respiratory acidosis than the use of nontitrated oxygen.[48] The predominant mechanism of hypoxemia in AECOPD is a ventilation-perfusion mismatch; therefore, it is easily correctable with low levels of oxygen supplementation. Hypoxemia in AECOPD not responding to a relatively low Fio_2 supplementation should prompt evaluation of alternative or concomitant diagnoses such as pulmonary emboli, acute respiratory distress syndrome, pulmonary edema, or pneumonia.

CARE IN THE INTENSIVE CARE UNIT

Indications for ICU admission in AECOPD include acute hypoxic or hypercapnic respiratory failure, nonresponse to low-flow supplemental oxygen, altered mental status with the inability to protect the airway, severe hemodynamic compromise, or impending respiratory failure. Along with the treatment modalities discussed previously, these patients require close monitoring and often noninvasive or invasive ventilatory support.

Bronchodilator Therapy

Nonintubated patients are usually provided intensive nebulized bronchodilator treatment with both SABAs and SAMAs. Ventilated patients are provided such treatment by puffs from an MDI delivered into the inspiratory limb of the ventilator circuit on a regular basis.

Corticosteroids

Large randomized controlled trials of systemic corticosteroids in AECOPD excluded patients requiring ventilatory support. A meta-analysis of smaller trials showed a nonsignificant difference in treatment success and mortality rates between steroids and placebo in both noninvasively or invasively ventilated patients.[49] Despite the lack of good quality data in the intensive care setting, given the significant benefits observed in hospitalized patients, the authors use systemic corticosteroids in AECOPD patients in the ICU. They use the parenteral route and a dose of 40 to 60 mg/d for 5 to 7 days. It is important to avoid high doses and prolonged durations, as that could make the benefit-risk ratio for this intervention unfavorable. ICU patients are highly prone to secondary infectious complications of steroid use, both bacterial and fungal. In fact, disseminated aspergillosis has been described in AECOPD patients in the ICU treated with high-dose steroids.[50]

Antibiotics

A single placebo-controlled randomized trial has been conducted with antibiotics in AECOPD patients in the ICU. In this study in 93 patients, patients who received a fluoroquinolone, ofloxacin, had a significant reduction in treatment failure, mortality, and length of hospital stay. The authors treat all AECOPD patients in the ICU with antibiotics, with antibiotic choices based on the considerations used for hospitalized patients (see **Fig. 3**).[25,51]

Ventilatory Support

Ventilatory support is needed in patients with severe AECOPD presenting with clinical signs of respiratory muscle fatigue, increased work of breathing, severe hypoxia, respiratory acidosis with pH no more than 7.35 and $Paco_2$ of at least 45 mm Hg or severe hemodynamic compromise.[1] Ventilatory support can be provided via noninvasive ventilation with bilevel positive airway pressure (BiPAP) with a face mask or by intubation and mechanical ventilation. High-flow nasal cannula has become an important modality to treat hypoxic respiratory failure; however, as most AECOPD patients are or can become hypercapnic, it is not useful in this setting.

AECOPD patients who receive noninvasive ventilation have a lower mortality rate and a shorter length of hospital and ICU stay. Additionally, they have had fewer complications, especially infections, compared with patients who received invasive ventilation.[52] Although these were not randomized controlled trials, a substantial body of evidence supports the use of noninvasive ventilation as the preferred modality in AECOPD patients. Noninvasive ventilation is contraindicated in patients who are unable to cooperate, unable to protect the airway or clear secretions, have altered mental status, have a facial deformity, are at high aspiration risk, or have had recent esophageal stenosis.[24] Patients who do not respond to noninvasive ventilation with worsening mental status or blood gases should be quickly escalated to mechanical ventilation.

Invasive ventilation is indicated in severe AECOPD patients with status postrespiratory or cardiac arrest, acute respiratory failure with an inability to tolerate noninvasive ventilation, increased respiratory secretions, altered mental status, inability to protect the airway, high risk of aspiration, cardiac arrhythmias, and severe hemodynamic stability.[1]

Adjunctive Care

AECOPD patients who are hospitalized should receive deep venous thrombosis prophylaxis, early physical therapy, and nutrition. Smoking cessation counseling and inhaler training prior to discharge and pulmonary rehabilitation commencing a few weeks after discharge are important.

SUMMARY

The management of AECOPD often still is a knee-jerk bundle approach of the standard interventions discussed previously. Emerging data are showing that except for bronchodilators, more selective and thoughtful use of treatment modalities in AECOPD is prudent. Universal prescription of systemic steroids and antibiotics can negate the potential benefits of these interventions. Newer modalities of diagnosis and treatment, such as better biomarkers, antibiotics, and anti-inflammatory agents are needed to improve the current success rates of AECOPD treatment. The profound influence of noninvasive ventilation in reducing mortality in critically ill AECOPD patients is a good example. In the interim, thoughtful application of antibiotics and corticosteroids is indicated.

REFERENCES

1. Global initiative for chronic obstructive lung disease 2020. Available at: https://goldcopd.org/wp-content/

uploads/2019/11/GOLD-2020-REPORT-ver1.0wms. pdf. Accessed May 30, 2020.

2. Jinjuvadia C, Jinjuvadia R, Mandapakala C, et al. Trends in outcomes, financial burden, and mortality for acute exacerbation of chronic obstructive pulmonary disease (COPD) in the United States from 2002 to 2010. COPD. J Chronic Obstr Pulm Dis 2017; 14(1):72–9.

3. Yawn BP, Wollan P, Rank M. Exacerbations in the pre- and post-COPD diagnosis periods. Pragmat Obs Res 2013;4:1–6.

4. Myint PK, Lowe D, Stone RA, et al. UK National COPD Resources and Outcomes Project 2008: patients with chronic obstructive pulmonary disease exacerbations who present with radiological pneumonia have worse outcome compared to those with non-pneumonic chronic obstructive pulmonary disease exacerbations. Respiration 2011;82(4): 320–7.

5. Zvezdin B, Milutinov S, Kojicic M, et al. A postmortem analysis of major causes of early death in patients hospitalized with COPD exacerbation. Chest 2009;136(2):376–80.

6. Werner AK, Koumans EH, Chatham-Stephens K, et al. Hospitalizations and deaths associated with EVALI. N Engl J Med 2020;382(17):1589–98.

7. Sethi S. Infectious etiology of acute exacerbations of chronic bronchitis. Chest 2000;117(5 Suppl 2): 380s–5s.

8. Desai H, Eschberger K, Wrona C, et al. Bacterial colonization increases daily symptoms in patients with chronic obstructive pulmonary disease. Ann Am Thorac Soc 2014;11(3):303–9.

9. Jacobs DM, Pandit U, Sethi S. Acute exacerbations in chronic obstructive pulmonary disease: should we use antibiotics and if so, which ones? Curr Opin Infect Dis 2019;32(2):143–51.

10. Sethi S, File TM, Dagan R. Acute exacerbations of chronic bronchitis: diagnosis and therapy; first, determine the cause of the worsening symptoms. J Respir Dis 2003;24(6):257–63.

11. Wilkinson TM, Hurst JR, Perera WR, et al. Effect of interactions between lower airway bacterial and rhinoviral infection in exacerbations of COPD. Chest 2006;129(2):317–24.

12. Niewoehner DE. Procalcitonin level-guided treatment reduced antibiotic use in exacerbations of COPD. ACP J Club 2007;146(3):57.

13. Stolz D, Christ-Crain M, Bingisser R, et al. Antibiotic treatment of exacerbations of COPD: a randomized, controlled trial comparing procalcitonin-guidance with standard therapy. Chest 2007; 131(1):9–19.

14. Anthonisen NR, Manfreda J, Warren CP, et al. Antibiotic therapy in exacerbations of chronic obstructive pulmonary disease. Ann Intern Med 1987; 106(2):196–204.

15. Stockley RA, O'Brien C, Pye A, et al. Relationship of sputum color to nature and outpatient management of acute exacerbations of COPD. Chest 2000; 117(6):1638–45.

16. Buist AS, McBurnie MA, Vollmer WM, et al. International variation in the prevalence of COPD (the BOLD Study): a population-based prevalence study. Lancet 2007;370(9589):741–50.

17. Jackson H, Hubbard R. Detecting chronic obstructive pulmonary disease using peak flow rate: cross sectional survey. BMJ 2003;327(7416): 653–4.

18. van Geffen WH, Douma WR, Slebos DJ, et al. Bronchodilators delivered by nebuliser versus pMDI with spacer or DPI for exacerbations of COPD. Cochrane Database Syst Rev 2016;(8):CD011826.

19. McCrory DC, Brown CD. Anticholinergic bronchodilators versus beta2-sympathomimetic agents for acute exacerbations of chronic obstructive pulmonary disease. Cochrane Database Syst Rev 2003;(1):CD003900.

20. Bleecker ER, Menzies-Gow AN, Price DB, et al. Systematic literature review of systemic corticosteroid use for asthma management. Am J Respir Crit Care Med 2020;201(3):276–93.

21. Bafadhel M, McKenna S, Terry S, et al. Blood eosinophils to direct corticosteroid treatment of exacerbations of chronic obstructive pulmonary disease: a randomized placebo-controlled trial. Am J Respir Crit Care Med 2012;186(1):48–55.

22. Bafadhel M, Davies L, Calverley PM, et al. Blood eosinophil guided prednisolone therapy for exacerbations of COPD: a further analysis. Eur Respir J 2014;44(3):789–91.

23. Huang YJ, Sethi S, Murphy T, et al. Airway microbiome dynamics in exacerbations of chronic obstructive pulmonary disease. J Clin Microbiol 2014;52(8):2813–23.

24. Wedzicha JA, Miravitlles M, Hurst JR, et al. Management of COPD exacerbations: a European Respiratory Society/American Thoracic Society guideline. Eur Respir J 2017;49(3):1600791.

25. Vollenweider DJ, Frei A, Steurer-Stey CA, et al. Antibiotics for exacerbations of chronic obstructive pulmonary disease. Cochrane Database Syst Rev 2018;(10):CD010257.

26. Sethi S, Murphy TF. Acute exacerbations of chronic bronchitis: new developments concerning microbiology and pathophysiology–impact on approaches to risk stratification and therapy. Infect Dis Clin North Am 2004;18(4):861–82, ix.

27. Balter MS, La Forge J, Low DE, et al. Canadian guidelines for the management of acute exacerbations of chronic bronchitis: executive summary. Can Respir J 2003;10(5):248–58.

28. Miravitlles M, Murio C, Guerrero T. Factors associated with relapse after ambulatory treatment of

acute exacerbations of chronic bronchitis. DAFNE Study Group. Eur Respir J 2001;17(5):928–33.

29. Wilson R, Anzueto A, Miravitlles M, et al. Moxifloxacin versus amoxicillin/clavulanic acid in outpatient acute exacerbations of COPD: MAESTRAL results. Eur Respir J 2012;40(1):17–27.

30. Wilson R, Jones P, Schaberg T, et al. Antibiotic treatment and factors influencing short and long term outcomes of acute exacerbations of chronic bronchitis. Thorax 2006;61(4):337–42.

31. Desai H, Richter S, Doern G, et al. Antibiotic resistance in sputum isolates of *Streptococcus pneumoniae* in chronic obstructive pulmonary disease is related to antibiotic exposure. COPD 2010;7(5): 337–44.

32. Sethi S, Breton J, Wynne B. Efficacy and safety of pharmacokinetically enhanced amoxicillin-clavulanate at 2,000/125 milligrams twice daily for 5 days versus amoxicillin-clavulanate at 875/125 milligrams twice daily for 7 days in the treatment of acute exacerbations of chronic bronchitis. Antimicrob Agents Chemother 2005;49(1): 153–60.

33. Daniels JM, Snijders D, de Graaff CS, et al. Antibiotics in addition to systemic corticosteroids for acute exacerbations of chronic obstructive pulmonary disease. Am J Respir Crit Care Med 2010;181(2): 150–7.

34. van Velzen P, Ter Riet G, Bresser P, et al. Doxycycline for outpatient-treated acute exacerbations of COPD: a randomised double-blind placebo-controlled trial. Lancet Respir Med 2017;5(6):492–9.

35. Rehman A, Patrick WM, Lamont IL. Mechanisms of ciprofloxacin resistance in *Pseudomonas aeruginosa*: new approaches to an old problem. J Med Microbiol 2019;68(1):1–10.

36. Walters JA, Tan DJ, White CJ, et al. Systemic corticosteroids for acute exacerbations of chronic obstructive pulmonary disease. Cochrane Database Syst Rev 2014;(9):CD001288.

37. Niewoehner DE, Erbland ML, Deupree RH, et al. Effect of systemic glucocorticoids on exacerbations of chronic obstructive pulmonary disease. N Engl J Med 1999;340(25):1941–7.

38. Leuppi JD, Schuetz P, Bingisser R, et al. Short-term vs conventional glucocorticoid therapy in acute exacerbations of chronic obstructive pulmonary disease: the REDUCE randomized clinical trial. JAMA 2013;309(21):2223–31.

39. Rothberg MB, Pekow PS, Lahti M, et al. Antibiotic therapy and treatment failure in patients hospitalized for acute exacerbations of chronic obstructive pulmonary disease. JAMA 2010;303(20):2035–42.

40. Stefan MS, Rothberg MB, Shieh MS, et al. Association between antibiotic treatment and outcomes in patients hospitalized with acute exacerbation of COPD treated with systemic steroids. Chest 2013; 143(1):82–90.

41. Gallego M, Pomares X, Espasa M, et al. Pseudomonas aeruginosa isolates in severe chronic obstructive pulmonary disease: characterization and risk factors. BMC Pulm Med 2014;14:103.

42. Garcia-Vidal C, Almagro P, Romani V, et al. Pseudomonas aeruginosa in patients hospitalised for COPD exacerbation: a prospective study. Eur Respir J 2009;34(5):1072–8.

43. Parameswaran GI, Sethi S. Pseudomonas infection in chronic obstructive pulmonary disease. Future Microbiol 2012;7(10):1129–32.

44. Boixeda R, Almagro P, Diez-Manglano J, et al. Bacterial flora in the sputum and comorbidity in patients with acute exacerbations of COPD. Int J Chron Obstruct Pulmon Dis 2015;10:2581–91.

45. Dobson J, Whitley RJ, Pocock S, et al. Oseltamivir treatment for influenza in adults: a meta-analysis of randomised controlled trials. Lancet 2015; 385(9979):1729–37.

46. Austin MA, Wills KE, Blizzard L, et al. Effect of high flow oxygen on mortality in chronic obstructive pulmonary disease patients in prehospital setting: randomised controlled trial. BMJ 2010;341:c5462.

47. Plant PK, Owen JL, Elliott MW. One year period prevalence study of respiratory acidosis in acute exacerbations of COPD: implications for the provision of non-invasive ventilation and oxygen administration. Thorax 2000;55(7):550–4.

48. Lellouche F, Bouchard PA, Roberge M, et al. Automated oxygen titration and weaning with FreeO2 in patients with acute exacerbation of COPD: a pilot randomized trial. Int J Chron Obstruct Pulmon Dis 2016;11:1983–90.

49. Abroug F, Ouanes I, Abroug S, et al. Systemic corticosteroids in acute exacerbation of COPD: a meta-analysis of controlled studies with emphasis on ICU patients. Ann Intensive Care 2014;4:32.

50. Bulpa PA, Dive AM, Garrino MG, et al. Chronic obstructive pulmonary disease patients with invasive pulmonary aspergillosis: benefits of intensive care? Intensive Care Med 2001;27(1):59–67.

51. Nouira S, Marghli S, Belghith M, et al. Once daily oral ofloxacin in chronic obstructive pulmonary disease exacerbation requiring mechanical ventilation: a randomised placebo-controlled trial. Lancet 2001;358(9298):2020–5.

52. Rochwerg B, Brochard L, Elliott MW, et al. Official ERS/ATS clinical practice guidelines: noninvasive ventilation for acute respiratory failure. Eur Respir J 2017;50(2):1602426.

Prevention of Chronic Obstructive Pulmonary Disease

Alberto Papi, MD*, Luca Morandi, MD, Leonardo M. Fabbri, MD

KEYWORDS

- Chronic bronchitis ● Emphysema ● Chronic diseases ● Asthma ● Vaccination

KEY POINTS

- Chronic obstructive pulmonary disease (COPD) is the pulmonary manifestation of multimorbidity caused by genetic susceptibility and interaction of environmental factors.
- COPD and multimorbidity are mainly caused by smoking/pollutants, unhealthy life style, and/or early events.
- The most important preventive interventions are smoking cessation and influenza and pneumococcal vaccination.
- Primary prevention may reduce the incidence and progression of COPD.

INTRODUCTION

Chronic obstructive pulmonary disease (COPD) is the third leading cause of death worldwide. In 2017, COPD was responsible for 3.2 million deaths, which is expected to reach an annual rate of 4.4 million by 2040. COPD has a worldwide prevalence of 10.1% and afflicts individuals across low-income, middle-income, and high-income countries. Further, the rate of years of life lost prematurely increased by 13.2% between 2007 and 2017.[1,2]

For a long time, COPD has been internationally recognized as a preventable condition[1] given the significant role played by environmental/nongenetic factors in the initiation and development of most of its clinical phenotypes. This article details the characteristics and relationships among these varying and heterogeneous preventable traits. In the latest GOLD (Global Initiative for Chronic Obstructive Lung Disease) version,[1] COPD is defined as "A common, preventable, and treatable disease characterized by persistent respiratory symptoms and airflow limitation, which result from airway and/or alveolar abnormalities usually caused by significant exposure to noxious particles or gases and influenced by host factors, including abnormal lung development. Comorbidities might have a significant impact on morbidity and mortality."

Prevention is usually classified as primal, primary, secondary, and tertiary (Table 1). Because current literature on COPD pathogenesis mainly discusses cigarette smoking and, to a lesser extent, exposure to outdoor, indoor, and occupational pollutants, this article primarily discusses the prevention, and particularly primary prevention.

General Chronic Obstructive Pulmonary Disease Prevention Concepts

The most recently updated consensus document[1] and review articles on COPD[2,3] indicate primary prevention as the most important and effective intervention for COPD development. However, they have limited discussions on primary

Section of Respiratory Diseases, Department of Morphology, Surgery and Experimental Medicine, University of Ferrara, Cona General Hospital, Via Aldo Moro 8, Ferrara 44124, Italy
* Corresponding author.
E-mail address: ppa@unife.it

Clin Chest Med 41 (2020) 453–462
https://doi.org/10.1016/j.ccm.2020.05.004

Table 1
Classification of preventive health care strategies

	Definition
Primal or primordial prevention	Any measure designed to help future parents provide their upcoming child with adequate attention, as well as secure physical and affective environments, from conception to the first birthday. Primordial prevention refers to measures designed to avoid initial early-life development of risk factors
Primary prevention	Measures for preventing disease establishment by eliminating disease causes or increasing resistance to disease. These measures include maintaining a healthy lifestyle, diet, and exercise regimen; avoiding smoking through prevention or cessation; and immunization against disease
Secondary prevention	Measures for preventing the disease from being symptomatic; for example, through blood pressure screening for hypertension (a risk factor for many cardiovascular diseases) and cancer screening
Tertiary prevention	Measures for reducing the harm of the disease, including symptoms, exacerbations, disability, or death, through treatment and rehabilitation

prevalence in the United States (www.healthdata.org/data-visualization/tobacco-visualization). However, although global estimates show a significant reduction in the prevalence of smoking between 1980 and 2012, the total number of smokers has increased in the same period from 721 million to 967 million, with a burden attributable to cigarette smoking exposure and secondhand smoking of 6.3 million deaths annually and 6.3% of disability-adjusted life-years.[5,6]

Moreover, preventing environmental, indoor, and occupational exposure, even in childhood, is important, which has been indicated by improved lung function in children from regions with reduced ambient pollution.[7] Previous studies have suggested that simple changes in cooking and heating methods, as well as in-house ventilation, in regions with indoor biomass use could improve lung health and reduce the COPD incidence.[8] Although the cause-effect relationship between cigarette smoking and COPD is well established, the relationship between other pollutants and COPD is supported by much weaker evidence.[9] In general, the strategy for COPD prevention is similar to that of all chronic diseases[10] involving chronic multimorbidity,[11] which is currently and increasingly the most important epidemic of the millennium.[12–15] In this context, appropriate vaccination (influenza and pneumococcal vaccines) plays an essential role because this has been associated with positive outcomes not only in COPD[1] but in all chronic diseases.[10,11]

PRIMAL AND PRIMARY PREVENTION

Currently available knowledge could be used to prevent and control chronic diseases, particularly COPD, which is likely both effective and cost-effective. Several approaches have been recommended for implementation of primal and primary prevention.[10]

Developmental Origins of Adult Chronic Diseases

Multiple longitudinal cohort studies have suggested that the origins of some chronic diseases, including asthma and COPD, could begin before and shortly after birth. Impaired lung function has been documented in infancy, with evidence indicating that this altered lung function trajectory remains well into adulthood. Further, reduced lung function in childhood predisposes the individual to accelerated lung function deterioration and COPD later in life.[16–18] Evidence relevant to both asthma and COPD indicates that early-life events, including environmental exposures, could alter the development of both immune function and lung mechanics, including lung injury and repair.[18,19]

prevention compared with those on tertiary prevention; that is, pharmacologic treatment and prevention of exacerbations, as well as self-management.[4] This limitation could be attributed to the limited evidence on primary prevention compared with that of other treatments; specifically, pharmacologic treatment.

In general, the most important approach for preventing COPD and chronic diseases is the primary prevention of the most important risk factor; specifically, but not exclusively for COPD, cigarette smoking. This approach has been indicated by the decreased mortality from smoking-induced diseases that have been associated with reduced smoking

This finding indicates that primary prevention of chronic obstructive respiratory diseases should be initiated before conception and continued during pregnancy and the first years of life.

Maternal smoking, particularly in the early stages of pregnancy (<27 weeks), premature birth with or without associated bronchopulmonary dysplasia development, and maternal malnutrition are among the most important early risk factors for lower lung function in later life.[18] Several longitudinal studies have reported that children with early-life lower respiratory tract illnesses are at an increased risk for subsequent chronic respiratory symptoms and forced expiratory volume in 1 second impairment, which often persist into adulthood.[18] This finding is particularly true for pneumonia, which is mostly caused by viruses; specifically, respiratory syncytial virus infections[20] and viral bronchiolitis obliterans.[21] Therefore, prevention of prematurity and bronchopulmonary dysplasia, as well as the implementation of effective vaccinations[22] and prevention strategies for childhood asthma, could help decrease the COPD risk. Similarly, efforts toward decreasing adolescent smoking and exposure to smoking, as well as environmental and indoor pollutants, during pregnancy and childhood could decrease the incidence of COPD.

Maternal Nutrition

Maternal nutrition is a potential risk factor for respiratory disease. Given that diet is modifiable, it provides an appealing approach for prevention strategies. Although there have been extensive studies on the impact of diet on asthma development with controversial results,[23] the relationship between diet and COPD is more difficult to study because of the long natural history of the disease. Thus, most of what is known rests on circumstantial evidence. Theoretically, the consumption of diets with antioxidants during adulthood might prevent the oxidant damage involved in COPD development.[24] However, the current reality is that, despite the prenatal period being a potentially critical development window, where interventions could contribute to the development of a healthy respiratory system and reduce the susceptibility to chronic respiratory diseases occurring later in life, it has been poorly studied and there remains a need for further active research.[18]

Primary Prevention: Lifestyle, Education, and Health Promotion

Physical activity
Physical inactivity is an important preventable trait of chronic diseases, including COPD. Receiving education regarding an active lifestyle[25] and improved access to exercise facilities, as well as walking and cycling paths, could promote physical activity. Individuals can be encouraged to use stairs instead of lifts or escalators in public places through signs, posters, and music; however, this has been reported to have small and short-lived effects.[10,26]

Advocacy
Various communication methods are available. They range from one-to-one conversations to mass media campaigns and are often more effective when applied together rather than individually. Common communication methods include information campaigns, publications, Web sites, press releases, lobbying, and peer-to-peer communication. Providing health education on cardiovascular and respiratory risk factors by broadcasting and print media has been reportedly to be cost-effective.[10]

Community-based interventions
Integrated community-based programs aim to reach the general population, as well as high-risk and priority segments such as workplaces, recreational areas, and religious/health care settings. Moreover, they enable active community participation in health decision making and simultaneous use of community resources and health services, as well as coordination of different activities through partnerships and coalitions. Successful community-based interventions require cooperation among community organizations, policy makers, businesses, health providers, and community residents. The successful implementation of such interventions for chronic diseases in developed countries shows that they could have considerable potential in developing countries.

School-based interventions
School health programs could be an effective means of reducing risks in a large susceptible population, the behavior of whom could determine future risk for chronic diseases such as COPD. These programs include 4 basic components: health policies, education, supportive environments, and health services. They make use of physical education, nutrition instruction and food services, health promotion among school personnel, and community outreach. Many school health programs focus on preventing risk factors associated with leading causes of death, disease, and disability, including tobacco and alcohol use, as well as dietary practices, physical activity, and sexual behavior. The World Bank reported that school health programs are highly cost-effective. For example, the annual cost of school health

programs was estimated to be US$0.03 and US$0.06 per capita in low-income and middle-income countries, respectively, with a resulting 0.1% and 0.4% reduction of future disease burden.[10,27]

Primary Prevention: Environmental Interventions

Recently, Abramson and colleagues[23] reviewed the role of outdoor, indoor, and workplace pollution as risk factors for chronic respiratory diseases, including COPD and asthma, as well as the related potential preventive measures.

Outdoor interventions

Outdoor air pollution is the result of a combination of primary sources, including wood and biomass smoke and vehicle exhaust, and secondary pollutants, including ozone (O_3) formed by atmospheric photochemical reactions. Monitored and regulated reference pollutants in many countries include particulate matter (PM 10 μm and PM 2.5 μm) and gaseous pollutants, including O_3, oxides of nitrogen (NOx), sulfur dioxide (SO_2), and carbon monoxide (CO). There have been extensive studies on the health effects of air pollutants, and their relationship with asthma and COPD have been well established,[28] with more limited evidence regarding the relationship between environmental pollution peaks and COPD/asthma exacerbations.[28]

Primary prevention of the adverse effects of air pollution is mainly focused on developing ambient air quality guidelines.[23] Although different approaches have been adopted across jurisdictions, legislated standards are typically based on environmental health risk assessment. In Dublin, banning the sale of coal reduced black smoke levels and was associated with significant reductions in both respiratory and cardiovascular deaths.[29] Implementation of emission control measures by Chinese authorities dramatically improved the air quality in Beijing during the 2008 Olympic Games,[30] which was associated with reduced respiratory inflammation among young adults.[31] However, many countries have not enforced such standards. Secondary prevention measures include advising individuals with preexisting cardiac and respiratory diseases to avoid heavy outdoor exertion on high-pollution days.

Indoor interventions

Biomass fuel (BMF) is the primary source of cooking and/or heating fuel for nearly 2.4 billion individuals worldwide, with most being from low-income countries; further, women and children are the most highly exposed during cooking and other domestic activities.[15] These countries have been reported to have higher levels of BMF air pollutants in homes than the corresponding levels in high-income countries.[32] A meta-analysis of 15 observational studies reported a dose-response association between BMF and COPD development,[33] which indicates the importance of BMF in primary COPD prevention. Further, there is recent evidence of decreased COPD incidence with improved cooking fuels, provision of support and instructions for installing household biogas digesters and kitchen ventilation, improving biomass stoves, and installing exhaust fans.[8] However, similar to environmental pollution, there is no solid evidence of the association between indoor pollution and increased COPD risk.[9]

Workplace interventions

Population studies have reported that 10% to 15% of the total COPD burden might be associated with workplace exposure. COPD prevention could be achieved through adequate control of harmful workplace exposure. The various specific COPD-related workplace exposures could be prevented by reducing work exposure to vapors, gases, dust, and fumes. It might be important to identify workers with rapidly declining lung function, irrespective of the specific exposure, through accurate annual lung function measures. Early identification of patients with COPD is important and should be considered for reducing causative exposures and to prevent further harm to the individual and other similarly exposed workers. This outcome can be achieved using a respiratory questionnaire, accurate lung function measurements, and controlling workplace exposure.[34]

Primary Prevention: Tobacco Smoking

Health policy: laws, regulations, and price interventions

International laws and treaties, as well as national and local legislation, regulations, ordinances, and other legal frameworks, are fundamental elements of effective public health policy and practice. Therefore, they should be considered while developing large-scale strategies for preventable diseases. Historically, laws have played a crucial role in several great achievements in public health, including environmental control laws, warnings on cigarette packs, and other tobacco control measures. Current laws related to chronic diseases, particularly COPD, have been shown to be effective and crucial components of comprehensive prevention and control strategies. Banning smoking in public places, as well as tobacco product advertisement, has been shown to be very cost-effective. There has been extensive use of legal frameworks regarding tobacco control; however, the World Health Organization (WHO) Framework Convention on Tobacco Control remains the only global framework. More effective use of legislation and regulations could reduce the burden of chronic disease (particularly COPD) and protect the rights of individuals with chronic diseases. For example, reducing nicotine levels in cigarettes could substantially reduce the enormous burden of smoking-related diseases and mortality.[35] A clear example of the importance of legislation for prevention is the recent tobacco bill passed in the United States, which increases the federal minimum age for buying cigarettes or other tobacco products (eg, e-cigarettes or other vaping products) from 18 to 21 years (The New York Times. Congress Approves Raising Age to 21 for E-Cigarette and Tobacco Sales, 19 December 2019).

Taxation policies could be used to reduce tobacco use and environmental exposure, as well as generate revenue for health promotion and disease prevention programs. Increasing the price of tobacco could encourage cessation from using tobacco products, prevent others from starting, and discourage relapsing of ex–tobacco users. A 10% price increase in tobacco products has been shown to reduce its demand by 3% to 5% in high-income countries and by 8% in low-income and middle-income countries, with young individuals and the poor being the most responsive to price changes.[36]

Secondhand smoke

A recent systematic review indicated significant variations in the studies conducted worldwide dealing with the potential effects of secondhand smoking and the associated disease burden across countries/regions. The variations observed could be attributed to different exposure levels, types of cigarettes, and smoking patterns leading to insufficient evidence in many areas.[37] Moreover, it highlighted relevant gaps in the data quality, which weakens any conclusions. This finding is consistent with the report by Burney and Amaral[9] on the validity of the evidence regarding outdoor and indoor pollution, a field that has the same methodological problems.

Smoking cessation

Active tobacco smoking is the single major COPD cause in large parts of the world; additionally, it might also cause fixed airflow limitation in patients with chronic asthma.[38] Smoking avoidance and cessation remain the only proven primary prevention strategy for chronic respiratory diseases, particularly COPD development. Primary prevention should seek to prevent smoking initiation

and promote smoking cessation. The WHO adopted a firm position and plan to increase smoking cessation and prevention, which has been ratified by several countries, including the European Union. However, 25 years after its publication, there is still no solid evidence of any global reduction in cigarette consumption attributable to this convention[39]; therefore, this approach remains only hypothetically preventable.

Smoking cessation using multiple approaches has the greatest potential for influencing the natural history of COPD. Long-term quitting success rates of up to 25% can be achieved[40] when individual approaches to smoking cessation and legislative smoking bans are instituted. These approaches are also effective not only at increasing the quitting rates but also in reducing harm from secondhand smoke exposure.[41] In addition, smoking cessation reduces the decline rate of lung function in early COPD and reduces all-cause mortality.[42,43] Various pharmacologic and behavioral approaches to smoking cessation are currently available.[1]

It remains unclear whether using electronic nicotine delivery systems (e-cigarettes) is an effective harm reduction strategy or a bridge to tobacco smoking among the youth. The Forum of International Respiratory Societies, which includes the International Union against Tuberculosis, issued a position statement calling for e-cigarette restriction or regulation.[44,45] In 2019, there was a lung-illness outbreak with deaths being associated with e-cigarette product use (devices, liquids, refill pods, and/or cartridges). Patients, mostly adolescents and young adults aged less than 35 years, often present with a history of using e-cigarettes or other vaping products, especially tetrahydrocannabinol (THC)-containing products.[46] Although the epidemic peak seems to have ended, it has attracted a lot of attention from health authorities and will possibly lead to some legislative controls on e-cigarette sales and use.[47] Taken together, current evidence indicates that e-cigarettes are not safe and, although they may be effective in improving smoking cessation rates, they are plagued by problems and are not a safe alternative to cigarette smoking. Recently, the European Respiratory Society released a position paper[48] stating the reasons why it does not recommend any product that may damage the lungs and human health, and therefore strongly supports the implementation of the WHO position, which also regulates the use of novel cigarette substitutive products.[49]

Pharmacotherapies for smoking cessation

There has been a recent review of smoking cessation strategies.[50] Nicotine replacement therapy (nicotine gums, inhalers, nasal sprays, transdermal patches, sublingual tablets, or lozenges) reliably increase the long-term smoking abstinence rates. Moreover, varenicline, bupropion, and nortriptyline, all of which have a safe therapeutic profile, have been shown to increase long-term quit rates; however, they should always be part of a supportive intervention program, rather than being provided as the sole intervention for smoking cessation. Counseling delivered by physicians and other health professionals significantly increases the quitting rates compared with self-initiated strategies. Even brief (3-minute) counseling periods urging smokers to quit improve the smoking cessation rates. Moreover, financial incentive models for smoking cessation have been shown to be more effective at facilitating persistent smoking cessation rates at 6 months than usual care. Combining pharmacotherapy and behavioral support increases smoking cessation rates.[1]

Vaccinations

Influenza
A recent Cochrane analysis on several randomized controlled trials (RCTs) concluded that inactivated vaccination of patients with COPD reduced influenza-induced exacerbations greater than or equal to 3 weeks after vaccination; further, the effect size was similar to that of previous observational studies. Coadministration of live attenuated virus with the inactivated vaccine did not confer additional benefit.[51] GOLD recommends influenza vaccinations for all patients with COPD.[1]

Pneumococcal
Although both the Centers for Disease Control and Prevention (CDC) and the GOLD acknowledge limited evidence stemming from the design and conduct of RCTs, they both recommend pneumococcal vaccination. In randomized, double-blind, placebo-controlled trial involving 84,496 adults 65 years of age or older, the 13-valent polysaccharide conjugate vaccine (PCV13) was effective in preventing vaccine-type pneumococcal, bacteremic, and nonbacteremic community-acquired pneumonia and vaccine-type invasive pneumococcal disease but not in preventing community-acquired pneumonia from any cause.[52] CDC recommends that individuals aged from 19 to 64 years should routinely receive PCV13 and the 23-valent pneumococcal polysaccharide vaccine (PPSV23).[53] GOLD recommends the aforementioned pneumococcal vaccinations for all patients aged greater than 65 years. Moreover, the PPSV23 is recommended for younger patients with COPD

with significant comorbid conditions, including chronic heart or lung disease.[1]

SECONDARY PREVENTION

In 2016, the US Preventive Services Task Force recommended against screening asymptomatic adults for COPD using spirometry.[54] GOLD has

---

Box 1
Recommendations for research priorities for the primary prevention of chronic obstructive pulmonary disease

Near-term priorities (next 5 years)

- Identification of existing National Heart Lung and Blood Institute (NHLBI) cohort studies with lung function data, allowing researchers to identify suitable material to address scientific gaps in primary prevention of COPD.

- Active engagement with other divisions and institutes to include pulmonary outcomes in cohort studies, the primary focus of which may be outside of COPD.

- Evaluation of maternal/fetal health interventions as they pertain to general lung health and COPD. This evaluation is likely to involve cohorts that follow individuals from the mother's pregnancy until children reach puberty.

- Identification of early biomarkers and imaging to detect preclinical disease.

- Intervention studies to determine whether progression of persistent chronic bronchitis to clinical COPD can be ameliorated or stopped.

- Interventions to prevent development of emphysema, including patients with alpha1-antitrypsin deficiency.

Long-term priorities (5–10 years)

- Extension of observational studies of adolescents and young adults into age ranges where incident COPD develops.

- Intervention studies of novel and established pharmacotherapies that may affect risk factors defined from observational studies.

- Interventional studies in preclinical COPD to reduce development of incident COPD.

Adapted from Drummond MB, Buist AS, Crapo JD, et al. Chronic obstructive pulmonary disease: NHLBI Workshop on the Primary Prevention of Chronic Lung Diseases. Annals of the American Thoracic Society. 2014;11 Suppl 3:S154-160; *Reprinted* with permission of the American Thoracic Society. Copyright © 2020 American Thoracic Society.

recommended case finding in symptomatic patients but not screening in asymptomatic populations.[1] The aforementioned recommendations are based on the absence of any evidence that screening helps in preventing risk factors. Further, early diagnosis is not useful because there is currently no available treatment that prevents the progression of early mild COPD in symptomatic patients to more severe COPD.[54,55] Thus the issue of screening for COPD remains highly controversial.[56,57] However, case finding is paramount so that interventions designed to reduce disease progression can be implemented.

TERTIARY PREVENTION

Tertiary prevention refers to reducing symptoms, exacerbations, disability, or death through pharmacologic treatment and rehabilitation. As detailed earlier, smoking cessation remains the most effective treatment to improve symptoms, alter disease progression, and reduce mortality in actively smoking patients with COPD. A recent study reported that 2-year treatment with tiotropium in early mild to moderate COPD improved lung function and quality of life and reduced exacerbations and lung function decline.[58] However, it remains unclear whether these findings indicate a treatment effect in the early natural history of COPD. There are similar ongoing bronchodilator studies on whether there is a pharmacologic treatment effect in symptomatic smokers without airflow limitation, a relevant patient population that might present another true early COPD or pre-COPD.[59,60]

SUMMARY

COPD is defined as a preventable condition given that environmental/nongenetic factors play a crucial role in the initiation and development of most of the disease's clinical expressions, which are possibly related to several interconnected preventable traits. Most of the current evidence on COPD pathogenesis originates from cigarette smoking, and to a lesser extent exposure to outdoor, indoor, and occupational pollutants. Therefore, currently available evidence regarding prevention strategies, and particularly primary prevention, is mainly related to these preventable traits. Smoking cessation has the greatest capacity for influencing the natural history of COPD, and smoking avoidance and cessation remains the only proven primary prevention strategy for chronic respiratory diseases. However, even 25 years after the publications of the WHO regarding cigarette smoking, there is still no solid evidence indicating that this convention has globally reduced cigarette consumption. Primary prevention of adverse air pollution effects has been focused on developing ambient air quality guidelines; however, many countries have lacked in the enforcement of standards. BMF air pollutants measured in homes in low-income countries have been greater than the corresponding values in high-income countries, with evidence of a consistent dose-response relationship. Improving cooking fuels and kitchen ventilation could potentially be effective in decreasing COPD incidence in these conditions. However, although primary prevention remains fundamental for COPD and for all chronic diseases, the evidence of its feasibility and effectiveness remains weak. This weakness is emphasized by a National Institutes of Health (NIH) workshop report that provides a detailed list of future research/actions necessary to properly address this important issue (**Box 1**).[61]

Many strategies have been developed for the many identified preventable trait; however, although these are effective in theory, there are no tangible changes in real-world/large-scale conditions.

In addition, there is current accumulating evidence highlighting that the origins of some chronic diseases, including COPD, could already be present shortly after birth and that primary prevention of chronic obstructive respiratory diseases should probably be started during pregnancy and the first years of life.

CONFLICTS OF INTEREST

A. Papi reports no conflict of interest for coauthoring this article. Outside the submitted work, Prof. A. Papi reports lecture fees and/or consultancies from AstraZeneca, Chiesi, Boehringer Ingelheim, GlaxoSmithKline, Merck, Novartis, Zambon, Mundipharma, Teva, Sanofi, and Elpen Pharmaceutical. L. Morandi reports no conflict of interest. L.M. Fabbri reports no conflict of interest for coauthoring this article. Outside the submitted work, Prof. L.M. Fabbri reports lecture fees and/or consultancies from AstraZeneca, Chiesi, Boehringer Ingelheim, GlaxoSmithKline Merck, Novartis, Zambon, Verona Pharma.

REFERENCES

1. Global Initiative for Chronic Obstructive Lung Disease. Global strategy for the diagnosis, management, and prevention of chronic obstructive pulmonary disease 2020. Available at: https://goldcopd.org/gold-reports/. Accessed June 24, 2020.

2. Celli BR, Wedzicha JA. Update on clinical aspects of chronic obstructive pulmonary disease. N Engl J Med 2019;381(13):1257–66.

3. Agusti A, Hogg JC. Update on the pathogenesis of chronic obstructive pulmonary disease. N Engl J Med 2019;381(13):1248–56.

4. Reddel HK, Jenkins CR, Partridge MR. Self-management support and other alternatives to reduce the burden of asthma and chronic obstructive pulmonary disease. Int J Tuberc Lung Dis 2014; 18(12):1396–406.

5. Lim SS, Vos T, Flaxman AD, et al. A comparative risk assessment of burden of disease and injury attributable to 67 risk factors and risk factor clusters in 21 regions, 1990-2010: a systematic analysis for the Global Burden of Disease Study 2010. Lancet 2012;380(9859):2224–60.

6. Morris PB, Ference BA, Jahangir E, et al. Cardiovascular effects of exposure to cigarette smoke and electronic cigarettes: clinical perspectives from the prevention of cardiovascular disease section leadership council and early career councils of the American College of Cardiology. J Am Coll Cardiol 2015;66(12):1378–91.

7. Gauderman WJ, Urman R, Avol E, et al. Association of improved air quality with lung development in children. N Engl J Med 2015;372(10):905–13.

8. Zhou Y, Zou Y, Li X, et al. Lung function and incidence of chronic obstructive pulmonary disease after improved cooking fuels and kitchen ventilation: a 9-year prospective cohort study. PLoS Med 2014; 11(3):e1001621.

9. Burney P, Amaral AFS. Air pollution and chronic airway disease: is the evidence always clear? Lancet 2019;394(10215):2198–200.

10. World Health Organization. Preventing chronic diseases: a vital investment. WHO global report. Switzerland (Geneva): World Health Organization; 2005.

11. National Institute for Health and Care Excellence. Multimorbidity: clinical assessment and management. NICE guideline [NG56]. 2016. Available at: nice.org.uk/guidance/ng56. Accessed June 24, 2020.

12. Hunter DJ, Reddy KS. Noncommunicable diseases. N Engl J Med 2013;369(14):1336–43.

13. Westney G, Foreman MG, Xu J, et al. Impact of comorbidities among medicaid enrollees with chronic obstructive pulmonary disease, United States, 2009. Prev Chronic Dis 2017;14:E31.

14. Landrigan PJ, Fuller R, Acosta NJR, et al. The Lancet Commission on pollution and health. Lancet 2018;391(10119):462–512.

15. Smith KR, Mehta S, Maeusezahl-Feuz M. Indoor air-pollution from solid fuel use. In: Ezzatti M, Lopez AD, Rodgers A, et al, editors. Comparative quantification of health risks: global and regional burden of diseases attributable to selected major risk factors.

Geneva (Switzerland): World Health Organization; 2004. p. 1435–93.

16. Whitney DG, Whitney RT, Kamdar NS, et al. Early-onset noncommunicable disease and multimorbidity among adults with pediatric-onset disabilities. Mayo Clin Proc 2020;95(2):274–82.

17. Lange P, Celli B, Agusti A, et al. Lung-function trajectories leading to chronic obstructive pulmonary disease. N Engl J Med 2015;373(2):111–22.

18. Martinez FD. Early-life origins of chronic obstructive pulmonary disease. N Engl J Med 2016;375(9): 871–8.

19. Joss-Moore LA, Albertine KH, Lane RH. Epigenetics and the developmental origins of lung disease. Mol Genet Metab 2011;104(1–2):61–6.

20. Edmond K, Scott S, Korczak V, et al. Long term sequelae from childhood pneumonia; systematic review and meta-analysis. PLoS One 2012;7(2): e31239.

21. Colom AJ, Maffey A, Garcia Bournissen F, et al. Pulmonary function of a paediatric cohort of patients with postinfectious bronchiolitis obliterans. A long term follow-up. Thorax 2015;70(2):169–74.

22. Higgins D, Trujillo C, Keech C. Advances in RSV vaccine research and development - a global agenda. Vaccine 2016;34(26):2870–5.

23. Abramson MJ, Koplin J, Hoy R, et al. Population-wide preventive interventions for reducing the burden of chronic respiratory disease. Int J Tuberc Lung Dis 2015;19(9):1007–18.

24. Romieu I. Nutrition and lung health. Int J Tuberc Lung Dis 2005;9(4):362–74.

25. Ambrosino N, Bertella E. Lifestyle interventions in prevention and comprehensive management of COPD. Breathe (Sheff) 2018;14(3):186–94.

26. Committee on Physical Activity, Health, Transportation, and Land Use, Transportation Research Board, Institute of Medicine of the National Academies. Does the built environment influence physical activity?: examining the evidence. Washington, D.C. 2005. Special report 282. Available at www.TRB.org.

27. World Bank. Focusing resources on effective school health: a FRESH start to enhancing the quality and equity of education. Focusing Resources on Effective School Health (FRESH) series. Washington, DC: World Bank. 2000. Available at: http://documents.worldbank.org/curated/en/722511468740994206/Focusing-resources-on-effective-school-health-a-FRESH-start-to-enhancing-the-quality-and-equity-of-education;jsessionid=CgEmr6gHG-jOMD9mE7wItYmZ. Accessed June 24, 2020.

28. Schraufnagel DE, Balmes JR, Cowl CT, et al. Air pollution and noncommunicable diseases: a review by the forum of international respiratory societies' environmental committee, part 2: air pollution and organ systems. Chest 2019;155(2):417–26.

29. Clancy L, Goodman P, Sinclair H, et al. Effect of air-pollution control on death rates in Dublin, Ireland: an intervention study. Lancet 2002;360(9341):1210–4.

30. Xin J, Wang Y, Wang L, et al. Reductions of PM2.5 in Beijing-Tianjin-Hebei urban agglomerations during the 2008 Olympic Games. Adv Atmos Sci 2012;29: 1330–42.

31. Huang W, Wang G, Lu SE, et al. Inflammatory and oxidative stress responses of healthy young adults to changes in air quality during the Beijing Olympics. Am J Respir Crit Care Med 2012;186(11): 1150–9.

32. Ezzati M, Kammen DM. The health impacts of exposure to indoor air pollution from solid fuels in developing countries: knowledge, gaps, and data needs. Environ Health Perspect 2002;110(11):1057–68.

33. Hu G, Zhou Y, Tian J, et al. Risk of COPD from exposure to biomass smoke: a metaanalysis. Chest 2010; 138(1):20–31.

34. Fishwick D, Sen D, Barber C, et al. Occupational chronic obstructive pulmonary disease: a standard of care. Occup Med (Lond) 2015;65(4):270–82.

35. Apelberg BJ, Feirman SP, Salazar E, et al. Potential public health effects of reducing nicotine levels in cigarettes in the United States. N Engl J Med 2018;378(18):1725–33.

36. Yeh CY, Schafferer C, Lee JM, et al. The effects of a rise in cigarette price on cigarette consumption, tobacco taxation revenues, and of smoking-related deaths in 28 EU countries– applying threshold regression modelling. BMC public health 2017; 17(1):676.

37. Carreras G, Lugo A, Gallus S, et al. Burden of disease attributable to second-hand smoke exposure: a systematic review. Prev Med 2019;129:105833.

38. Lange P, Parner J, Vestbo J, et al. A 15-year follow-up study of ventilatory function in adults with asthma. N Engl J Med 1998;339(17):1194–200.

39. Hoffman SJ, Poirier MJP, Rogers Van Katwyk S, et al. Impact of the WHO Framework Convention on Tobacco Control on global cigarette consumption: quasi-experimental evaluations using interrupted time series analysis and in-sample forecast event modelling. BMJ 2019;365:l2287.

40. van Eerd EA, van der Meer RM, van Schayck OC, et al. Smoking cessation for people with chronic obstructive pulmonary disease. Cochrane Database Syst Rev 2016;(8):CD010744.

41. Frazer K, Callinan JE, McHugh J, et al. Legislative smoking bans for reducing harms from secondhand smoke exposure, smoking prevalence and tobacco consumption. Cochrane Database Syst Rev 2016;(2):CD005992.

42. Anthonisen NR, Connett JE, Kiley JP, et al. Effects of smoking intervention and the use of an inhaled anticholinergic bronchodilator on the rate of decline of FEV1. The Lung Health Study. JAMA 1994;272(19):1497–505.

43. Anthonisen NR, Skeans MA, Wise RA, et al. The effects of a smoking cessation intervention on 14.5-year mortality: a randomized clinical trial. Ann Intern Med 2005;142(4):233–9.

44. Ferkol TW, Farber HJ, La Grutta S, et al. Electronic cigarette use in youths: a position statement of the Forum of International Respiratory Societies. Eur Respir J 2018;51(5):1800278.

45. Schraufnagel DE, Blasi F, Drummond MB, et al. Electronic cigarettes. A position statement of the forum of international respiratory societies. Am J Respir Crit Care Med 2014;190(6):611–8.

46. Kalininskiy A, Bach CT, Nacca NE, et al. E-cigarette, or vaping, product use associated lung injury (EVALI): case series and diagnostic approach. Lancet Respir Med 2019;7(12):1017–26.

47. Jaffe S. Will Trump snuff out e-cigarettes? Lancet 2019;394(10213):1977–8.

48. Pisinger C, Dagli E, Filippidis FT, et al. ERS and tobacco harm reduction. Eur Respir J 2019;54(6).

49. World Health Organization. The Convention Secretariat calls Parties to remain vigilant towards novel and emerging nicotine and tobacco products. Geneva (Switzerland): World Health Organization; 2019.

50. Garcia-Gomez L, Hernandez-Perez A, Noe-Diaz V, et al. Smoking cessation treatments: current psychological and pharmacological options. Rev Invest Clin 2019;71(1):7–16.

51. Kopsaftis Z, Wood-Baker R, Poole P. Influenza vaccine for chronic obstructive pulmonary disease (COPD). Cochrane Database Syst Rev 2018;(6): CD002733.

52. Bonten MJ, Huijts SM, Bolkenbaas M, et al. Polysaccharide conjugate vaccine against pneumococcal pneumonia in adults. N Engl J Med 2015;372(12): 1114–25.

53. Centers for Disease Control and Prevention, National Center for Immunization and Respiratory Diseases (NCIRD). Adult immunization schedule 2017. Atlanta (GA). 2017. Available at: https://www.cdc.gov/vaccines/schedules/easy-to-read/adult.html. Accessed January 20, 2020.

54. Guirguis-Blake JM, Senger CA, Webber EM, et al. Screening for chronic obstructive pulmonary disease: evidence report and systematic review for the US Preventive Services Task Force. JAMA 2016;315(13):1378–93.

55. Kaplan A, Thomas M. Screening for COPD: the gap between logic and evidence. Eur Respir Rev 2017; 26(143):160113.

56. Mannino DM, Thomashow B. COUNTERPOINT: can screening for COPD Improve Outcomes? No. Chest 2020;157(1):9–12.

57. Yawn BP, Martinez FJ. POINT: can screening for COPD improve outcomes? Yes. Chest 2020;157(1): 7–9.

58. Zhou Y, Zhong NS, Li X, et al. Tiotropium in early-stage chronic obstructive pulmonary disease. N Engl J Med 2017;377(10):923–35.

59. Lambert AA, Bhatt SP. Respiratory symptoms in smokers with normal spirometry: clinical significance and management considerations. Curr Opin Pulm Med 2019;25(2):138–43.

60. Celli BR, Agusti A. COPD: time to improve its taxonomy? ERJ Open Res 2018;4(1).

61. Drummond MB, Buist AS, Crapo JD, et al. Chronic obstructive pulmonary disease: NHLBI Workshop on the primary prevention of chronic lung diseases. Ann Am Thorac Soc 2014;11(Suppl 3): S154–60.

Section IV: Pharmacologic Therapy in COPD

Long-Acting Bronchodilators for Chronic Obstructive Pulmonary Disease
Which One(S), How, and When?

Alexander G. Mathioudakis, MD[a,b], Jørgen Vestbo, DMSc[a,b,*],
Dave Singh, PhD[a,b,c]

KEYWORDS

- COPD • Bronchodilators • LAMA • LABA • Dual bronchodilators • LABA/LAMA combination
- Inhaler devices • Randomized controlled trials

KEY POINTS

- Maintenance management of chronic obstructive pulmonary disease (COPD) should be guided by patients' symptoms and exacerbations.
- Long-acting beta-2 agonists (LABAs), long-acting muscarinic antagonists (LAMAs), and fixed combinations of a LAMA with a LABA are safe and effective and represent the first line of COPD maintenance treatment.
- Compared with LABAs, LAMAs are more effective in preventing exacerbations.
- A low threshold is suggested for the addition of a second long-acting bronchodilator (LABD).
- The most important consideration when making a choice within LABD drug class is the selection of the inhaler device that is most suitable for each patient.

INTRODUCTION

Chronic obstructive pulmonary disease (COPD) is characterized by chronic respiratory symptoms, such as breathlessness and chronic productive cough, limited exercise tolerance, poor quality of life, and acute exacerbations.[1] COPD is characterized by an abnormal, chronic inflammatory response in the airways to the inhalation of tobacco smoke or other noxious particles.[2] This results in the development of fixed obstruction of the small airways, due to airway wall thickening and fibrosis. Other pathologic features include mucus hypersecretion and emphysema, due to destruction of the lung parenchyma.[2]

Bronchodilators hold the first line and second line of maintenance pharmacologic treatment of COPD for most patients, conferring significant health benefits and limited adverse events.[1] There are 2 classes of long-acting bronchodilators (LABDs), with different pharmacologic targets. Long-acting muscarinic antagonists (LAMAs)

Funding: A.G. Mathioudakis, J. Vestbo and D. Singh are supported by the NIHR Manchester Biomedical Research Centre (BRC). The views expressed are those of the author(s) and not necessarily those of the NHS, the NIHR or the Department of Health.

[a] Division of Infection, Immunity and Respiratory Medicine, School of Biological Sciences, The University of Manchester, Manchester Academic Health Science Centre, UK; [b] North West Lung Centre, Wythenshawe Hospital, Manchester University NHS Foundation Trust, 2nd Floor ERC Building, Southmoor Road, Manchester M23 9LT, UK; [c] Medicines Evaluation Unit, Manchester, UK
* Corresponding author. Wythenshawe Hospital, 2nd Floor ERC Building, Southmoor Road, Manchester M23 9LT, UK.
E-mail address: jorgen.vestbo@manchester.ac.uk

Clin Chest Med 41 (2020) 463–474
https://doi.org/10.1016/j.ccm.2020.05.005
0272-5231/20/© 2020 Elsevier Inc. All rights reserved.

inhibit the action of acetylcholine at muscarinic receptors, whereas long-acting beta-2 adrenoreceptor agonists (LABAs) stimulate beta-2 adrenergic receptors, enhancing cyclic adenosine monophosphate pathway signaling.[3] Both LABAs and LAMAs mediate airway smooth muscle relaxation, exerting potent, prolonged bronchodilator effects, that are to some extent additive. Other beneficial effects of LABAs, mediated through their action on beta-adrenoreceptors in various cell types, include an enhanced mucociliary clearance and attenuation of the recruitment of neutrophils, of the release of mast cell mediators, and of the inhibition of smooth muscle cells proliferation.[4] Anti-inflammatory effects also are attributed to LAMAs that appear to inhibit airway neutrophilia, eosinophilia, MUC5AC expression, and fibrosis.[5,6] These anti-inflammatory effects, however, are supported only by in vitro studies and have not been proved in clinical trials in COPD.

This review (1) summarizes data on the safety and clinical efficacy/effectiveness of LABDs from systematic reviews, randomized controlled trials (RCTs), and real-life studies, and (2) describes their role in COPD management, as defined by current national and international clinical guidelines. Although narrative, this review is based on thorough searches of PubMed, the Cochrane Library, and Google Scholar for relevant RCTs, real-life studies, systematic reviews, and clinical practice guidelines.

SAFETY AND CLINICAL EFFECTIVENESS OF LONG-ACTING BRONCHODILATORS

Data on the safety and clinical effectiveness of LABAs, LAMAs, and dual combinations of a LABA and a LAMA are summarized in the following paragraphs and in **Fig. 1**. In preparation of this review, patient-important effectiveness outcomes, including mortality, frequency of exacerbations, quality of life, symptoms severity, and exercise tolerance, have been prioituized.[7] To a lesser extent, forced expiratory volume in the first second of expiration (FEV_1) has been included, which is a favored surrogate endpoint for regulators. FEV_1, a traditional lung function parameter that correlates with disease progression and mortality,[8] is related only weakly to patient-reported outcomes. Where good systematic reviews are used, information has been added on individual large trials with particular impact.

Minimal clinically important differences (MCIDs) have been defined for several of the outcomes. For patient-reported outcomes, however, it is well established that there is a marked placebo effect[9] and, therefore, treatment effects may be more

difficult to evaluate for these outcomes than for traditional physiologic measures. Responder analyses, describing the proportion of patients exceeding the MCIDs during the treatment period, are more appropriate measures and are used in this article.[10]

Reports from the ECLIPSE and other studies have demonstrated patients at risk of exacerbations have distinct clinical characteristics and a worse prognosis.[11] When possible, data are presented in this group of patients separately.

LONG-ACTING BETA-2 ADRENORECEPTOR AGONIST VERSUS PLACEBO

The safety and clinical efficacy of LABA versus placebo were evaluated in a Cochrane review of 26 RCTs, totaling 14,939 participants with moderate or severe airflow limitation.[12] The median treatment period was 6 months and only a small number of the studies were enriched with patients experiencing exacerbations. Overall, LABA monotherapy was found to improve quality of life as measured by the St. George's Respiratory Questionnaire (SGRQ), but the mean difference (MD −2.32 units [−3.09 to −1.54]) did not exceed the MCID of 4 units. LABAs also were associated with a decreased risk of moderate (odds ratio [OR] 0.73 [0.61–0.87]) and severe (OR 0.73 [0.56–0.95]) exacerbations. No impact was observed on the risk of mortality (OR 0.90 [0.75–1.08]) or severe adverse events (OR 0.97 [0.83–1.14]).

This Cochrane review did not include a responder analysis. Many of the older trials did not include such analyses. Newer trials demonstrated a significant proportion of responders in the LABA group compared with placebo.[13]

TRISTAN[14] (n=733, study duration of 12 months) and TORCH[15] (n = 3,087, 36 months) were the largest double-blind trials to compare salmeterol to placebo, whereas SHINE[16] (n = 584, 6 months) and INVOLVE[17] (n = 867, 12 months) compared formoterol to placebo. Apart from patient-important outcomes, they also evaluated FEV_1 longitudinally and demonstrated a decelerated FEV_1 decline rate over time (MD 13.0 mL [4.3–21.7] per year in the TORCH trial). Moreover, TRISTAN and SHINE recruited patients with a history of exacerbations, whereas the remaining trials were not enriched for exacerbations. Their results were consistent with the Cochrane review findings, confirming the efficacy of LABAs in this group of patients.

Newer LABA molecules (indacaterol, vilanterol, and olodaterol) have a duration of action that exceeds 24 hours and for this reason they can be administered once a day and, therefore, have

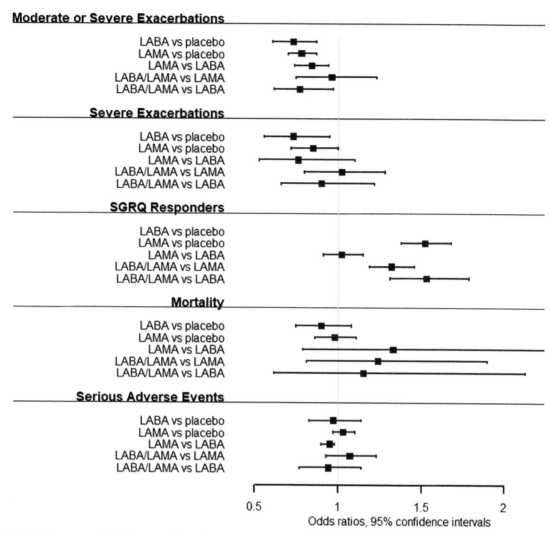

Fig. 1. Summary of the impact of bronchodilators on patient-important outcomes. (*Data from* Refs.[33,46,48,50])

been called ultra-LABAs. Their safety and efficacy profiles are comparable with the older LABAs.[17–22]

LONG-ACTING MUSCARINIC ANTAGONIST VERSUS PLACEBO

Tiotropium was for many years the only commercially available LAMA and, for this reason, it is the most thoroughly evaluated. Data from RCTs comparing tiotropium with placebo were pooled in a recent Cochrane meta-analysis of 22 RCTs with a study duration that varied between 3 months and 4 years (median: 6 months), with an overall population exceeding 23,000 participants.[23] Most RCTs were of good methodological quality and included patients with severe or very severe airflow limitation. Only 2 studies selected patients with a history of exacerbations. Tiotropium was

associated with a decrease in the number of patients experiencing 1 or more moderate or severe exacerbations (OR 0.78 [0.70–0.87]) or severe exacerbations (OR 0.85 [0.72–1.00]). It also was associated with an improved quality of life, evaluated by the SGRQ (MD −2.89 units [−3.35 to −2.44]). Although the MD did not exceed the MCID of 4 units, the number of participants that experienced such a positive change was higher in the tiotropium group (OR 1.52 [1.38–1.68]). Tiotropium did not appear to decrease mortality (OR 0.98 [0.86–1.11]). From a safety perspective, it was not associated with increased risk of serious adverse events.

Aclidinium, a newer LAMA compound, was evaluated in another Cochrane review, based on 12 good-quality RCTs, involving 9547 participants with moderate or severe COPD, not necessarily exacerbators, who were followed for 4 weeks to 52 weeks.[24] Compared with placebo, aclidinium was found to decrease the proportion of severe exacerbations (OR 0.64 [0.46–0.88]), whereas there also was a trend over decreased proportion of moderate exacerbations (OR 0.88 [0.74–1.04]). It also increased the number of people who achieved a clinically meaningful improvement in their quality of life (OR 1.49 [1.31–1.7]) but did not appear to affect mortality (OR 0.92 [0.43–1.94]) or the risk of serious adverse events.

Similar results also were found for umeclidinium, which was evaluated in 4 studies of 12 weeks' to 52 weeks' duration and good methodological quality, involving 3798 participants with COPD.[25] Umeclidinium decreased the proportion of participants experiencing at least 1 moderate or severe exacerbation (OR 0.61 [0.46–0.80]) and increased the number of people who achieved a clinically meaningful improvement (SGRQ; OR 1.45 [1.16–1.82]), although it was not associated with frequent serious adverse events (OR 1.33 [0.89–2.00]). Umeclidinium did not appear, however, to have an impact on the number of participants experiencing severe exacerbations (OR 0.86 [0.25–2.92]).

Tiotropium did not reduce the rate of decline in FEV_1 in the UPLIFT trial.[26] The TIE-COPD trial (n = 841) evaluated longitudinal impact of tiotropium on FEV_1 decline over 24 months, in patients with mild or moderate airflow limitation[27] and demonstrated a decrease in post-bronchodilator FEV_1 decline rate (22 mLs preserved per year [6–37]; P = .006) and a trend over decreased pre-bronchodilator FEV_1 decline rate (15 mLs [−1, 31] per year; P = .06). The conflicting results between the 2 trials might be explained by the earlier spirometric stage of the TIE-COPD participants, because FEV_1 decline is more pronounced during earlier stages of COPD and, therefore, more amenable to therapeutic interventions.[28] The impact of LAMAs on mortality has been evaluated extensively, although none of the available RCTs was powered to identify a potential survival benefit. A focused meta-analyses of 28 RCTs involving greater than 33,500 participants, who were followed between 6 weeks and 4 years, evaluated the impact of tiotropium versus placebo or any control on mortality.[26] Data from all available studies were homogeneous and suggested tiotropium may be associated with a significant decrease in all-cause mortality (relative risk [RR] 0.86 [0.76–0.98]). This positive result was driven mainly from the UPLIFT trial, which recruited approximately 6000 participants, who were followed for 4 years,[29] because all remaining studies had significantly more limited study population, duration, and fatalities. Decreased mortality associated with LAMAs also was observed in several extensive, well-conducted, real-life studies.[30–34] Currently available evidence, however, cannot confidently confirm this hypothesis.

LONG-ACTING BETA-2 AGONIST VERSUS LONG-ACTING MUSCARINIC ANTAGONIST

The comparative safety and efficacy of LAMA versus LABA were evaluated in a meta-analysis of 16 good-quality RCTs involving 22,872 participants, who were followed between 12 weeks and 52 weeks.[35] Similar to other RCTs evaluating LABAs or LAMAs as monotherapies, exacerbations history rarely were considered inclusion criteria. LAMAs achieved a greater decrease in the rate of moderate or severe exacerbations (OR 0.84 [0.74–0.94]) and were associated with a lower risk of adverse events (OR 0.92 [0.86–0.97]) compared with LABA. No significant differences were observed in quality-of-life measures, transitional dyspnea index, or the trough FEV_1.

The POET-COPD and INVIGORATE trials compared LAMA versus LABA among patients experiencing exacerbations. The POET-COPD study, a 1-year trial involving 7384 patients, compared tiotropium with salmeterol.[36] Compared with salmeterol, tiotropium increased the time to first moderate or severe exacerbation (187 days vs 145 days, respectively; hazard ratio [HR] 0.83 [0.77–0.90]) and the time to first severe exacerbation (HR 0.72 [0.61–0.85]). It also decreased the frequency of moderate or severe (RR 0.89 [0.83–0.96]) and severe (RR 0.73 [0.66–0.82]) exacerbations, compared with salmeterol. The INVIGORATE trial compared tiotropium with the ultra-LABA indacaterol and found the latter to have a noninferior impact on trough FEV_1, health status (SGRQ), or the degree of dyspnea (TDI total score). Time to first exacerbation, however, was longer with tiotropium (HR 1.20 [0.73–1.33]) and indacaterol was associated with a higher rate of exacerbations (RR 1.24 [1.12–1.37]).

LONG-ACTING BETA-2 AGONIST/LONG-ACTING MUSCARINIC ANTAGONIST VERSUS MONOCOMPONENTS

Results of early studies evaluating the combination of tiotropium with a LABA as 2 separate inhalers versus the monocomponents were pooled in a Cochrane review of 10 good-quality RCTs, evaluating 10,894 participants.[37] The addition of a LABA to tiotropium was associated with an increase in the proportion of patients achieving the

MCID for SGRQ (OR 1.32 [1.19–1.46]) and a small increase in the trough FEV_1 [MD 0.06 L [0.05–0.07]). No differences were observed in the rate of severe exacerbations, hospitalization for any cause, or mortality. The addition of tiotropium to a LABA led to an increase in the proportion of patients achieving the MCID for SGRQ (OR 1.53 [1.31–1.79]) and in the trough FEV_1 (MD 0.07 L [0.06–0.09]) but did not appear to have a significant impact on the rate of severe exacerbations, hospital admission for any cause, or mortality. Newer meta-analyses, involving more RCTs, have confirmed these findings and also suggest that the addition of a LAMA to a LABA might lead to a significant decrease in the proportion of patients experiencing an exacerbation (OR 0.77 [0.62–0.97]).[38–40]

The addition of a LAMA to a LABA in patients at risk of exacerbations has not been evaluated in any trials, whereas only 3 trials (DYNAGITO,[41] SPARK,[42] and ISRCTN29870041[43]) have tested the addition of LABA to a LAMA in this population. In the DYNAGITO trial, comparing the combination of tiotropium with olodaterol versus tiotropium monotherapy in more than 9000 participants,[41] dual bronchodilator therapy was not associated with a decreased rate of moderate or severe exacerbations at the prospectively targeted 0.01 significance level (RR 0.93; 99% CI [0.85–1.02]; $P = .05$). In addition, it failed to demonstrate a decrease in the frequency of severe exacerbations (RR 0.89; 95% CI [0.78–1.02]) or a prolongation in the time to the first severe and moderate or severe exacerbation. Similar findings were observed in the SPARK trial, where the combination of indacaterol with glycopyrronium was compared with glycopyrronium monotherapy or tiotropium monotherapy in 741 participants.[42] Dual bronchodilation therapy was associated with a small but statistically significant decrease in the rate of moderate or severe exacerbations compared with glycopyrronium (RR 0.88 [0.77–0.99]) and only a trend over decreased exacerbations rate compared with tiotropium (RR 0.90 [0.79–1.02]). Moreover, compared with LAMA monotherapies, dual bronchodilation did not appear to decrease the rate of severe exacerbations. Similar results also were observed in the ISRCTN29870041 study.[43] These findings suggest that a LABA/LAMA combination is likely to have only a modest impact on the frequency of moderate or severe exacerbations compared with LAMA monotherapy.

This observation is validated further by a well-designed real-life study from the Optum research database.[44] This study comparing the impact of dual bronchodilator therapy versus LABA or LAMA monotherapies (mostly LAMA), involved 2572 participants and used propensity score matching to improve the comparability of the participants. Dual therapy was not associated with decreased risk of moderate or severe exacerbations but only with a modestly decreased risk of exacerbations leading to hospitalization.

Early introduction of a LAMA/LABA combination over monocomponents has been evaluated in several RCTs. A post hoc analysis of the ACLIFORM COPD[45] and AUGMENT[46] trials evaluated the introduction of aclidinium/formoterol compared with the monocomponents or placebo in 1056 treatment-naïve patients with COPD and moderate or severe airflow limitation.[47] LABA/LAMA combination was associated with a modest improvement in quality-of-life and symptoms scores that did not exceed the MCID and improved postdose FEV_1 compared with all comparators. In addition, the combination also improved trough FEV_1 compared with LABA monotherapy or placebo. The role of LABA/LAMA combination for patients with a significant symptoms burden but no history of frequent exacerbations and no background inhaled corticosteroid (ICS) use was prospectively evaluated in the EMAX trial, which compared the efficacy of the combination of umeclidinium and vilanterol versus umeclidinium and salmeterol monotherapies.[48] LABA/LAMA combination led to an increase in trough FEV_1 compared with LAMA (MD 66 mL [43–89]) and LABA (MD 141 mL [118–164]) monotherapy. It also was associated with an improved TDI total score compared with LAMA (MD 0.37 [0.06–0.68]) and LABA (MD 0.45 [0.15–0.76]), which did not, however, exceed the MCID. In the TDI responder analysis, LABA/LAMA combination was superior to LAMA (OR 1.43 [1.17–1.75]) and LABA (OR 1.48 [1.21–1.81]). Exacerbations frequency and incidence of severe adverse events were similar in all groups. Overall, in this group of patients, addition of a second bronchodilator may limit the burden of respiratory symptoms to some extent, without posing an additional risk of adverse events.

LONG-ACTING MUSCARINIC ANTAGONIST VERSUS LONG-ACTING BETA-2 AGONIST/INHALED CORTICOSTEROID

Few RCTs have compared the combination of LABA/ICS with a LAMA. Pooled results of 2 RCTs of unclear methodological quality, comparing once-daily administration of LABA/ICS versus LAMA, involving 880 participants, did not reveal any between-treatment difference on the rate of exacerbations, mortality, risk of pneumonia, or quality of life.[49]

Twice-daily administration of fluticasone/salmeterol versus once-daily tiotropium was compared in the INSPIRE trial, a 2-year RCT involving 1323 participants with severe airflow limitation and a clinical history of COPD exacerbations.[50] Although no difference was found on the annual rate of moderate or severe exacerbations (RR 0.97 [0.84–1.12]), LABA/ICS was associated with a decrease in SGRQ total score (MD 2.1 units [0.1–4.0]), with a corresponding increase in the proportion of participants achieving the MCID (OR 1.30 [1.05–1.61]) compared with LAMA. From a safety perspective, LABA/ICS was associated with an increased risk of pneumonia (HR 1.94 [1.19–3.17]), but lower risk of death (RR 0.56 [0.33–0.94]).

These findings need to be interpreted with caution because COPD is a heterogeneous disease and patients have a differential response to ICS. Several studies have demonstrated ICS are effective only for patients with higher blood eosinophil count[51,52] and this was not accounted for. Accordingly, a post hoc analysis of the INSPIRE trial suggested superiority of LABA/ICS in reducing the rate of moderate or severe exacerbations in patients with blood eosinophils of greater than or equal to 2% of total white cell count at presentation (25% reduction [8% to 40%]) and a trend toward inferiority of LABA/ICS in the remaining patients (18% increase [−8% to 51%]).[53]

LONG-ACTING BETA-2 AGONIST/LONG-ACTING MUSCARINIC ANTAGONIST VERSUS LONG-ACTING BETA-2 AGONIST/INHALED CORTICOSTEROID

The Cochrane review comparing LABA/LAMA versus LABA/ICS combinations included 11 RCTs of good methodological quality, comprising 9839 participants.[54] Study duration varied between 6 weeks and 52 weeks. Only 1 of the included studies was enriched in patients experiencing exacerbations. Compared with LABA/ICS, LAMA/LAMA led to a decrease in the proportion of patients who experienced at least 1 moderate or severe exacerbation (OR 0.82 [0.70–0.96]) and the risk of pneumonia (OR 0.57 [0.42–0.79]). More people receiving LABA/LAMA achieved the MCID in SGRQ (OR 1.25 [1.09–1.44]), whereas there were no significant between group differences in the risk of serious adverse events or all-cause mortality.

An important limitation of this review and the included RCTs is that they did not account for the presence of airway eosinophilic inflammation, a trait that is known to be associated with ICS treatment response.[55] A post hoc analysis from the FLAME,[56,57] the largest of the included RCTs

(n = 3362), explored if blood eosinophils could predict treatment response. LABA/LAMA combination was more effective than LABA/ICS in preventing exacerbations (all severities, or moderate or severe) at lower eosinophil counts, whereas there was no treatment difference at higher eosinophil counts.[50] Contrasting findings were reported in a prespecified analysis from the IMPACT trial, where LABA/LAMA were compared with LABA/ICS for 1 year in 6204 participants.[58,59] LABA/LAMA was more effective than LABA/ICS in reducing the rate of exacerbations among patients with lower blood eosinophil counts, whereas LABA/ICS was more effective among patients with a higher eosinophil count. Differences in the inclusion criteria of the trials may be partly responsible for these differences. Importantly, IMPACT included more patients with 2 exacerbations in the previous year (54% vs 19%, respectively) compared with FLAME; this suggests that the effects of ICS are increased in patients at higher exacerbation risk. Additionally, FLAME excluded patients with any asthmatic characteristics (including those with a current or previous history of asthma, any other respiratory disease or symptoms prior to the age of 40, very high eosinophils, and allergic rhinitis), who are more likely to respond to ICS. On the contrary, IMPACT only excluded subjects with a current diagnosis of asthma. In addition, FLAME included a run-in period of 1 month, whereas all participants were receiving only tiotropium. Patients who potentially could benefit from ICS might have experienced a disease deterioration during this period, potentially leading to a discontinuation and exclusion from the trial.

IMPACT OF BRONCHODILATORS ON DYNAMIC HYPERINFLATION AND EXERCISE PERFORMANCE

Several trials have evaluated the impact of dual bronchodilation on exercise performance. MORACTO 1 and MORACTO 2, two replicate, double-blind, 6-week crossover trials involving 585 patients with moderate or severe airflow limitation, assessed the impact of the combination of tiotropium with olodaterol compared with the monocomponents or placebo.[60] Compared with placebo, exercise endurance time during constant work-rate cycle ergometry was improved by all active treatments: LAMA (MD 65.60 seconds [63.94–67.26]), LABA (MD 50.50 seconds [48.83–52.17]), and LABA/LAMA combination (MD 83.90 seconds [82.25–85.55]). Tiotropium also improved exercise endurance time compared with olodaterol (MD 15.10 seconds [13.44, 16.76]). Finally,

LABA/LAMA combination significantly improved the exercise endurance time 5.6% compared with olodaterol (MD 33.4 seconds [31.75–35.05]), but no significant difference was observed between LABA/LAMA and LAMA monotherapy.

Change in the inspiratory capacity from baseline was used to evaluate the impact of treatments on hyperinflation. LABA/LAMA combination was superior to LAMA (MD 87 mL [34–141]), LABA (MD 92 mL [38–145]), and placebo (MD 218 mL [164–271]). LABA and LAMA monotherapies also were superior to placebo.

Two other 12-week trials involving 657 patients with moderate or severe airflow limitation (NCT01323660 and NCT01328444) assessed the impact of the combination of indacaterol with glycopyrronium compared with the monocomponents or placebo on exercise tolerance.[61] Dual bronchodilation initially appeared to significantly improve exercise endurance time compared with placebo. This effect was not maintained at 12 weeks, however, mainly because of a significant treatment effect in the placebo group.

An 8-week study comparing aclidinium/formoterol to placebo, the ACTIVATE trial, also included a behavioral intervention for all participants, aiming at enhancing their exercise endurance.[62] In this trial, LABA/LAMA combination achieved a maintained improvement in exercise tolerance, demonstrated by 55.2 seconds' ($P = .03$) increase in the exercise endurance time, daily activity (treatment difference of 731 steps per day; $P = .002$), trough FEV_1, and different measures of lung hyperinflation. The behavioral intervention might have been the key success factor in the ACTIVATE trial. More specifically, the challenge in these studies often is that patients are deconditioned and, unless exercise is trained and maintained along treatment initiation and/or escalation, it will be difficult to translate any improvement in lung function into an effect on exercise capacity.

BRONCHODILATORS AND COMORBIDITIES

Although the safety of LABAs and LAMAs has been confirmed in numerous RCTs, there still is ongoing discussion regarding their cardiovascular safety, owing to their mechanisms of action. As a result, cardiovascular safety was evaluated in a meta-analysis involving 43 RCTs, which did not find any association between cardiovascular death and the use of LAMA (RR 0.92 [0.81–1.04]), LABA (RR 0.93 [0.75–1.15]), or LAMA/LABA combination (RR 1.03 [0.38–2.80]).[63] No impact on the frequency of overall cardiovascular adverse events was found either. Use of LABA appeared

associated with an increased risk of cardiac failure (RR 1.71 [1.04–2.84]).

Cardiovascular safety of introducing a second LABD for COPD was evaluated in a real-life study from the UK Clinical Practice Research Datalink, involving 62,348 patients receiving single or dual bronchodilators, who were matched using high-dimensional propensity scores.[64] Adding a second LABD was associated with a small increase in the risk of heart failure (HR 1.16 [1.03–1.30]), but it did not have an impact on the risk of myocardial infarction, stroke or any arrhythmia. The increase in the risk of heart failure was confined to the subgroup where patients receiving LABA/LAMA were compared with matched patients receiving LAMA monotherapy (HR 1.28 [1.07–1.54]).

Moreover, cardiovascular safety of LABAs versus LAMAs was compared in 52,884 propensity matched patients with COPD from the same database.[65] There were no significant differences in the risk of myocardial infarction, stroke, or arrhythmia, but there was a trend over increased risk of heart failure associated with the use of LABAs. The LABA population, however, included in these 2 real-life observational studies was overlapping. Therefore, the results of these studies were not independent and could have been driven by an unexpectedly high risk of heart failure in the included LABA population.

These findings were not confirmed, however, in SUMMIT, an extensive RCT of 16,590 participants with COPD and heightened cardiovascular risk, where the combination of fluticasone furoate and vilanterol was compared with the monocomponents and placebo.[66,67] This RCT, specifically designed to evaluate the cardiovascular safety, did not reveal between-group differences in cardiovascular outcomes, including sudden death, acute coronary syndrome, arrhythmia, cardiac failure, stroke, transient ischemic attack, or any adverse cardiovascular event. More specifically, heart failure was reported in 4% of the participants who received the LABA vilanterol and in 5% of the participants in the placebo group.

Overall, cardiovascular safety of LABA, LAMA, and LABA/LAMA combination is strongly supported by these findings. The potential association between LABA and heart failure found in some studies is more likely the result of type 1 statistical error.

FACTORS TO BE CONSIDERED WHEN CHOOSING MOLECULES AND DEVICES

There now are a wide range of different LABD molecules available for clinicians to choose from, administered though different inhaler devices.

Although this offers patient choice, allowing individuals to choose a suitable inhaler device, it also poses challenges to clinicians faced with making optimum treatment recommendations. Once a clinician has decided on the class of drug to be prescribed (eg, a LAMA), then the choice of molecule and inhaler device has to be made. This should be done based on considerations of efficacy, safety, once-a-day versus twice-a-day dosing, inhaler device characteristics, and local cost issues.

In general, there is little to differentiate between molecules within a class when considering efficacy and safety. There is evidence that indacaterol has greater efficacy than twice-a-day LABAs.[17,68,69] The reported differences, however, between other molecules within a class are small; for example, a 12-week study comparing tiotropium and umeclidinium reported a 53-mL difference in trough FEV_1 in favor of the latter but without any treatment differences in symptom scores.[70] Similarly, the combination treatment umeclidinium/vilanterol caused a 52-mL greater trough FEV_1 increase compared with tiotropium/olodaterol but again with no differences in symptoms.[71]

The profile of bronchodilation over 24 hours caused by once-a-day versus twice-a-day LABDs is different.[72] Accordingly, the choice of LABDs may be tailored to individual patient choice based on requirements for additional bronchodilation in the evening. This may be important particularly for patients who suffer with respiratory symptoms at night or in the early morning.

Perhaps the most important consideration when making a choice within LABD drug class is the selection of inhaler device. In general, pressurized metered dose inhalers require more coordination of operation and inhalation but are not dependent on the inspiratory flow generated. In contrast, breath-activated dry powder inhalers are difficult for some patients to use because they cannot reach the required inspiratory flow rates.

In summary, the choice of drug within LABD class should be driven mainly by tailoring treatment to individual needs regarding inhaler type and the suitability of once-a-day versus twice-a-day delivery. This is influenced by local cost issues.

PLACE OF LONG-ACTING BRONCHODILATORS IN GUIDELINES AND THE CLINICAL PRACTICE

In the strategy document from the Global Initiative for Chronic Obstructive Lung Disease (GOLD), the introduction of a single LABD followed by a dual combination of LABDs is recommended as the initial maintenance therapy for all patients, apart from those experiencing frequent exacerbations, who have raised blood eosinophils. An option to use a combination of LABDs as first line of treatment of patients with GOLD group B or group D with more severe symptoms also is offered. For these patients, early introduction of an ICS also may be considered. Overall, GOLD recommends LABDs as the mainstay of COPD treatment of all patients experiencing symptoms and/or exacerbations.

The Australian and New Zealand guidelines (COPD-X) follow a similar approach, suggesting the use of a LABD in case short-acting bronchodilators are insufficient, with LABA/LAMA combination the next step.[73] A combination of a LABA with an ICS without the addition of a LAMA is suggested as only an option in cases of severe airflow limitation (FEV_1 <50% predicted), with frequent exacerbations, although the associated risks of pneumonia and inferiority of LABA/ICS in reducing the frequency of exacerbations are highlighted.

The National Institute for Health and Care Excellence (NICE), in the United Kingdom, recommends the introduction of a LABA/LAMA combination for all patients who do not have asthmatic features and experience symptoms or exacerbations, despite using a short-acting bronchodilator as needed.[74] This contrasts with previous guidelines suggesting a step-up approach, starting from a single bronchodilator, and may appear counterintuitive, given that many patients respond well to a single LABD. Given their demonstrated safety, even a modest effect of adding a second bronchodilator is considered acceptable probably because the costs of LAMA monotherapy and dual bronchodilation therapy are similar and NICE recommendations are based on cost-effectiveness analyses. Despite the positive group level data, however, there is a wide variability between individual patients in the magnitude of clinical response to LABDs.[75] Therefore, in real life, not every patient gains benefit from the introduction of a second LABD and it still is not clear which individuals would benefit. Moreover, patients with mild airflow limitation, many of whom are classified in GOLD group A, have not been included in any of the trials evaluating dual bronchodilator combinations; thus, the evidence base supporting treatment decisions is thin in this group. Overall, based on currently available evidence, a stepwise approach might be more appropriate. For patients exerting asthmatic features, NICE recommends the use of LABA/ICS combination. Asthmatic features are defined as a confirmed diagnosis of asthma or atopy, higher blood eosinophil count, a substantial variation of FEV_1 over time or substantial diurnal variation in the peak expiratory flow. Many of these criteria appear arbitrary and have not been tested in RCTs; only blood eosinophil counts have evidence that supports prediction of ICS effects.

Spanish guidelines (GesEPOC) also suggest the use of single or dual bronchodilators as first-line treatment of the majority of patients with COPD.[76] LABA/ICS combination is recommended as a first-line treatment for those with asthma-COPD overlap.

SUMMARY

The management of COPD should be guided by patients' symptoms and exacerbations. LABA, LAMA, and their combinations represent safe and effective options for maintenance therapy. Introduction of a single LABD should be considered the first step in the maintenance treatment of all patients, apart from those with more severe symptoms and frequent exacerbations (GOLD group D). Compared with a LABA, a LAMA is more effective in preventing exacerbations, and, for this reason, LABA monotherapy should be avoided in patients experiencing frequent exacerbations. The threshold for adding a second LABD should be low because dual bronchodilator therapy has shown greater effect on lung function and quality of life and an excellent safety profile. The most important consideration when making a choice within a LABD drug class is the selection of inhaler device and clinicians must devote adequate time to demonstrate use of the inhaler device and periodically check and reinforce the correct technique.

DISCLOSURE

A.G. Mathioudakis has received grant support from Boehringer-Ingelheim. J. Vestbo has received personal fees from AstraZeneca, Boehringer-Ingelheim, Chiesi, GSK, and Novartis and grant support from Boehringer-Ingelheim. D. Singh has received personal fees from AstraZeneca, Boehringer Ingelheim, Chiesi, Cipla, Genentech, Glenmark, GSK, Menarini, Mundipharma, Novartis, Peptinnovate, Pfizer, Pulmatrix, Theravance, and Verona and grant support from AstraZeneca, Boehringer Ingelheim, Chiesi, Glenmark, Menarini, Mundipharma, Novartis, Pfizer, Pulmatrix, Theravance, and Verona.

REFERENCES

1. Vogelmeier CF, Criner GJ, Martinez FJ, et al. Global strategy for the diagnosis, management, and prevention of chronic obstructive lung disease 2017 report: GOLD executive summary. Eur Respir J 2017;53:128–49.

2. Barnes PJ, Burney PG, Silverman EK, et al. Chronic obstructive pulmonary disease. Nat Rev Dis Primers 2015;1:15076.

3. Singh D. New combination bronchodilators for chronic obstructive pulmonary disease: current evidence and future perspectives. Br J Clin Pharmacol 2015;79:695–708.

4. Ejiofor S, Turner AM. Pharmacotherapies for COPD. Clin Med Insights Circ Respir Pulm Med 2013;7: 17–34.

5. Pera T, Zuidhof A, Valadas J, et al. Tiotropium inhibits pulmonary inflammation and remodelling in a Guinea pig model of COPD. Eur Respir J 2011;38:789–96.

6. Buels KS, Jacoby DB, Fryer AD. Non-bronchodilating mechanisms of tiotropium prevent airway hyperreactivity in a Guinea-pig model of allergic asthma. Br J Pharmacol 2012;165:1501–14.

7. Zhang Y, Morgan RL, Alonso-Coello P, et al. A systematic review of how patients value COPD outcomes. Eur Respir J 2018;52:1800222.

8. Schunemann HJ, Dorn J, Grant BJ, et al. Pulmonary function is a long-term predictor of mortality in the general population: 29-year follow-up of the Buffalo Health Study. Chest 2000;118:656–64.

9. Hrobjartsson A, Gotzsche PC. Placebo interventions for all clinical conditions. Cochrane Database Syst Rev 2010;(1):CD003974.

10. Zysman M, Chabot F, Devillier P, et al. Pharmacological treatment optimization for stable chronic obstructive pulmonary disease. Proposals from the Societe de Pneumologie de Langue Francaise. Rev Mal Respir 2016;33:911–36.

11. Hurst JR, Vestbo J, Anzueto A, et al. Susceptibility to exacerbation in chronic obstructive pulmonary disease. N Engl J Med 2010;363:1128–38.

12. Kew KM, Mavergames C, Walters JA. Long-acting beta2-agonists for chronic obstructive pulmonary disease. Cochrane Database Syst Rev 2013;(10): CD010177.

13. Bogdan MA, Aizawa H, Fukuchi Y, et al. Efficacy and safety of inhaled formoterol 4.5 and 9 mug twice daily in Japanese and European COPD patients: phase III study results. BMC Pulm Med 2011;11:51.

14. Calverley P, Pauwels R, Vestbo J, et al. Combined salmeterol and fluticasone in the treatment of chronic obstructive pulmonary disease: a randomised controlled trial. Lancet 2003;361:449–56.

15. Calverley PM, Anderson JA, Celli B, et al. Salmeterol and fluticasone propionate and survival in chronic obstructive pulmonary disease. N Engl J Med 2007;356:775–89.

16. Tashkin DP, Rennard SI, Martin P, et al. Efficacy and safety of budesonide and formoterol in one pressurized metered-dose inhaler in patients with moderate

to very severe chronic obstructive pulmonary disease: results of a 6-month randomized clinical trial. Drugs 2008;68:1975–2000.

17. Dahl R, Chung KF, Buhl R, et al. Efficacy of a new once-daily long-acting inhaled beta2-agonist indacaterol versus twice-daily formoterol in COPD. Thorax 2010;65:473–9.

18. Ferguson GT, Feldman GJ, Hofbauer P, et al. Efficacy and safety of olodaterol once daily delivered via Respimat(R) in patients with GOLD 2-4 COPD: results from two replicate 48-week studies. Int J Chron Obstruct Pulmon Dis 2014;9:629–45.

19. Koch A, Pizzichini E, Hamilton A, et al. Lung function efficacy and symptomatic benefit of olodaterol once daily delivered via Respimat(R) versus placebo and formoterol twice daily in patients with GOLD 2-4 COPD: results from two replicate 48-week studies. Int J Chron Obstruct Pulmon Dis 2014;9:697–714.

20. Martinez FJ, Boscia J, Feldman G, et al. Fluticasone furoate/vilanterol (100/25; 200/25 mug) improves lung function in COPD: a randomised trial. Respir Med 2013;107:550–9.

21. Dransfield MT, Bourbeau J, Jones PW, et al. Once-daily inhaled fluticasone furoate and vilanterol versus vilanterol only for prevention of exacerbations of COPD: two replicate double-blind, parallel-group, randomised controlled trials. Lancet Respir Med 2013;1:210–23.

22. Geake JB, Dabscheck EJ, Wood-Baker R, et al. Indacaterol, a once-daily beta2-agonist, versus twice-daily beta(2)-agonists or placebo for chronic obstructive pulmonary disease. Cochrane Database Syst Rev 2015;(1):CD010139.

23. Karner C, Chong J, Poole P. Tiotropium versus placebo for chronic obstructive pulmonary disease. Cochrane Database Syst Rev 2014;(7):CD009285.

24. Ni H, Soe Z, Moe S. Aclidinium bromide for stable chronic obstructive pulmonary disease. Cochrane Database Syst Rev 2014;(9):CD010509.

25. Ni H, Htet A, Moe S. Umeclidinium bromide versus placebo for people with chronic obstructive pulmonary disease (COPD). Cochrane Database Syst Rev 2017;(6):CD011897.

26. Mathioudakis AG, Kanavidis P, Chatzimavridou-Grigoriadou V, et al. Tiotropium HandiHaler improves the survival of patients with COPD: a systematic review and meta-analysis. J Aerosol Med Pulm Drug Deliv 2014;27:43–50.

27. Zhou Y, Zhong NS, Li X, et al. Tiotropium in early-stage chronic obstructive pulmonary disease. N Engl J Med 2017;377:923–35.

28. Vestbo J, Edwards LD, Scanlon PD, et al. Changes in forced expiratory volume in 1 second over time in COPD. N Engl J Med 2011;365:1184–92.

29. Tashkin DP, Celli B, Senn S, et al. A 4-year trial of tiotropium in chronic obstructive pulmonary disease. N Engl J Med 2008;359:1543–54.

30. Lee TA, Wilke C, Joo M, et al. Outcomes associated with tiotropium use in patients with chronic obstructive pulmonary disease. Arch Intern Med 2009;169: 1403–10.

31. Verhamme KM, Afonso AS, van Noord C, et al. Tiotropium Handihaler and the risk of cardio- or cerebrovascular events and mortality in patients with COPD. Pulm Pharmacol Ther 2012;25:19–26.

32. Short PM, Williamson PA, Elder DHJ, et al. The impact of tiotropium on mortality and exacerbations when added to inhaled corticosteroids and long-acting beta-agonist therapy in COPD. Chest 2012; 141:81–6 {Short, 2012 #1679}.

33. Gershon AS, Wang L, To T, et al. Survival with tiotropium compared to long-acting beta-2-agonists in chronic obstructive pulmonary disease. COPD 2008;5:229–34.

34. Rebordosa C, Aguado J, Plana E, et al. Use of aclidinium did not increase the risk of death in a noninterventional cohort study in the Clinical Practice Research Datalink (CPRD), United Kingdom. Respir Med 2019;152:37–43.

35. Chen WC, Huang CH, Sheu CC, et al. Long-acting beta2-agonists versus long-acting muscarinic antagonists in patients with stable COPD: a systematic review and meta-analysis of randomized controlled trials. Respirology 2017;22:1313–9.

36. Vogelmeier C, Hederer B, Glaab T, et al. Tiotropium versus salmeterol for the prevention of exacerbations of COPD. N Engl J Med 2011;364:1093–103.

37. Farne HA, Cates CJ. Long-acting beta2-agonist in addition to tiotropium versus either tiotropium or long-acting beta2-agonist alone for chronic obstructive pulmonary disease. Cochrane Database Syst Rev 2015;(10):CD008989.

38. Miravitlles M, Urrutia G, Mathioudakis AG, et al. Efficacy and safety of tiotropium and olodaterol in COPD: a systematic review and meta-analysis. Respir Res 2017;18:196.

39. Oba Y, Keeney E, Ghatehorde N, et al. Dual combination therapy versus long-acting bronchodilators alone for chronic obstructive pulmonary disease (COPD): a systematic review and network meta-analysis. Cochrane Database Syst Rev 2018;(12): CD012620.

40. Ni H, Moe S, Soe Z, et al. Combined aclidinium bromide and long-acting beta2-agonist for chronic obstructive pulmonary disease (COPD). Cochrane Database Syst Rev 2018;(12):CD011594.

41. Calverley PMA, Anzueto AR, Carter K, et al. Tiotropium and olodaterol in the prevention of chronic obstructive pulmonary disease exacerbations (DYNAGITO): a double-blind, randomised, parallel-

group, active-controlled trial. Lancet Respir Med 2018;6:337–44.

42. Wedzicha JA, Decramer M, Ficker JH, et al. Analysis of chronic obstructive pulmonary disease exacerbations with the dual bronchodilator QVA149 compared with glycopyrronium and tiotropium (SPARK): a randomised, double-blind, parallel-group study. Lancet Respir Med 2013;1:199–209.

43. Aaron SD, Vandemheen KL, Fergusson D, et al. Tiotropium in combination with placebo, salmeterol, or fluticasone-salmeterol for treatment of chronic obstructive pulmonary disease: a randomized trial. Ann Intern Med 2007;146:545–55.

44. Strange C, Walker V, Tong J, et al. A retrospective claims analysis of dual bronchodilator fixed-dose combination versus bronchodilator monotherapy in patients with chronic obstructive pulmonary disease. Chronic Obstr Pulm Dis 2019;6:221–32.

45. Singh D, Jones PW, Bateman ED, et al. Efficacy and safety of aclidinium bromide/formoterol fumarate fixed-dose combinations compared with individual components and placebo in patients with COPD (ACLIFORM-COPD): a multicentre, randomised study. BMC Pulm Med 2014;14:178.

46. D'Urzo AD, Rennard SI, Kerwin EM, et al. Efficacy and safety of fixed-dose combinations of aclidinium bromide/formoterol fumarate: the 24-week, randomized, placebo-controlled AUGMENT COPD study. Respir Res 2014;15:123.

47. Singh D, D'Urzo AD, Donohue JF, et al. An evaluation of single and dual long-acting bronchodilator therapy as effective interventions in maintenance therapy-naive patients with COPD. Int J Chron Obstruct Pulmon Dis 2019;14:2835–48.

48. Maltais F, Bjermer L, Kerwin EM, et al. Efficacy of umeclidinium/vilanterol versus umeclidinium and salmeterol monotherapies in symptomatic patients with COPD not receiving inhaled corticosteroids: the EMAX randomised trial. Respir Res 2019;20:238.

49. Sliwka A, Jankowski M, Gross-Sondej I, et al. Once-daily long-acting beta(2)-agonists/inhaled corticosteroids combined inhalers versus inhaled long-acting muscarinic antagonists for people with chronic obstructive pulmonary disease. Cochrane Database Syst Rev 2018;(8):CD012355.

50. Wedzicha JA, Calverley PM, Seemungal TA, et al. The prevention of chronic obstructive pulmonary disease exacerbations by salmeterol/fluticasone propionate or tiotropium bromide. Am J Respir Crit Care Med 2008;177:19–26.

51. Siddiqui SH, Guasconi A, Vestbo J, et al. Blood eosinophils: a biomarker of response to extrafine beclomethasone/formoterol in chronic obstructive pulmonary disease. Am J Respir Crit Care Med 2015;192:523–5.

52. Mathioudakis AG, Bikov A, Foden P, et al. Change in blood eosinophils following treatment with inhaled corticosteroids may predict long-term clinical response in COPD. Eur Respir J 2020;55(5): 1902119.

53. Pavord ID, Lettis S, Locantore N, et al. Blood eosinophils and inhaled corticosteroid/long-acting beta-2 agonist efficacy in COPD. Thorax 2016;71: 118–25.

54. Horita N, Goto A, Shibata Y, et al. Long-acting muscarinic antagonist (LAMA) plus long-acting beta-agonist (LABA) versus LABA plus inhaled corticosteroid (ICS) for stable chronic obstructive pulmonary disease (COPD). Cochrane Database Syst Rev 2017;(2):CD012066.

55. Agusti A, Bel E, Thomas M, et al. Treatable traits: toward precision medicine of chronic airway diseases. Eur Respir J 2016;47:410–9.

56. Wedzicha JA, Banerji D, Chapman KR, et al. Indacaterol-glycopyrronium versus salmeterol-fluticasone for COPD. N Engl J Med 2016;374:2222–34.

57. Roche N, Chapman KR, Vogelmeier CF, et al. Blood eosinophils and response to maintenance chronic obstructive pulmonary disease treatment. Data from the FLAME trial. Am J Respir Crit Care Med 2017;195:1189–97.

58. Lipson DA, Barnhart F, Brealey N, et al. Once-daily single-inhaler triple versus dual therapy in patients with COPD. N Engl J Med 2018;378: 1671–80.

59. Pascoe S, Barnes N, Brusselle G, et al. Blood eosinophils and treatment response with triple and dual combination therapy in chronic obstructive pulmonary disease: analysis of the IMPACT trial. Lancet Respir Med 2019;7:745–56.

60. O'Donnell DE, Casaburi R, Frith P, et al. Effects of combined tiotropium/olodaterol on inspiratory capacity and exercise endurance in COPD. Eur Respir J 2017;49:1601348.

61. Maltais F, Singh S, Donald AC, et al. Effects of a combination of umeclidinium/vilanterol on exercise endurance in patients with chronic obstructive pulmonary disease: two randomized, double-blind clinical trials. Ther Adv Respir Dis 2014;8:169–81.

62. Watz H, Troosters T, Beeh KM, et al. ACTIVATE: the effect of aclidinium/formoterol on hyperinflation, exercise capacity, and physical activity in patients with COPD. Int J Chron Obstruct Pulmon Dis 2017; 12:2545–58.

63. Li C, Cheng W, Guo J, et al. Relationship of inhaled long-acting bronchodilators with cardiovascular outcomes among patients with stable COPD: a meta-analysis and systematic review of 43 randomized trials. Int J Chron Obstruct Pulmon Dis 2019;14: 799–808.

64. Suissa S, Dell'Aniello S, Ernst P. Concurrent use of long-acting bronchodilators in COPD and the risk of adverse cardiovascular events. Eur Respir J 2017;49:1602245.

65. Suissa S, Dell'Aniello S, Ernst P. Long-acting bronchodilator initiation in COPD and the risk of adverse cardiopulmonary events: a population-based comparative safety study. Chest 2017;151:60–7.

66. Vestbo J, Anderson JA, Brook RD, et al. Fluticasone furoate and vilanterol and survival in chronic obstructive pulmonary disease with heightened cardiovascular risk (SUMMIT): a double-blind randomised controlled trial. Lancet 2016;387:1817–26.

67. Brook RD, Anderson JA, Calverley PM, et al. Cardiovascular outcomes with an inhaled beta2-agonist/corticosteroid in patients with COPD at high cardiovascular risk. Heart 2017;103:1536–42.

68. Kornmann O, Dahl R, Centanni S, et al. Once-daily indacaterol versus twice-daily salmeterol for COPD: a placebo-controlled comparison. Eur Respir J 2011;37:273–9.

69. Korn S, Kerwin E, Atis S, et al. Indacaterol once-daily provides superior efficacy to salmeterol twice-daily in COPD: a 12-week study. Respir Med 2011;105:719–26.

70. Feldman G, Maltais F, Khindri S, et al. A randomized, blinded study to evaluate the efficacy and safety of umeclidinium 62.5 mug compared with tiotropium 18 mug in patients with COPD. Int J Chron Obstruct Pulmon Dis 2016;11:719–30.

71. Feldman GJ, Sousa AR, Lipson DA, et al. Comparative efficacy of once-daily umeclidinium/vilanterol and tiotropium/olodaterol therapy in symptomatic chronic obstructive pulmonary disease: a randomized study. Adv Ther 2017;34:2518–33.

72. Fuhr R, Magnussen H, Sarem K, et al. Efficacy of aclidinium bromide 400 mug twice daily compared with placebo and tiotropium in patients with moderate to severe COPD. Chest 2012;141:745–52.

73. Yang IA, Brown JL, George J, et al. COPD-X Australian and New Zealand guidelines for the diagnosis and management of chronic obstructive pulmonary disease: 2017 update. Med J Aust 2017;207:436–42.

74. National Institute for Health and Care Excellence (NICE). Chronic obstructive pulmonary disease in over 16s: diagnosis and management. NICE guideline [NG115]. 2018. Available at: https://www.nice.org.uk/guidance/ng115. Accessed June 28, 2020.

75. Donohue JF, Singh D, Munzu C, et al. Magnitude of umeclidinium/vilanterol lung function effect depends on monotherapy responses: results from two randomised controlled trials. Respir Med 2016;112:65–74.

76. Miravitlles M, Soler-Cataluna JJ, Calle M, et al. Spanish guidelines for management of chronic obstructive pulmonary disease (GesEPOC) 2017. Pharmacological treatment of stable phase. Arch Bronconeumol 2017;53:324–35.

Inhaled Corticosteroids in Chronic Obstructive Pulmonary Disease
Benefits and Risks

Takudzwa Mkorombindo, MD[a], Mark T. Dransfield, MD[b],*

KEYWORDS

- Inhaled corticosteroids • COPD • Pneumonia • Exacerbations

KEY POINTS

- Inhaled corticosteroids (ICSs) should not be prescribed as monotherapy in chronic obstructive pulmonary disease (COPD).
- Combination therapy with ICS and long-acting beta-agonist (LABA) results in reduced exacerbations compared with bronchodilator treatment alone and triple therapy with ICS/LABA, and a long-acting muscarinic antagonist offers further benefit, including a possible survival advantage in some patients.
- In patients with higher blood eosinophil counts, the use of ICSs is associated with a greater reduction in COPD exacerbations risk.
- ICSs are associated with an increased risk of pneumonia. COPD patients with the highest pneumonia risk are those with low body mass index, advanced age, male gender, and greater airflow obstruction, and ICS-containing treatments should be used with caution in these groups.

INTRODUCTION

The Global Burden of Disease Study recently has reported that chronic obstructive pulmonary disease (COPD) is the third leading cause of death worldwide, reaching this threshold approximately 10 years earlier than predicted.[1,2] Explanations for this rise are multifactorial and include the aging population and improved outcomes for cardiovascular disease and cancer. Additionally, no pharmacologic treatment has been definitively shown to improve COPD mortality, which also contributes. Other treatment goals for COPD include reducing the burden of disease by alleviating symptoms, improving health-related quality of life, reducing exacerbation frequency and severity, and preservation of lung function.[1,3] Achieving these goals is challenging due to the heterogeneity and complex pathobiology of the disease, which include dysregulation in immune activation, airflow obstruction due to bronchoconstriction, small airway fibrosis, emphysema and muco-obstruction, and dysfunction of the mucociliary escalator.[4,5] The presence of lung inflammation also promotes airway and alveolar tissue damage, airway remodeling, and airflow obstruction and contributes to the risk of exacerbations of COPD (ECOPD), which cause life-limiting symptoms and also are associated with loss of lung function, poor quality of life, and significant health care costs.[2,6–8]

Anti-inflammatory therapeutics evaluated in COPD include inhaled corticosteroids (ICSs), oral

a Division of Pulmonary, Allergy and Critical Care Medicine, Lung Health Center, University of Alabama at Birmingham, 1720 2nd Avenue South, THT 422, Birmingham, AL 35294-0006, USA; b Division of Pulmonary, Allergy and Critical Care Medicine, Lung Health Center, University of Alabama at Birmingham, 526 20th Street South, Birmingham, AL 35294-0006, USA
* Corresponding author.
E-mail address: mdransfield@uabmc.edu

Clin Chest Med 41 (2020) 475–484
https://doi.org/10.1016/j.ccm.2020.05.006

glucocorticoids, phosphodiesterase inhibitors, antibiotics, statins, mucolytics, and monoclonal antibodies targeting inflammatory mediators, such as benralizumab and mepolizumab that target interleukin (IL)-5, among other drugs.[4,9,10] The best studied of these approaches is the use of ICSs, alone and in combination with a long-acting beta-agonist (LABA) and with long-acting muscarinic antagonists (LAMAs). Although targeting lung inflammation with ICSs can have clinical benefits, including reducing the risk of exacerbations, it also can be associated with untoward effects.

INHALED CORTICOSTEROID MONOTHERAPY

Although ICS therapy has a well-established role in the management of asthma, early studies in COPD patients were small and resulted in conflicting results.[11–14] Subsequent more extensive studies suggested modest benefits on lung function, symptoms, and exacerbation risk but did not demonstrate effects on the rate of forced expiratory volume in the in the first second of expiration (FEV_1) decline and raised the possibility of a mortality disadvantage with long-term use.[15–17]

Paggiaro and colleagues[15] reported that 6 months of monotherapy with fluticasone propionate (FP) resulted in increased 6-minute walking distance, improved symptom scores for cough and sputum production, and a reduction in the number of patients who suffered moderate or severe exacerbations compared with placebo (60% vs 86%, respectively; $P<.001$). Pauwels and colleagues[16] reported that in COPD patients who continued to smoke, monotherapy with budesonide resulted in initial improvement in FEV_1 in the first 6 months of treatment compared with placebo but that the rates of decline in FEV_1 over 3 years in the 2 groups were similar. These studies were followed by a 3-year single-center, double-blind, randomized placebo-controlled study nested in the Copenhagen City Heart Study. In this trial, Vestbo and colleagues[18] evaluated the effect of budesonide on the rate of FEV_1 decline in COPD patients and again found no clear treatment benefit at 3 years with ICS monotherapy. The Inhaled Steroids in Obstructive Lung Disease in Europe (ISOLDE) study also reported no statistical difference in decline in FEV_1 with FP compared with placebo, although there was a 25% reduction in median annual exacerbation rate and lower decline in health status as measured by St George's Respiratory Questionnaire with ICS therapy.[19] The Towards a Revolution in COPD Health (TORCH) trial randomized more than 6000 patients with COPD to FP/salmeterol (SAL), SAL, FP, or placebo. FP monotherapy again was shown to reduce the rate

of exacerbations versus placebo, but the risk of death at 3 years with FP actually was increased vs placebo (15.2% versus 16.0%, respectively; [hazard ratio (HR) 1.060; 95% CI, 0.886–1.268; $P = .53$]) and statistically significantly higher when FP compared with FP/SAL (16.0% versus 12.6%, respectively; $P = .007$). Although there have been additional studies of ICS monotherapy in subpopulations of COPD, including those with heightened cardiovascular risk, and there has been a suggestion that they may have an impact on lung function decline in those with elevated blood eosinophils, the results of the TORCH study strongly suggested that this strategy should not be used routinely.[20,21]

INHALED CORTICOSTEROID/LONG-ACTING BETA-AGONIST THERAPY

Numerous studies have compared ICS/LABA to LABA or LAMA alone as well as to dual bronchodilator therapy and have examined a range of clinical outcomes, although the effects of ICS/LABA on exacerbations and mortality have been of greatest interest.

Exacerbations

Inhaled corticosteroid/long-acting beta-agonist versus long-acting beta-agonist

In TORCH, FP/SAL was associated with a reduction in moderate or severe ECOPD compared with placebo, FP, and SAL, with FP/SAL compared to SAL alone being the most clinically relevant comparison with a risk ratio of 0.88 (95% CI, 0.81–0.95) favoring combination treatment. Although there are differences in the ICSs tested as well as trial methodology and the populations enrolled, ICS/LABA repeatedly has been shown to reduce the rate of ECOPD by 10% to 25%.[17,22–33]

Inhaled corticosteroid/long-acting beta-agonist versus long-acting muscarinic antagonist

The Investigating New Standards for Prophylaxis in Reducing Exacerbations (INSPIRE) trial evaluated tiotropium therapy compared with FP/SAL for patients with severe and very severe COPD (mean FEV_1 39%) over 2 years and found no difference in annual exacerbation rate (rate ratio [RR] 0.967; 95% CI, 0.836–1.119; $P = .656$). FP/SAL was associated with better health status and a lower withdrawal rate, suggesting an overall advantage to ICS/LABA.

Inhaled corticosteroid/long-acting beta-agonist versus long-acting muscarinic antagonist/long-acting beta-agonist

The Indacaterol–Glycopyrronium versus Salmeterol–Fluticasone for COPD (FLAME) trial demonstrated the superiority of the LABA/LAMA for the endpoint of annual rate of moderate or severe COPD exacerbations (RR 0.83; 95% CI, 0.75–0.91; P<.001). These results contrast with those from the IMPACT study, which showed an exacerbation benefit of fluticasone furoate (FF)/vilanterol (VI) compared with umeclidinium (UMEC)/VI. This difference in outcome likely is explained by methodological differences between the trials, including the inclusion of a run-in period on tiotropium in FLAME and the fact that the population in IMPACT was at much higher exacerbation risk, with 54% have greater than or equal to 2 moderate to severe exacerbations and 26% with greater than or equal to 1 severe exacerbation requiring hospitalization.[34,35]

Survival/Mortality

In TORCH, FP/SAL was associated with a trend toward a reduction in mortality (HR 0.825; 95% CI, 0.68–1.00; P = .052). Although the results did not reach statistical significance, a prespecified secondary analysis using Cox proportional hazard testing did suggest a survival advantage with FP/SAL compared with placebo (HR 0.811; 95% CI, 0.670–0.982; P = .03).[17] There are several possible explanations for the study failing to definitively establish a mortality benefit, including lower than expected mortality and differential dropout in the placebo arm.[36]

A post hoc analysis of the TORCH study did demonstrate that in those patients treated for cardiovascular disease and with moderate airflow limitation (FEV$_1$ >50%), FP/SAL reduced the risk of cardiovascular adverse events compared with placebo. These data suggested the possibility of ICS/LABA being especially beneficial to those with heightened cardiovascular risk.[37] This hypothesis was tested in the Study to Understand Mortality and Morbidity in COPD (SUMMIT) that enrolled patients with moderate COPD and heightened cardiovascular risk and randomized them to FF, VI, their combination (FF/VI), or placebo. The study was designed to evaluate the effect of FF/VI on all-cause mortality, but cardiovascular events and exacerbations also were examined. All-cause mortality was unaffected by FF/VI compared with placebo (HR 0.88; 95% CI, 0.74–1.04) and although there was also no impact of any active treatment on cardiovascular outcomes, there was no evidence of an adverse effect.[38] Prespecified secondary analyses demonstrated that FF/VI reduced the risk of exacerbations compared with placebo and that FF-containing treatments might slow the rate of FEV$_1$ decline.[39,40] The study also demonstrated an important link between exacerbations and cardiovascular events as the HR

for cardiovascular events after ECOPD was increased, particularly in the first 30 days (HR 3.8; 95% CI, 2.7–5.5) and remained elevated for up to 1 year.[41]

The INSPIRE trial examined survival as a safety endpoint and demonstrated that FP/SAL was associated with a reduction in mortality compared with tiotropium (3% vs 6%, respectively; P = .032). Additionally, Cox proportional hazards model for time to death on treatment showed a 52% reduction in the risk of death in those randomized to FP/SAL (HR 0.48; 95% CI, 0.27–0.85; P = .012).[42,43]

TRIALS OF TRIPLE THERAPY WITH INHALED CORTICOSTEROID/LONG-ACTING BETA-AGONIST/LONG-ACTING MUSCARINIC ANTAGONIST

The recent development of single-inhaler triple therapies has prompted a series of clinical trials testing the effects of maximal inhaled treatment with an emphasis on exacerbations.

Exacerbations

The Informing the Pathway of COPD Treatment (IMPACT) trial evaluated the effect of triple therapy with FF/VI/UMEC versus both FF/VI and UMEC/VI in more than 10,000 patients with symptomatic COPD and a history of exacerbations.[35] There was a lower rate of moderate and severe COPD exacerbations with triple therapy compared with UMEC/VI (RR 0.75; 95% CI, 0.70–0.81; P<.001) as well as a lower rate of COPD-related hospitalizations (RR 0.66; 95% CI, 0.56–0.78; P<.001). The efficacy and safety of fixed triple inhaler therapy also was demonstrated in TRILOGY as well as TRINITY, where the combination of beclometasone dipropionate (BDP), formoterol fumarate (FF), and glycopyrronium (G) showed a 23% reduction in moderate/severe exacerbations versus ICS/LABA (BDP/FF) (RR 0.77; 95% CI, 0.65–0.92; P = .005) and 20% reduction versus LAMA (tiotropium) (RR 0.80; 95% CI 0.69–0.92; P = 0.0025) in symptomatic severe/very severe COPD patients with an exacerbation history.[44,45]

Similar to IMPACT, the Extrafine Inhaled Triple Therapy versus Dual Bronchodilator Therapy in Chronic Obstructive Pulmonary Disease (TRIBUTE) study also compared triple ICS-containing therapy versus LABA/LAMA in patients with severe/very severe COPD at risk for ECOPD.[35,46] BDP/FF/G reduced the risk of moderate/severe exacerbations compared with indacaterol/GLY (annual exacerbation rate of 0.50 vs 0.59 events, respectively, per patient-year: RR 0.848; 95% CI, 0.723–0.995; P = .043). Although the overall rate of exacerbations and the relative benefit of triple therapy were less than observed in IMPACT, the results still suggest a clinically relevant advantage.[46]

Survival/Mortality

In IMPACT, triple inhaled therapy with ICFF/VI/UMEC was associated with a signal toward a reduction in all-cause mortality compared with UMEC/VI. Although assessment of the mortality signal in IMPACT should be interpreted with caution because it was not the primary outcome, the trial is invaluable because of its meticulous adjudication of clinical events and the assessment of outcomes both on and off treatment and after capture of the vital status on all but 42 (0.4%) patients. With time to on-treatment all-cause mortality as a prespecified endpoint, the HR for FF/VI/UMEC versus UMEC/VI was 0.58 (95% CI, 0.38–0.88; unadjusted $P = .011$). Similar results were observed when the analysis included data after patients stopped treatment (HR 0.71; 95% CI, 0.51–0.99; $P = .043$) and when the vital status was available for 99.6% of randomized subjects (HR 0.72; 95% CI, 0.53–0.99; $P = .042$).[35,43] A pooled analysis of the TRILOGY, TRINITY, and TRIBUTE studies evaluated mortality as a safety outcome and found that the risk of nonrespiratory mortality was lower with ICS-containing treatments compared with treatment without ICSs (HR 0.65%; 95% CI; 0.43–0.97; $P = .037$)[44–48]

Although no study has demonstrated an advantage to ICS-containing therapy with mortality as the primary endpoint, the weight of the evidence suggests that there may be a benefit in a subset of patients, likely those with more severe disease, significant symptoms, and exacerbation risk.

RISKS/SAFETY

Population-based studies and analyses of randomized controlled trials (RCTs) have shown that ICS therapy has untoward effects that include changes in bone density, oral candidiasis, insulin resistance, skin changes, and adrenal suppression as well as increased risk of pneumonia and mycobacterial infections (**Table 1**).[49–56]

Pneumonia Risk

COPD patients are at increased risk of community-acquired pneumonia as well as increased risk of death from pneumonia.[57] Risk factors for pneumonia in COPD include older age, lower body mass index (BMI), male gender, lower FEV_1, prior pneumonia, and ICS use, although the magnitude of additional risk attributable to ICSs is uncertain.[58] There also has been substantial interest in the use of blood eosinophils as a predictor of pneumonia, but most studies have shown either no association or an association only with very low eosinophil counts.[59,60] There also is significant variability in pneumonia rates across studies with differences in study populations, study design, the ICS included, and varied definitions of pneumonia that complicate comparisons. Despite these challenges, a Cochrane review has concluded that pneumonia is a class-related risk of ICS.[61]

The TORCH study reported increased pneumonia risk in the FF-containing treatment groups, and although this was not a prespecified outcome and chest radiographs were not required for diagnosis, the same trend has been observed in subsequent RCTs of ICS-containing therapies, including those where pneumonia events were adjudicated.[17,35,62]

Although the weight of the evidence suggests that ICSs increase the risk of any pneumonia, this does not seem to increase pneumonia-related or all-cause mortality. There also are data to suggest that outcomes for COPD patients admitted with pneumonia are better in those taking ICSs as outpatients and that there may be a double effect of the drugs, including both an adverse effect and an additional unidentified mitigating effect.[63] Additionally, in order to determine overall risk-benefit, the risk of ICS-related pneumonia has to be compared and counterbalanced with the ICS-related reduction in acute exacerbations. Data from IMPACT[35] and TRIBUTE[46] show that the rate of ECOPD is approximately 10-fold higher than the rate of pneumonia and, thus, the small increase in pneumonia risk with ICSs may be offset by the exacerbation benefit, although the decision to use ICSs must be individualized.

Mycobacterial Risk

Recent population-based studies suggest that COPD patients on ICSs are at an increased risk of nontuberculous mycobacterial (NTM) infections.[64,65] In a large population-based study in Canada, Brode and colleagues[65] found that there was an association between NTM and ICS use in patients with obstructive lung disease (asthma, COPD, and asthma-COPD overlap). When selected for COPD patients, the investigators found an adjusted odds ratio of 1.96 (95% CI, 1.62–2.36).[65] Similar findings were seen in a population-based case-control study in Denmark that verified that COPD is a risk factor for NTM, and ICS therapy further increases the risk.[64] This effect of ICSs on mycobacterial risk has not been demonstrated in a randomized clinical trial.

Table 1
Side effects of inhaled corticosteroids in chronic obstructive pulmonary disease and strength of evidence

	Randomized Controlled Trial	Observational/Case-Control Study	Systematic Review
Pneumonia	✔✔✔	✔✔✔	✔✔✔
Mycobacterial infections		✔	✔
Diabetes		✔	
Bone density	(No effect on fracture risk)	✔✔	✔✔

Fractures and Bone Density

A long-standing concern for ICS therapy is an effect on bone density and fracture risk. Osteoporosis is significant comorbidity in COPD, and patients not on ICS therapy are estimated to have a prevalence of ranging from 10% to 33%.[66] The systemic bioavailability of most ICS molecules is believed to be minimal, but the effects of very long exposure have not been studied adequately. In the Lung Health Study, after 3 years of ICS therapy with triamcinolone, a significant number of patients had reduced bone density in the femoral neck and lumbar spine compared with placebo.[67] These findings were not observed in other studies, and no RCT has demonstrated a significant increase in fracture risk.[68–71] The effects of ICSs on bone density likely are both dose dependent and time dependent and many patients started on the drugs take them for far longer than has been studied. It, therefore, is advisable that ICS dose and duration be minimized, therapy limited to those who will receive benefit, and individuals monitored for adverse bone effects.

Glycemic Control/Insulin Resistance

Diabetes is a common comorbid condition in patients with COPD; thus, understanding the effect of ICSs on glycemic control is essential. A case-control study in patients with asthma or COPD reported that ICS use was associated with an increased risk of new-onset diabetes and diabetes progression, with a clear dose-response relationship.[72] In a UK-based historical matched cohort study, Price and colleagues[73] evaluated the change in hemoglobin (Hb) A_{1c} in COPD patients with coexisting diabetes who were taking ICSs over 12 months to 18 months relative to a non-ICS cohort. The adjusted difference in change in HbA_{1c} was 0.16% (95% CI, 0.05%–0.27%), suggesting that patients using ICSs had worse diabetes control.[73] Another cohort study noted small changes in serum glucose (ranging from 2 mg/dL to 5 mg/dL) without an increased risk of developing diabetes, even though the clinical relevance of this effect is unclear.[74] Additional studies are needed to determine the overall impact of ICSs on long-term glycemic control.

Adrenal Suppression

Systemic administration of glucocorticoids causes hypothalamic-pituitary-adrenal (HPA) axis suppression by reducing corticotropin production, which reduces cortisol secretion by the adrenal gland. The degree of HPA suppression is dependent on dose, duration, frequency, and timing of glucocorticoid administration; however, there have been no data to suggest that doses delivered with inhaled corticosteroids have a meaningful clinical impact on the HPA axis for most patients.[75–77]

RISK-BENEFIT CONSIDERATIONS

The selection of patients for ICS-containing therapy requires an assessment of their likelihood of receiving a benefit, most clearly in reducing exacerbation risk and the risk of hospitalization, and their propensity to suffer ICS-related side effects. As discussed previously, older age, low BMI, lower lung function, and male sex increase the risk of pneumonia in COPD but may not preclude treatment with ICSs if the potential for exacerbation prevention is more significant. Several studies suggest that sputum eosinophilia, although not readily available in most clinical settings, may serve as a predictive biomarker of response to corticosteroids in patients with COPD.[3,78–81] Although sputum eosinophils correlate well with exacerbations and ICS benefit, findings from the Subpopulations and Intermediate Outcome Measures in COPD Study (SPIROMICS) suggest that the use of blood eosinophils as a surrogate may perform poorly due to weak association between sputum and blood eosinophilia.[82] This contrasts with data from several RCTs that demonstrate a clear association between greater eosinophil count and both the risk of exacerbations and the magnitude of ICS benefit. A post hoc analysis of pooled phase III data also showed that patients with a peripheral blood eosinophil count of at least 100 cells/μL with at least 1 exacerbation in the preceding year had a reduction in exacerbations with ICS/LABA therapy (RR 0.75; 95% CI, 0.57–0.99; $P = .015$), with the most significant treatment effect noted in those with the highest level of blood eosinophils.[82,83] IMPACT and TRIBUTE had a predefined analysis based on blood eosinophilia that showed more significant treatment effects to ICSs with eosinophil level greater than 150 cells/μL to 200 cells/μL, although in smokers the threshold for benefit may be higher.[35,46] Pascoe and colleagues[84] redemonstrated a direct relationship between ECOPD reduction and higher peripheral eosinophil count; however, there was not a clear association between pneumonia with baseline blood eosinophils. Based on available data, it is reasonable to consider ICS use in those patients with frequent and severe exacerbations and consider avoiding in patients with a history of frequent cases of pneumonia. There also may be a role for examining sputum culture data to select ICS candidates, because chronic bronchial infection also may increase pneumonia risk (**Box 1**).[60]

ICS WITHDRAWAL

There have been concerns about the risk of abrupt discontinuation of ICSs in patients who are tolerating the drugs. During the run-in period of the ISOLDE trial, there was an increased rate of ECOPD after the withdrawal of ICS.[19] The Withdrawal of Inhaled Steroids during Optimized Bronchodilator Management (WISDOM) study assessed response to de-escalation of ICS

therapy in patients on triple inhaled therapy. When the ICS dose gradually was decreased over 12 weeks, there was not an increased risk of exacerbations compared with the group that remained on triple ICS-containing therapy (HR 1.06; 95% CI, 0.94–1.19). There was a small decline in FEV_1 (approximately 40 mL) and mild worsening in health status in the ICS withdrawal group.[85] Subgroup analysis showed that the subset of the study population who had eosinophil counts greater than 4% had an increased risk of exacerbations when ICSs were withdrawn (HR 1.63; 95% CI, 1.19–2.24), and a similar pattern was noted for an absolute eosinophil count greater than 300 cells/μL.[85–90] The recent SUNSET (Study to Understand the Safety and Efficacy of ICS Withdrawal from Triple Therapy in COPD) trial confirmed that the patients that fair best with ICS withdrawal are those with stable disease, low eosinophils, and infrequent exacerbations.[91]

DISCUSSION

As more is understood about COPD and its varying endotypes, it is becoming increasingly clear that a standardized approach to this heterogeneous disease is inadequate and that it is essential to personalize care. ICS-based therapy continues to play an important role in COPD care as it results in improvements in lung function, health care–related quality of life, and reduced exacerbations compared with bronchodilator treatment alone. Triple therapy with ICS/LAMA/LABA may offer further benefit, including a potential survival advantage in select patients. It is evident, however, that these ICS-containing regimens are associated with adverse effects, with pneumonia garnering the most attention. Factors associated with highest pneumonia risk are male sex, low BMI, low lung function, and advanced age but should not preclude ICS treatment if the exacerbation benefits exceed this risk. Practical factors to assist in determining patient suitability for long-term pharmacotherapy with ICS-containing compounds should include evaluating exacerbation history, including the frequency and severity of prior events, blood eosinophils, history of pneumonia, and history of concomitant illnesses, such as asthma.

DISCLOSURE

M.T. Dransfield reports grants support from the American Lung Association, NIH, Department of Defense, and Department of Veterans Affairs; consulting   fees   from   AstraZeneca,

Box 1 Selecting inhaled corticosteroid candidates	
Consider Inhaled Corticosteroid Use	**Avoid Inhaled Corticosteroid Use**
• Frequent and severe exacerbations (>2 moderate exacerbations or one hospitalization) • Eosinophilia • Concomitant asthma	• Infrequent exacerbations/stable disease • Frequent pneumonia events • Significant fractures in stable disease • Low BMI <21

GlaxoSmithKline, Mereo, Pulmonx, PneumRx/BTG, and Quark; and contracted clinical trial support from AstraZeneca, Boehringer Ingelheim, Boston Scientific, GALA, GlaxoSmithKline, Nuvaira, Pulmonx, and PneumRx/BTG.

REFERENCES

1. Singh D, Agusti A, Anzueto A, et al. Global strategy for the diagnosis, management, and prevention of chronic obstructive lung disease: the GOLD science committee report 2019. Eur Respir J 2019;53(5): 1900164.

2. GBD 2015 Chronic Respiratory Disease Collaborators. Global, regional, and national deaths, prevalence, disability-adjusted life years, and years lived with disability for chronic obstructive pulmonary disease and asthma, 1990-2015: a systematic analysis for the Global Burden of Disease Study 2015. Lancet Respir Med 2017;5(9):691–706.

3. Bafadhel M, Davies L, Calverley PM, et al. Blood eosinophil guided prednisolone therapy for exacerbations of COPD: a further analysis. Eur Respir J 2014;44(3):789–91.

4. Barnes PJ, Pedersen S, Busse WW. Efficacy and safety of inhaled corticosteroids. New developments. Am J Respir Crit Care Med 1998;157(3 Pt 2):S1–53.

5. Barnes PJ. Inflammatory mechanisms in patients with chronic obstructive pulmonary disease. J Allergy Clin Immunol 2016;138(1):16–27.

6. Dransfield MT, Kunisaki KM, Strand MJ, et al. Acute exacerbations and lung function loss in smokers with and without chronic obstructive pulmonary disease. Am J Respir Crit Care Med 2017;195(3):324–30.

7. Berry CE, Wise RA. Mortality in COPD: causes, risk factors, and prevention. COPD 2010;7(5):375–82.

8. Moldoveanu B, Otmishi P, Jani P, et al. Inflammatory mechanisms in the lung. J Inflamm Res 2009;2:1.

9. Criner GJ, Celli BR, Singh D, et al. Predicting response to benralizumab in chronic obstructive pulmonary disease: analyses of GALATHEA and TERRANOVA studies. Lancet Respir Med 2019; 8(2):158–70.

10. Xia Y, Li W, Shen H. Mepolizumab for eosinophilic COPD. N Engl J Med 2018;378(7):680–1.

11. Engel T, Heinig J, Madsen O, et al. A trial of inhaled budesonide on airway responsiveness in smokers with chronic bronchitis. Eur Respir J 1989;2(10): 935–9.

12. Auffarth B, Postma D, De Monchy J, et al. Effects of inhaled budesonide on spirometric values, reversibility, airway responsiveness, and cough threshold in smokers with chronic obstructive lung disease. Thorax 1991;46(5):372–7.

13. Wardman A, Simpson F, Knox A, et al. The use of high dose inhaled beclomethasone dipropionate as a means of assessing steroid responsiveness in obstructive airways disease. Br J Dis Chest 1988; 82:168–71.

14. Thompson AB, Mueller MB, Heires AJ, et al. Aerosolized beclomethasone in chronic bronchitis: improved pulmonary function and diminished airway inflammation. Am Rev Respir Dis 1992;146(2): 389–95.

15. Paggiaro PL, Dahle R, Bakran I, et al. Multicentre randomised placebo-controlled trial of inhaled fluticasone propionate in patients with chronic obstructive pulmonary disease. Lancet 1998;351(9105): 773–80.

16. Pauwels RA, Lofdahl CG, Laitinen LA, et al. Long-term treatment with inhaled budesonide in persons with mild chronic obstructive pulmonary disease who continue smoking. European Respiratory Society Study on Chronic Obstructive Pulmonary Disease. N Engl J Med 1999;340(25): 1948–53.

17. Calverley PM, Anderson JA, Celli B, et al. Salmeterol and fluticasone propionate and survival in chronic obstructive pulmonary disease. N Engl J Med 2007;356(8):775–89.

18. Leigh R, Pizzichini MM, Morris MM, et al. Stable COPD: predicting benefit from high-dose inhaled corticosteroid treatment. Eur Respir J 2006;27(5): 964–71.

19. Burge PS, Calverley P, Jones PW, et al. Randomised, double blind, placebo controlled study of fluticasone propionate in patients with moderate to severe chronic obstructive pulmonary disease: the ISOLDE trial. BMJ 2000;320(7245):1297–303.

20. Barnes NC, Sharma R, Lettis S, et al. Blood eosinophils as a marker of response to inhaled corticosteroids in COPD. Eur Respir J 2016;47(5):1374–82.

21. Vestbo J, Anderson JA, Brook RD, et al. Fluticasone furoate and vilanterol and survival in chronic obstructive pulmonary disease with heightened cardiovascular risk (SUMMIT): a double-blind randomised controlled trial. Lancet 2016;387(10030): 1817–26.

22. Calverley P, Pauwels R, Vestbo J, et al. Combined salmeterol and fluticasone in the treatment of chronic obstructive pulmonary disease: a randomised controlled trial. Lancet 2003;361(9356): 449–56.

23. Dransfield MT, Bourbeau J, Jones PW, et al. Once-daily inhaled fluticasone furoate and vilanterol versus vilanterol only for prevention of exacerbations of COPD: two replicate double-blind, parallel-group, randomised controlled trials. Lancet Respir Med 2013;1(3):210–23.

24. Anzueto A, Ferguson GT, Feldman G, et al. Effect of fluticasone propionate/salmeterol (250/50) on COPD exacerbations and impact on patient outcomes. COPD 2009;6(5):320–9.

25. Kardos P, Wencker M, Glaab T, et al. Impact of salmeterol/fluticasone propionate versus salmeterol on exacerbations in severe chronic obstructive pulmonary disease. Am J Respir Crit Care Med 2007; 175(2):144–9.

26. Calverley P, Boonsawat W, Cseke Z, et al. Maintenance therapy with budesonide and formoterol in chronicobstructive pulmonary disease. Eur Respir J 2003;22(6):912–9.

27. Ferguson GT, Anzueto A, Fei R, et al. Effect of fluticasone propionate/salmeterol (250/50 μg) or salmeterol (50 μg) on COPD exacerbations. Respir Med 2008;102(8):1099–108.

28. Papi A, Dokic D, Tzimas W, et al. Fluticasone propionate/formoterol for COPD management: a randomized controlled trial. Int J Chron Obstruct Pulmon Dis 2017;12:1961.

29. Rennard SI, Tashkin DP, McElhattan J, et al. Efficacy and tolerability of budesonide/formoterol in one hydrofluoroalkane pressurized metered-dose inhaler in patients with chronic obstructive pulmonary disease. Drugs 2009;69(5):549–65.

30. Sharafkhaneh A, Southard JG, Goldman M, et al. Effect of budesonide/formoterol pMDI on COPD exacerbations: a double-blind, randomized study. Respir Med 2012;106(2):257–68.

31. Szafranski W, Cukier A, Ramirez A, et al. Efficacy and safety of budesonide/formoterol in the management of chronic obstructive pulmonary disease. Eur Respir J 2003;21(1):74–81.

32. Wedzicha J, Singh D, Vestbo J, et al. Extrafine beclomethasone/formoterol in severe COPD patients with history of exacerbations. Respir Med 2014; 108(8):1153–62.

33. Agusti A, Fabbri LM, Singh D, et al. Inhaled corticosteroids in COPD: friend or foe? Eur Respir J 2018; 52(6).

34. Singh D. Double combination inhalers in COPD: how to get your head around this data. Respirology 2018; 23(12):1088–9.

35. Lipson DA, Barnhart F, Brealey N, et al. Once-Daily single-inhaler triple versus dual therapy in patients with COPD. N Engl J Med 2018;378(18):1671–80.

36. Rabe KF. Treating COPD–the TORCH trial, P values, and the Dodo. N Engl J Med 2007;356(8):851–3.

37. Calverley PM, Anderson JA, Celli B, et al. Cardiovascular events in patients with COPD: TORCH study results. Thorax 2010;65(8):719–25.

38. Brook RD, Anderson JA, Calverley PM, et al. Cardiovascular outcomes with an inhaled beta2-agonist/corticosteroid in patients with COPD at high cardiovascular risk. Heart 2017;103(19):1536–42.

39. Calverley PMA, Anderson JA, Brook RD, et al. Fluticasone furoate, vilanterol, and lung function decline in patients with moderate chronic obstructive pulmonary disease and heightened cardiovascular risk. Am J Respir Crit Care Med 2018;197(1):47–55.

40. Martinez FJ, Vestbo J, Anderson JA, et al. Effect of fluticasone furoate and vilanterol on exacerbations of chronic obstructive pulmonary disease in patients with moderate airflow obstruction. Am J Respir Crit Care Med 2017;195(7):881–8.

41. Kunisaki KM, Dransfield MT, Anderson JA, et al. Exacerbations of chronic obstructive pulmonary disease and cardiac events. A post hoc cohort analysis from the SUMMIT randomized clinical trial. Am J Respir Crit Care Med 2018;198(1):51–7.

42. Wedzicha JA, Calverley PM, Seemungal TA, et al. The prevention of chronic obstructive pulmonary disease exacerbations by salmeterol/fluticasone propionate or tiotropium bromide. Am J Respir Crit Care Med 2008;177(1):19–26.

43. Lipson D, Barnhart F, Brealey N, et al. Reduction in all-cause mortality with single inhaler triple therapy (FF/UMEC/VI) versus dual therapy (FF/VI and UMEC/VI) in symptomatic patients with COPD: prespecified analysis of the Phase III IMPACT Trial. In: A15. ICS IN COPD: the pendulum keeps swinging. American Thoracic Society; 2018. p. A1015.

44. Singh D, Papi A, Corradi M, et al. Single inhaler triple therapy versus inhaled corticosteroid plus long-acting beta2-agonist therapy for chronic obstructive pulmonary disease (TRILOGY): a double-blind, parallel group, randomised controlled trial. Lancet 2016;388(10048):963–73.

45. Vestbo J, Papi A, Corradi M, et al. Single inhaler extrafine triple therapy versus long-acting muscarinic antagonist therapy for chronic obstructive pulmonary disease (TRINITY): a double-blind, parallel group, randomised controlled trial. Lancet 2017; 389(10082):1919–29.

46. Papi A, Vestbo J, Fabbri L, et al. Extrafine inhaled triple therapy versus dual bronchodilator therapy in chronic obstructive pulmonary disease (TRIBUTE): a double-blind, parallel group, randomised controlled trial. Lancet 2018;391(10125):1076–84.

47. Vestbo J, Fabbri L, Papi A, et al. Inhaled corticosteroid containing combinations and mortality in COPD. Eur Respir J 2018;52(6):1801230.

48. Fabbri L, Singh D, Roche N, et al. Reduction in fatal events with extrafine inhaled corticosteroid (ICS)-containing medications: results of stratified safety pooled analysis of the TRILOGY, TRINITY and TRIBUTE studies. Eur Respiratory Soc 2018;52 (SUPPLEMENT 62 OA 1659).

49. Derendorf H. Pharmacokinetic and pharmacodynamic properties of inhaled corticosteroids in relation to efficacy and safety. Respir Med 1997;91: 22–8.

50. Almirall J, Bolibar I, Serra-Prat M, et al. New evidence of risk factors for community-acquired pneumonia: a population-based study. Eur Respir J 2008; 31(6):1274–84.

51. Johnson M. Pharmacodynamics and pharmacokinetics of inhaled glucocorticoids. J Allergy Clin Immunol 1996;97(1):169–76.

52. Garbe E, LeLorier J, Boivin J-F, et al. Inhaled and nasal glucocorticoids and the risks of ocular hypertension or open-angle glaucoma. JAMA 1997; 277(9):722–7.

53. Fukushima C, Matsuse H, Tomari S, et al. Oral candidiasis associated with inhaled corticosteroid use: comparison of fluticasone and beclomethasone. Ann Allergy Asthma Immunol 2003;90(6):646–51.

54. Alsaeedi A, Sin DD, McAlister FA. The effects of inhaled corticosteroids in chronic obstructive pulmonary disease: a systematic review of randomized placebo-controlled trials. Am J Med 2002;113(1):59–65.

55. Suissa S, Patenaude V, Lapi F, et al. Inhaled corticosteroids in COPD and the risk of serious pneumonia. Thorax 2013;68(11):1029–36.

56. Tashkin DP, Murray HE, Skeans M, et al. Skin manifestations of inhaled corticosteroids in COPD patients: results from Lung Health Study II. Chest 2004;126(4):1123–33.

57. Restrepo MI, Mortensen EM, Pugh JA, et al. COPD is associated with increased mortality in patients with community-acquired pneumonia. Eur Respir J 2006;28(2):346–51.

58. Williams NP, Coombs NA, Johnson MJ, et al. Seasonality, risk factors and burden of community-acquired pneumonia in COPD patients: a population database study using linked health care records. Int J Chron Obstruct Pulmon Dis 2017;12:313.

59. Pascoe S, Locantore N, Dransfield MT, et al. Blood eosinophil counts, exacerbations, and response to the addition of inhaled fluticasone furoate to vilanterol in patients with chronic obstructive pulmonary disease: a secondary analysis of data from two parallel randomised controlled trials. Lancet Respir Med 2015;3(6):435–42.

60. Martinez-Garcia MA, Faner R, Oscullo G, et al. Inhaled steroids, circulating eosinophils, chronic airway infection and pneumonia risk in chronic obstructive pulmonary disease: a network analysis. Am J Respir Crit Care Med 2020;201(9):1078–85.

61. Kew KM, Seniukovich A. Inhaled steroids and risk of pneumonia for chronic obstructive pulmonary disease. Cochrane Database Syst Rev 2014;(3): CD010115.

62. Crim C, Dransfield MT, Bourbeau J, et al. Pneumonia risk with inhaled fluticasone furoate and vilanterol compared with vilanterol alone in patients with COPD. Ann Am Thorac Soc 2015;12(1):27–34.

63. Festic E, Scanlon PD. Incident pneumonia and mortality in patients with chronic obstructive pulmonary disease. A double effect of inhaled corticosteroids? Am J Respir Crit Care Med 2015;191(2):141–8.

64. Andrejak C, Nielsen R, Thomsen VO, et al. Chronic respiratory disease, inhaled corticosteroids and risk of non-tuberculous mycobacteriosis. Thorax 2013;68(3):256–62.

65. Brode SK, Campitelli MA, Kwong JC, et al. The risk of mycobacterial infections associated with inhaled corticosteroid use. Eur Respir J 2017;50(3): 1700037.

66. Sin DD, Man JP, Man SP. The risk of osteoporosis in Caucasian men and women with obstructive airways disease. Am J Med 2003;114(1):10–4.

67. Scanlon PD, Connett JE, Wise RA, et al. Loss of bone density with inhaled triamcinolone in Lung Health Study II. Am J Respir Crit Care Med 2004; 170(12):1302–9.

68. Johnell O, Pauwels R, Löfdahl C-G, et al. Bone mineral density in patients with chronic obstructive pulmonary disease treated with budesonide Turbuhaler®. Eur Respir J 2002;19(6):1058–63.

69. Ferguson GT, Calverley PM, Anderson JA, et al. Prevalence and progression of osteoporosis in patients with COPD: results from the TOwards a Revolution in COPD Health study. Chest 2009;136(6): 1456–65.

70. Waljee AK, Rogers MA, Lin P, et al. Short term use of oral corticosteroids and related harms among adults in the United States: population based cohort study. BMJ 2017;357:j1415.

71. Loke YK, Cavallazzi R, Singh S. Risk of fractures with inhaled corticosteroids in COPD: systematic review and meta-analysis of randomised controlled trials and observational studies. Thorax 2011;66(8): 699–708.

72. Suissa S, Kezouh A, Ernst P. Inhaled corticosteroids and the risks of diabetes onset and progression. Am J Med 2010;123(11):1001–6.

73. Price DB, Russell R, Mares R, et al. Metabolic effects associated with ICS in patients with COPD and comorbid type 2 diabetes: a historical matched cohort study. PLoS One 2016;11(9):e0162903.

74. Slatore CG, Bryson CL, Au DH. The association of inhaled corticosteroid use with serum glucose concentration in a large cohort. Am J Med 2009; 122(5):472–8.

75. Drescher T, Duerring U, Henzen C, et al. Prospective analysis of adrenal function in patients with acute exacerbations of COPD: the Reduction in the Use of Corticosteroids in Exacerbated COPD (REDUCE) trial. Endocrinology 2015;173:19–27.

76. Fan Y, Ma L, Pippins J, et al. Impact of study design on the evaluation of inhaled and intranasal corticosteroids' effect on hypothalamic–pituitary–adrenal Axis function. J Pharm Sci 2014;103(10):2963–79.

77. Heffler E, Madeira LNG, Ferrando M, et al. Inhaled corticosteroids safety and adverse effects in patients with asthma. J Allergy Clin Immunol Pract 2018;6(3):776–81.

78. Brightling CE, Monteiro W, Ward R, et al. Sputum eosinophilia and short-term response to

prednisolone in chronic obstructive pulmonary disease: a randomised controlled trial. Lancet 2000; 356(9240):1480–5.

79. Pizzichini E, Pizzichini MM, Gibson P, et al. Sputum eosinophilia predicts benefit from prednisone in smokers with chronic obstructive bronchitis. Am J Respir Crit Care Med 1998;158(5):1511–7.

80. Bafadhel M, McKenna S, Terry S, et al. Blood eosinophils to direct corticosteroid treatment of exacerbations of chronic obstructive pulmonary disease: a randomized placebo-controlled trial. Am J Respir Crit Care Med 2012;186(1):48–55.

81. Siddiqui SH, Guasconi A, Vestbo J, et al. Blood eosinophils: a biomarker of response to extrafine beclomethasone/formoterol in chronic obstructive pulmonary disease. Am J Respir Crit Care Med 2015;192(4):523–5.

82. Hastie AT, Martinez FJ, Curtis JL, et al. Association of sputum and blood eosinophil concentrations with clinical measures of COPD severity: an analysis of the SPIROMICS cohort. Lancet Respir Med 2017; 5(12):956–67.

83. Bafadhel M, Peterson S, De Blas MA, et al. Predictors of exacerbation risk and response to budesonide in patients with chronic obstructive pulmonary disease: a post-hoc analysis of three randomised trials. Lancet Respir Med 2018;6(2):117–26.

84. Pascoe S, Barnes N, Brusselle G, et al. Blood eosinophils and treatment response with triple and dual combination therapy in chronic obstructive pulmonary disease: analysis of the IMPACT trial. Lancet Respir Med 2019;7(9):745–56.

85. Magnussen H, Disse B, Rodriguez-Roisin R, et al. Withdrawal of inhaled glucocorticoids and exacerbations of COPD. N Engl J Med 2014;371(14): 1285–94.

86. Watz H, Tetzlaff K, Wouters EF, et al. Blood eosinophil count and exacerbations in severe chronic obstructive pulmonary disease after withdrawal of inhaled corticosteroids: a post-hoc analysis of the WISDOM trial. Lancet Respir Med 2016;4(5):390–8.

87. Kunz LI, Ten Hacken NH, Lapperre TS, et al. Airway inflammation in COPD after long-term withdrawal of inhaled corticosteroids. Eur Respir J 2017;49(1): 1600839.

88. Vogelmeier C, Worth H, Buhl R, et al. "Real-life" inhaled corticosteroid withdrawal in COPD: a subgroup analysis of DACCORD. Int J Chron Obstruct Pulmon Dis 2017;12:487.

89. van der Valk P, Monninkhof E, van der Palen J, et al. Effect of discontinuation of inhaled corticosteroids in patients with chronic obstructive pulmonary disease: the COPE study. Am J Respir Crit Care Med 2002;166(10):1358–63.

90. Vestbo J, Anderson JA, Brook RD, et al. Effect of treatment withdrawal on outcomes in the Summit study. In: C41. Long acting bronchodilator therapy in COPD II. American Thoracic Society; 2017. p. A5483.

91. Chapman KR, Hurst JR, Frent S-M, et al. Long-term triple therapy de-escalation to indacaterol/glycopyrronium in patients with chronic obstructive pulmonary disease (SUNSET): a randomized, double-blind, triple-dummy clinical trial. Am J Respir Crit Care Med 2018;198(3):329–39.

Systemic Medications in Chronic Obstructive Pulmonary Disease
Use and Outcomes

Nicolas Roche, MD, PhD, FERS

KEYWORDS

- COPD • Theophylline • Phosphodiesterase inhibitors • Oral corticosteroids • Macrolides
- Mucoactive agents • Alpha1-antitrypsin • Morphine

KEY POINTS

- Systemic treatments of chronic obstructive pulmonary disease (COPD) are not first-line therapeutic options.
- The benefit/risk ratio of oral beta2-adrenergic agonists and xanthines is not favorable.
- Azithromycin, phosphodiesterase 4 inhibitors, and mucomodifiers can contribute to exacerbation prevention in patients on inhaled therapy.
- The long-term use of systemic corticosteroids in COPD should be strongly discouraged.
- Several biologics are currently in development for COPD therapy and may prove useful in particular subpopulations identified through the use of specific biomarkers.

INTRODUCTION

Chronic obstructive pulmonary disease (COPD) is now defined by the coexistence of chronic respiratory symptoms and permanent (ie, not fully reversible) airflow limitation, caused by airways and parenchymal disease.[1] The development of airflow obstruction and emphysema is the consequence of a close interplay between inflammation, innate and adaptive immune reactions, protease-antiprotease imbalance, and oxidative stress, leading to airway wall and parenchymal remodeling and mucus hypersecretion.[2–6] Associated phenomena include chronic infection/colonization/microbiota modifications, autoimmunity, senescence, and systemic inflammation.[7,8]

Although some decades ago systemic treatments (ie, theophylline and oral corticosteroids for very severe cases) represented the main therapeutic approach for patients with COPD, inhaled medications are now the cornerstone of COPD treatment.[1] They have the obvious advantage of delivering high local concentrations of effective medication, while minimizing systemic absorption and side effects. However, because of these properties, they do not exert any significant effect on the systemic components of the disease, which have been repeatedly emphasized in the last 15 years.[9] The comorbidities and systemic features frequently seen in patients with COPD include muscle deconditioning, malnutrition, osteoporosis, psychological distress (anxiety-depression), cognitive impairment, metabolic and cardiovascular diseases, anemia, and lung cancer.[10–12] In the mid 2000s there was great enthusiasm around the concept of systemic

Dr N. Roche reports grants and personal fees from Boehringer Ingelheim, Novartis, and Pfizer, and personal fees from Teva, GSK, AstraZeneca, Chiesi, Mundipharma, Cipla, Sanofi, Sandoz, 3M, Trudell, and Zambon.
Respiratory Medicine, Pneumologie et Soins Intensifs Respiratoires, APHP Centre, Cochin Hospital, Université de Paris (Descartes), Institut Cochin (UMR 1016), 27, rue du Fbg St Jacques, Paris 75014, France
E-mail address: nicolas.roche@aphp.fr

Clin Chest Med 41 (2020) 485–494
https://doi.org/10.1016/j.ccm.2020.05.007
0272-5231/20/© 2020 Elsevier Inc. All rights reserved.

inflammation as a common trigger for all of these conditions, with many studies showing increases in several systemic inflammatory biomarkers. However, the exact relation between COPD and underlying pathophysiologic mechanisms remained uncertain. At present, decreased physical activity (also associated with systemic inflammation) is viewed as a major common contributor to most systemic aspects of COPD.[13] The increased frequency of cardiovascular events and treatments in patients with COPD also led to some interest in the possible interaction between inflammatory bursts and/or increases in lung hyperinflation with COPD outcomes, and this is the most plausible mechanism helping explain the increased risk of major cardiovascular events following acute exacerbations.[10]

In addition to their lack of effects on the systemic component of COPD, inhaled treatments may not be sufficiently effective to deliver pharmaceutical agents to the small airways, where most of the disease processes outlined earlier reside.[14]

This article reviews the effects of systemic agents with a main focus on clinical outcomes and long-term maintenance use. Pharmaceutical families of interest include oral beta2 agonists, theophylline, phosphodiesterase (PDE) inhibitors, macrolides with antiinflammatory properties and other antibiotics, mucoactive agents, corticosteroids, antileukotrienes, cardiovascular drugs, and biologics.

ORAL BETA2-ADRENERGIC AGONISTS

The benefit/risk ratio of oral beta2 agonists is much less favorable than that of their inhaled counterparts, because high systemic levels are required to achieve sufficient local concentrations leading to bronchodilation. At therapeutic doses, side effects (tremor, tachycardia) are more frequent and intense, whereas bronchodilation is similar[15] or less pronounced[16] than the inhaled presentation. In addition, these agents have been assessed only in small short-term studies with no patient-reported outcome end points. As a consequence, they are not recommended for COPD treatment except when the use of any inhaled treatment is impossible.

XANTHINES, THEOPHYLLINE

Theophylline is a xanthine structurally similar to caffeine that was initially developed for asthma in the late 1930s, at a time when COPD was not even well recognized.[17–19] Its main mechanisms of action are adenosine receptor (A1 and A2) inhibition (high potency at therapeutic concentrations) and (weak) PDE-3 and PDE-4 selective inhibition at higher and poorly tolerated concentrations.[20] Through these pathways, it exerts numerous immunomodulatory and antiinflammatory effects and has weak bronchodilator properties. Interestingly, theophylline decreases neutrophilic and eosinophilic airways inflammation, which can both be involved in patients with COPD, depending on the underlying endotype (ie, pathophysiologic profile). It also modulates lymphocytes functions.

The acute physiologic effects of theophylline include bronchodilation, lung deflation, improved gas exchanges, increased diaphragmatic function, reduced work of breathing, and improved mucociliary clearance. How these numerous demonstrable effects translate into clinical improvements is less clear, which is largely explained by the narrow therapeutic index of the drug; for instance, bronchodilation and diaphragmatic improvements need high doses to be clinically meaningful, which exposes patients to risks of serious dose/concentration-dependent side effects such as gastrointestinal (GI) perturbations (nausea, vomiting, exacerbated gastroesophageal reflux), tremor, sleep disturbance, headache, seizures, arrhythmias, and heart failure. In addition, many factors can interact with theophylline serum concentrations, including diseases that are frequently seen in patients with COPD, such as heart failure, liver disease, and smoking. In addition, theophylline serum concentrations vary depending on its interaction with several concomitant drugs (including antibiotics used in COPD exacerbations), the elimination of which is modulated by the cytochrome P (CYP) 1A2 or CYP3A4 coenzymatic activity (**Table 1**). Thus, using theophylline often requires monitoring its blood concentrations, further influencing its ease of use. As a consequence, and particularly in acute situations, the acute use of theophylline has been widely abandoned because of the need for high serum concentrations to achieve clinically meaningful bronchodilation or diaphragmatic improvement, and the associated risk of significant toxicity.

Regarding long-term use, there has been some interest in one particular property of theophylline: restoration of histone-deacetylase 2 (HDAC2) activity.[21] HDAC2 is an important cofactor of corticosteroids effects because it interacts with the corticosteroid-glucocorticoid receptor, contributing to chromatin condensation and thereby inhibiting the transcription and subsequent expression of proinflammatory genes (transrepression).[22] In smokers, and even more in patients with COPD, the oxidative stress impairs HDAC2 function, representing 1 of the numerous

Table 1
Main modulators of theophylline's pharmacokinetics

Effect	Increased Bioavailability	Reduced Bioavailability
Disease/condition	Viral infections Congestive heart failure Liver diseases	—
Age	—	Children<16 y
Toxic agents	—	Cigarette and marijuana smoking
Medications (through CYP1A2 and CYP3A4 modulation)	Erythromycin, clarithromycin (not azithromycin), ciprofloxacin (not ofloxacin), cimetidine (not ranitidine) allopurinol, serotonin uptake inhibitors, flu vaccination	Phenytoin, phenobarbitone, rifampicin

Data from Refs.[18,20]

mechanisms of corticosteroid resistance.[23] Thus, conceptually theophylline could restore the effects of corticosteroids, which are reduced in smokers and in COPD. This mode of action could be of particular interest because it occurs at serum concentrations that are approximately half the threshold of toxicity. Following encouraging results from in vitro experiments on HDAC2 activity and corticosteroid cellular effects, this hypothesis has been clinically tested in 2 randomized controlled trials, with disappointing results regarding all variables of clinical interest (ie, lung function, exacerbations, symptoms, and quality of life).[24,25]

As a consequence, the use of theophylline has been largely abandoned as part of long-term maintenance therapy. However, in some areas of the world, Cost-issues are such that theophylline is one of a few affordable options, together with a few low-cost (but still very effective) inhaled drugs such as salbutamol and beclomethasone.

The theophylline/xanthines family includes not only theophylline but also its derivatives aminophylline (the oldest one), bamiphylline, and doxophylline. The main potential difference between these agents is the efficacy/safety profile, which might be better for doxophylline according to a recent network meta-analysis.[19] How this translates into clinical superiority at the individual patient level is not fully clear.

PHOSPHODIESTERASE 4 INHIBITORS

PDE-4 inhibitors are often wrongly considered as modern theophyllines. This concept is not valid because most of the clinical effect of theophylline observed at nontoxic doses are linked to adenosine receptor antagonism, whereas effective PDE inhibition occurs only at toxic or close-to-toxic doses. Real selective PDE inhibitors commercially available at present are limited to one agent, roflumilast, which is not authorized or reimbursed in all countries. Another agent, cilomilast, was provisionally approved in the early 2000s but its development has been abandoned because of concerns about its efficacy/safety profile.[26]

There are many subtypes of PDE-4 (A, B, C, and D) and more than 25 isoforms, many of which are expressed in various inflammatory and resident cell types in the airways.[17,27,28] The potential beneficial effects of PDE-4 inhibition are numerous because PDE-4 is involved in cyclic AMP (cAMP) degradation. Thus, PDE-4 inhibition increases cellular levels of cAMP, which acts as an antiinflammatory second messenger decreasing the release of inflammatory mediators and the expression of proinflammatory surface receptors (eg, adhesion molecules) by neutrophils and other cell types, including macrophages, eosinophils, and T lymphocytes. Roflumilast (through its active metabolite roflumilast N-oxide) reduces the recruitment of inflammatory cells in the airways. cAMP is also involved in smooth muscle relaxation, but the bronchodilator effect of roflumilast at therapeutic concentrations is limited. In animal models, roflumilast prevents cigarette smoke–induced lung inflammation and emphysema.[18]

In humans, following the first studies and their subgroup analyses, roflumilast has been shown to reduce the risk of exacerbations in patients with COPD and frequent exacerbations (or previous hospitalization), severe airflow obstruction (Global initiative on Obstructive Lung Disease [GOLD] 3–4, postbronchodilator forced expiratory volume in 1 second [FEV_1] <50% predicted), symptoms of chronic bronchitis, and receiving bronchodilator therapy.[29] This beneficial effect occurs even in patients receiving concomitant treatment with inhaled long-acting bronchodilators and corticosteroids and is accompanied by an improvement in lung function, although the increase in FEV$_1$ (mean, 51 mL) does not reach the classic (but debatable for therapies administered on top of active medications) threshold for clinical significance (100 mL).[30] These effects have been confirmed by Cochrane systematic reviews collating data from 20 studies using roflumilast in more than 17,000 participants,[29] in which small improvements in symptoms and quality of life were also noted.

Roflumilast shares GI side effects with xanthines but, in contrast with those agents, it is not associated with an increased risk of cardiovascular effects. It can induce moderate weight loss (3 kg on average), mostly related to a decrease in fat mass. GI side effects can lead to treatment interruption.

Compounds with both PDE-3 and PDE-4 inhibitory activity have been assessed in humans with no success because of lack or safety and/or unacceptable side effects. A new agent of this family administered through the inhaled route, ensifentrine, is currently being tested in clinical trials.[31] Currently available data are insufficient to draw conclusions.

MACROLIDES AND OTHER ANTIBIOTICS

The most studied macrolide for long-term maintenance therapy in COPD is azithromycin,[32,33] although earlier clinical studies were reported using erythromycin.[34] Antiinflammatory and immune-modulating properties are a feature of these macrolides.[18,35] Their first applications were the successful treatment of diffuse panbronchiolitis with erythromycin, and cystic fibrosis colonized by *Pseudomonas aeruginosa* with azithromycin. Animal models have confirmed the antiinflammatory effects of this agent, which can also prevent cigarette smoke–induced development of emphysema.[18,35] Macrolides also have the potential to augment HDAC2 expression, thereby potentially restoring corticosteroid sensitivity.

During the late 2000s, 3 studies showed the preventive effect of erythromycin on exacerbation occurrences. Subsequent trials showed a similar effect using azithromycin. Although some individual studies failed to achieve the same success, an overall positive effect was shown in a meta-analysis.[36] Studies with roxithromycin and clarithromycin did not provide convincing evidence but did not have a sufficiently robust design because they had a low sample size and were of limited duration.[35]

Considering the beneficial effect of both erythromycin and azithromycin (although they have never been directly compared), 4 main questions arise. First, selection of the best agent and the best scheme of administration. In terms of convenience of use, azithromycin is clearly the preferred drug: once versus twice or 3 times a day for erythromycin. Trials used a 250 mg/d or greater than 500 mg 3 times a week scheme,[35] although 250 mg 3 times a week is probably used more often in clinical practice as in cystic fibrosis (in which the efficacy of this protocol was shown), despite a lack of formal evaluation in COPD.

Second, the most appropriate target population. The largest study with erythromycin recruited 109 patients in a single center. There were no exacerbation-related inclusion criteria, but more than one-third of the population reported at least 3 exacerbations during the 12 months preceding inclusion, and median exacerbation frequency in the placebo group was 2, suggesting a population of frequent exacerbators.[37] The rate reduction of exacerbations in the active arm was 36% and, in addition, erythromycin reduced not only the rate but also the duration of exacerbations. Responders analysis was not performed and would have been difficult considering the limited sample size. The effect on exacerbation was not associated with effects on biomarkers of inflammation or bacterial loads in the airways, preventing any firm conclusions regarding the mechanisms of observed efficacy. Azithromycin was studied over 12 months in the largest macrolide trial (n = 1142).[32] Patients were on supplemental oxygen, had received systemic corticosteroids, or had been hospitalized for an exacerbation during the previous year. There was a 17% overall risk reduction in exacerbations. Responders analysis found the greatest benefit in ex-smokers, older patients, and milder GOLD stages.[38] However this analysis was post hoc, requiring further confirmation before drawing firm conclusions. The other 12-month study on azithromycin was performed in patients with a history of 3 or more exacerbations in the previous year, most of whom received triple inhaled therapy. Overall it remains difficult to define a specific target subgroup, although baseline exacerbation risk is an appropriate selection criterion.

The third question relates to risks associated with long-term macrolide therapy.[35] GI side effects (diarrhea), impairments in liver function, and a minimal increase in hearing loss have been reported. Although there is a theoretic risk of increased cardiac arrhythmias, caused by the potential increase in the corrected QT (QTc) electrocardiographic interval, this was not observed in any of the trials. However, patients with prolonged QTc interval were excluded from those trials. In practice, it may be important to consider its use primarily in patients with normal electrocardiograms. An increase in the proportion of macrolide-resistant microorganisms in nasal swabs has been observed, although the absolute number of patients colonized by such bacteria did not change. The bacteriologic consequences of long-term macrolide use in COPD populations remains unknown. The last important question is the duration of treatment. For this question, there is no firm answer at present. Conclusive trials have lasted 6 to 12 months, and no trial of sequential administration (eg, during the winter period) has been performed.

Regarding other (nonmacrolide) antibiotics, the only sufficiently powered trial was performed with pulsed moxifloxacin (400 mg/d 5 days every 8 weeks), which produced a nonsignificant trend toward a reduction in exacerbations and is thus considered a negative trial.[39]

MUCOMODIFIERS

There are 2 main potential reasons for considering the use of mucoactive agents in COPD[40]: first, chronic mucus hypersecretion is thought to play an important role in the pathophysiology and natural course of the disease. The mucus is more abundant and viscous in many patients with COPD and is responsible for small airways obstruction, which is associated with poor prognosis in patients undergoing lung volume reduction surgery. In smokers and patients with COPDs, chronic mucus hypersecretion is also associated with several prognostic variables (FEV_1 decline and development of COPD, exacerbation and hospitalization risk, and mortality). Mucin concentrations (MUC5B, MUC5AC) seem to play a key role in the pathogenesis of chronic bronchitis.[5]

Several mucoactive agents have antioxidant properties, and oxidative stress is thought to be involved in the pathobiology of COPD, both at local (airways) and systemic levels.[6] Its consequences include inflammatory cells recruitment, protease-antiprotease imbalance, and production of proinflammatory mediators. Paradoxically, there has been no firm demonstration of an effect of most mucoactive agents on mucociliary clearance in vivo in humans. In vitro data and animal models found effects on airway wall remodeling, chemotaxis, and activation of neutrophils and monocytes/macrophages as well as decreasing bacterial adherence. In vivo during acute exacerbations, a reduction in levels of inflammatory markers and an improvement in bacterial elimination and symptoms has been found but was not accompanied by effects on hard end points such as lung function or length of stay in the hospital, questioning the clinical relevance of biological effects. Some mucoactive agents (carbocysteine, N-acetylcysteine, erdosteine, and ambroxol) have reduced the occurrence of COPD exacerbations in several trials, a finding that is supported by the results of a meta-analysis.[41] One of those trials found a reduction in exacerbation rate only in patients not taking inhaled corticosteroids (ICS), whereas the other found a reduction in the overall population, in which only a minority (<20%) of patients received ICS, suggesting that mucoactive agents may prove effective only in patients with suboptimal inhaled therapy. This point was further tested in a specifically designed large study that did not find any interaction between ICS and effects of N-acetylcysteine on exacerbations occurrence. This finding was confirmed in a more recent network meta-analysis in which a metaregression was performed to identify factors associated with treatment response.[41] Surprisingly, this analysis identified a trend toward less response in Chinese populations. This finding needs to be interpreted with caution considering the significant heterogeneity observed in the meta-analysis.

ORAL CORTICOSTEROIDS

The long-term use of oral corticosteroids is discouraged in COPD because of the well-known burden of side effects,[42] contrasting with the lack of evidence of clinically relevant beneficial effects.

Systemic dose-dependent side effects include fractures, diabetes, cataracts, hypertension, open-angle glaucoma, skin bruising, muscular weakness, cardiovascular events, and cerebrovascular events. Many of these effects can have major consequences leading to severe health status impairment. In addition, the use of oral corticosteroids has been linked to increased mortality and reduced efficacy of nutritional supplementation, a component of pulmonary rehabilitation.[43,44] The combination of COPD and oral corticosteroids also increases the risk of infections that may have particularly disastrous consequences in patients with severe lung function impairment, such as mycobacteria, *Aspergillus* spp, and various types of bacteria involved in chronic airways colonization/infection and pneumonia.

The most recent meta-analysis by the Cochrane Collaboration on oral corticosteroids for stable COPD was published in 2005.[45] Treatment lasted more than 3 weeks in only 5 studies among the 24 that were identified. Combining all studies, the mean FEV_1 improvement was 53 mL, half the minimal clinically important difference. The proportion of FEV_1 responders (>20% increase relative to baseline) was approximately 2.5 times higher with oral steroids than on placebo. Effects were more prominent with higher dosages (>30 mg/d vs 7–15 mg/d), associated with more risks of side effects. Increases in walking distance were statistically significant but not clinically relevant (29 m with the 12-minute walk test), and most of these studies were short term. Some symptomatic and health status differences were reported but considered insignificant from a clinical perspective. Oral corticosteroids did not prevent exacerbations but the studies were not designed to test this end point in a robust manner.

The considerations presented here are valid only for patients with COPD and no associated asthma. The situation may be different in patients with COPD associated with predominating severe asthma, the subject of another article in this issue.

ANTILEUKOTRIENES

Antileukotriene agents are not recommended in COPD.[1] Only very few properly designed studies have been performed to assess their effects in this population. There are 2 types of available agents[18]: 5-lipoxygenase (LO) or 5-LO–activating protein inhibitors and cysteinyl-leukotrienes (Cys-LTs: LT-C4, D4, E4) receptor antagonists. Their purpose is to reduce the production of leukotrienes with proinflammatory activity (LTB4, product of the 5-LO pathway) or to decrease effects on airway smooth muscle, mucus secretion, vascular permeability, and mucociliary clearance (Cys-LTs). In 2015, 7 studies were identified, 3 of which were nonrandomized (2 with montelukast, 1 with zafirlukast). Among the 4 others, 1 dealt with zileuton (for acute exacerbations), 1 with montelukast, and 2 with products that have been secondarily abandoned. All these randomized trials were short term, whereas 2 observational studies (1 prospective, 1 retrospective) had a duration of at least 12 months.[46] Thus, from a review of all of these studies, it is clear that anti-LTs have not been properly assessed in COPD. In only 1 (short-term) randomized controlled trial (RCT) with montelukast, some nonsignificant effects on symptoms (dyspnea, sputum production) and lung function were reported.[46]

CARDIOVASCULAR/METABOLIC TREATMENTS

There is a strong interaction between COPD and cardiovascular diseases, both sharing common risk factors[10]; however, the increased cross-prevalence of these conditions is not explained simply by smoking. As mentioned earlier, this association may relate to systemic inflammation and/or decreased daily physical activity, both of which are interrelated. Impairment of cardiac function caused by lung hyperinflation may also play a role, as well as chronic or intermittent hypoxia. In addition, the burden (eg, in terms of dyspnea and exacerbations) and prognosis of COPD is impaired in the presence of cardiovascular diseases. Reciprocally, there is an increased frequency of COPD in patients with cardiovascular conditions, and COPD impairs their prognosis. Consequently, cardiovascular drugs are frequently used in patients with COPD. In addition, cardiovascular events are more frequent during and after COPD exacerbations, of which they can represent either complications or part of differential diagnoses. Because of these strong interactions, there has been a lot of interest in the potential effects of cardiovascular drugs in patients with COPD.

The first question that was raised related to the safety of β-blockers in patients with COPD: these agents, especially those with poor beta1-adrenoreceptor selectivity, can enhance airway smooth muscle contractions and, thereby worsen airflow limitation, through beta2-adrenoreceptor antagonism. In clinical trials of β-blockers for ischemic heart disease, patients with COPD were found to benefit as much as, or even more than, those with no COPD in terms of survival.[47] The effect of cardioselective β1-blockers on lung function seems very limited, if any, and these agents do not increase the occurrence of respiratory symptoms. In addition, they do not impair respiratory outcomes when continued during acute exacerbations. Observational studies had even suggested that β-blockers could decrease the risk of COPD exacerbations and related hospitalizations and mortality. However, a recent large controlled trial in the United States did not confirm this hypothesis, and found a worse outcome, including risk of death in patients randomized to receive β-blockers and who had no cardiovascular indication of beta1-blockade.[48]

Similarly, retrospective database or prospective cohort studies suggested some benefits from statins in terms of exacerbation risk. Such effects could be explained by the pleiotropic antiinflammatory effects of statins, which could control the systemic inflammation observed in many patients with COPD. However, again a randomized controlled trial did not report any effect on exacerbation rate or mortality in patients with no cardiovascular or metabolic indication.[49]

Renin-angiotensin-aldosterone system inhibitors can have antiinflammatory, antifibrotic, and antioxidant effects that could be of interest in COPD.[10] It has even been suggested that these agents have some potential to prevent emphysema progression.[50] However, no clinical advantage related to the use of these agents has ever been formally established in adequately designed studies.

BIOLOGICS

Inflammation, oxidative stress, and airway and parenchymal remodeling, including fibrosis, all represent potential targets for biologics directed at modulating (upstream or downstream) their mediators, biological triggers, or signaling pathways. Their intimate mechanisms are involved in the clinical manifestations of COPD, including dyspnea and exacerbations, as well as in disease progression. However, this involvement is highly heterogeneous and the disease biology is still incompletely deciphered, making it difficult to identify the most relevant targets and define the corresponding patient populations. Heterogeneity applies not only to stable state but also to exacerbations. In addition, COPD is a slowly evolutive disease with an overall low reactivity to any pharmacologic intervention to date. These properties create additional hurdles when testing new agents clinically. Although clinical phenotypes correspond with clinical features or combinations of features associated with disease progression and/or treatment responses, endotypes are underlying biological mechanisms that can be identified through biomarkers.[51,52] How the disease can be split into phenotypes and endotypes is much less clear in COPD than in asthma.[53] In addition, because there is some marked overlap and discrepancies between phenotypes and between them and endotypes, the current trend is to adopt the concept of individual treatable traits that can be independently targeted by dedicated interventions.[54] Altogether, these traits cover the entire spectrum of asthma, COPD, and complex overlapping/intricate situations. Among them, eosinophilic COPD triggers particular interest.

The central role of systemic and local inflammation in COPD pathophysiology suggested that anti–tumor necrosis factor (THF) agents could have some potential to influence the natural history of the disease. In addition, TNF-alpha has been shown to induce emphysema in animal models. However, clinical trials gave disappointing results, in terms of both effects on markers of local (sputum) and systemic inflammation, and clinical outcomes.[55,56]

More recently, anti–interleukin-5 (IL-5) agents have been tested in COPD. These agents (IL-5 inhibitor or IL-5 receptor blocker) primarily target eosinophilic inflammation. In 2 parallel RCTs using mepolizumab (IL-5 inhibitor), 1 of the trials showed a reduction in the risk of COPD exacerbations (−23%) in patients with higher (>300/μL) blood eosinophil counts (considered as a reliable surrogate for sputum eosinophils).[57] However, these results were not significant in the other study. Further, there was no difference in lung function or health status in either study compared with the placebo arm. The larger and more recent study using benralizumab (IL-5 receptor blocker) did not reduce exacerbation rate in patients with eosinophilic COPD (>220 cells/μL). Therefore, additional data need to be gathered before these treatments can be recommended.

ALPHA1-ANTITRYPSIN AUGMENTATION THERAPY

Because severe alpha1-antitrypsin (AAT) deficiency is a rare disease, RCTs are difficult to conduct. A European Respiratory Society taskforce recently performed a systematic review that identified 8 RCTs and 17 observational studies (11 of which were uncontrolled) assessing the effects of augmentation therapy on various clinical and imaging outcomes.[58] Only 3 RCTs were placebo controlled. There was a beneficial effect on emphysema progression as assessed by computed tomography (CT) scan, but efficacy could not be shown in terms of clinical outcomes. However, such efficacy (although subject to more biases) was suggested by some observational studies. In addition, emphysema progression on CT scan is associated with mortality and quality of life, suggesting that it may represent a clinically relevant outcome. Therefore, several guidelines recommend augmentation therapy in AAT-deficient patients with emphysema and progressive disease.[1]

SYSTEMIC TREATMENTS FOR DYSPNEA

Dyspnea is the most important and relevant symptom of patients with COPD. It is the limiting element of exercise capacity/tolerance and daily activity. Therefore, relieving dyspnea is one of the major goals of COPD care. First-line approaches include bronchodilators and rehabilitation. Interventional techniques such as lung volume reduction can be considered in highly selected patient populations. In some patients, dyspnea remains refractory to those therapies. In such instances, benzodiazepines and morphine have been considered, but they remain seldom prescribed as part of routine practice.[59] In 2016, a Cochrane Review identified 26 RCTs with more than 500 patients with refractory breathlessness in the context of advanced disease and terminal illness. In 14 studies, recruited subjects were

Table 2
Examples of systemic treatments targeting specific subpopulations/treatable traits in chronic obstructive pulmonary disease

Treatment	Subpopulation/Treatable Trait
Established	
PDE-4 inhibitors (roflumilast)	Severe airflow obstruction, repeated exacerbations, chronic mucus hyperproduction, on top of long-acting bronchodilators
AAT	AAT deficiency
Putative	
Azithromycin	Ex-smokers, older patients, milder airflow obstruction Airway bacterial colonization/chronic infection Repeated bacterial exacerbations
Anti–IL-5 agents	Eosinophilic COPD
Mucoactive agents	Chronic mucus hyperproduction

primarily or exclusively patients with COPD. Altogether, the quality of evidence was deemed low or very low, but some evidence of dyspnea alleviation was found. In parallel, drowsiness, nausea and vomiting, and constipation were frequent (13%, 20%, and 18%, respectively).[60] Thus, the benefit/risk ratio needs to be carefully considered on an individual basis, balancing the risk of side effects and the burden of dyspnea. In summary, for very breathless patients, a trial can be initiated under close monitoring and stopped if the benefits are not evident or if side effects limit its use.

In a similar way, the last Cochrane Review on benzodiazepines for dyspnea was performed in 2016 and included 8 studies in patients with advanced cancer or COPD, in which benzodiazepines were compared with placebo, promethazine, or morphine. No demonstration of positive effects was found, although the investigators found less drowsiness than with morphine.

SUMMARY

Although numerous systemic treatments for COPD exist, they are positioned late in treatment algorithms, with inhaled therapy remaining the cornerstone of treatment. However, when inhaled therapy is not sufficient to control the burden of disease, oral therapies such as PDE-4 inhibitors, azithromycin, or mucoactive agents can be of help in some patients (**Table 2**), especially to reduce the risk of exacerbations. The major difficulty here is to choose the appropriate responder and how these treatments should be positioned in the global treatment algorithm. For instance, should they be prescribed in addition to other anti-inflammatory agents (ie, corticosteroids) or should they replace them in some specific subgroups of patients? Some currently available biologics used in severe asthma could also be effective in

some patient categories (eosinophilic COPD), but additional studies centered on well-selected candidates are needed. Some oral agents, such as beta2-adrenergic agents and particularly theophylline, remain widely used in some countries because of their low cost, although their benefit/risk profiles are unfavorable compared with inhaled therapy. AAT augmentation therapy is useful in patients with AAT deficiency and progressive emphysema. Cardiovascular drugs should be used in COPD only if those patients have underlying cardiovascular condition supporting their indication. Ongoing research aims at identifying new therapeutic targets and agents in inflammation, destruction/repair mechanisms, immune regulation, microbiota homeostasis, mucus modulation, and lung regeneration.

REFERENCES

1. Global Initiative for Chronic Obstructive Lung Disease. Global strategy for the diagnosis, management and prevention of chronic obstructive lung disease. Available at: https://goldcopd.org.
2. Bagdonas E, Raudoniute J, Bruzauskaite I, et al. Novel aspects of pathogenesis and regeneration mechanisms in COPD. Int J Chron Obstruct Pulmon Dis 2015;10:995–1013.
3. Eapen MS, Myers S, Walters EH, et al. Airway inflammation in chronic obstructive pulmonary disease (COPD): a true paradox. Expert Rev Respir Med 2017;11:827–39.
4. Hussell T, Lui S, Jagger C, et al. The consequence of matrix dysfunction on lung immunity and the microbiome in COPD. Eur Respir Rev 2018;27. https://doi.org/10.1183/16000617.0032-2018.
5. Kesimer M, Ford AA, Ceppe A, et al. Airway mucin concentration as a marker of chronic bronchitis. N Engl J Med 2017;377:911–22.

6. Fischer BM, Voynow JA, Ghio AJ. COPD: balancing oxidants and antioxidants. Int J Chron Obstruct Pulmon Dis 2015;10:261–76.

7. Barnes PJ. Senescence in COPD and its comorbidities. Annu Rev Physiol 2017;79:517–39.

8. Caramori G, Ruggeri P, Di Stefano A, et al. Autoimmunity and COPD: clinical implications. Chest 2018;153:1424–31.

9. Barnes PJ, Celli BR. Systemic manifestations and comorbidities of COPD. Eur Respir J 2009;33:1165–85.

10. Rabe KF, Hurst JR, Suissa S. Cardiovascular disease and COPD: dangerous liaisons? Eur Respir Rev 2018;27. https://doi.org/10.1183/16000617.0057-2018.

11. Pelgrim CE, Peterson JD, Gosker HR, et al. Psychological co-morbidities in COPD: targeting systemic inflammation, a benefit for both? Eur J Pharmacol 2019;842:99–110.

12. Corlateanu A, Covantev S, Mathioudakis AG, et al. Prevalence and burden of comorbidities in chronic obstructive pulmonary disease. Respir Investig 2016;54:387–96.

13. Gimeno-Santos E, Frei A, Steurer-Stey C, et al. Determinants and outcomes of physical activity in patients with COPD: a systematic review. Thorax 2014. https://doi.org/10.1136/thoraxjnl-2013-204763.

14. Higham A, Quinn AM, Cançado JED, et al. The pathology of small airways disease in COPD: historical aspects and future directions. Respir Res 2019;20:49.

15. Cazzola M, Calderaro F, Califano C, et al. Oral bambuterol compared to inhaled salmeterol in patients with partially reversible chronic obstructive pulmonary disease. Eur J Clin Pharmacol 1999;54:829–33.

16. Shim CS, Williams MH. Bronchodilator response to oral aminophylline and terbutaline versus aerosol albuterol in patients with chronic obstructive pulmonary disease. Am J Med 1983;75:697–701.

17. Spina D, Page CP. Xanthines and phosphodiesterase inhibitors. Handb Exp Pharmacol 2017;237:63–91.

18. Pleasants RA. Clinical pharmacology of oral maintenance therapies for obstructive lung diseases. Respir Care 2018;63:671–89.

19. Cazzola M, Calzetta L, Barnes PJ, et al. Efficacy and safety profile of xanthines in COPD: a network meta-analysis. Eur Respir Rev 2018;27. https://doi.org/10.1183/16000617.0010-2018.

20. Barnes PJ. Theophylline. Am J Respir Crit Care Med 2013;188:901–6.

21. Cosio BG, Tsaprouni L, Ito K, et al. Theophylline restores histone deacetylase activity and steroid responses in COPD macrophages. J Exp Med 2004;200:689–95.

22. Barnes PJ, Adcock IM. Glucocorticoid resistance in inflammatory diseases. Lancet 2009;373:1905–17.

23. Ito K, Ito M, Elliott WM, et al. Decreased histone deacetylase activity in chronic obstructive pulmonary disease. N Engl J Med 2005;352:1967–76.

24. Devereux G, Cotton S, Fielding S, et al. Effect of theophylline as adjunct to inhaled corticosteroids on exacerbations in patients with COPD: a randomized clinical trial. JAMA 2018;320:1548–59.

25. Cosío BG, Shafiek H, Iglesias A, et al. Oral low-dose theophylline on top of inhaled fluticasone-salmeterol does not reduce exacerbations in patients with severe COPD: a pilot clinical trial. Chest 2016. https://doi.org/10.1016/j.chest.2016.04.011.

26. Compton CH, Gubb J, Nieman R, et al. Cilomilast, a selective phosphodiesterase-4 inhibitor for treatment of patients with chronic obstructive pulmonary disease: a randomised, dose-ranging study. Lancet 2001;358(9278):265–70, 358:265–70.

27. Lipworth BJ. Phosphodiesterase-4 inhibitors for asthma and chronic obstructive pulmonary disease. Lancet 2005;365:167–75.

28. Contreras S, Milara J, Morcillo E, et al. Selective inhibition of phosphodiesterases 4A, B, C and D isoforms in chronic respiratory diseases: current and future evidences. Curr Pharm Des 2017;23:2073–83.

29. Chong J, Leung B, Poole P. Phosphodiesterase 4 inhibitors for chronic obstructive pulmonary disease. Cochrane Database Syst Rev 2017;(9):CD002309.

30. Martinez FJ, Rabe KF, Sethi S, et al. Effect of roflumilast and inhaled corticosteroid/long-acting β2-agonist on chronic obstructive pulmonary disease exacerbations (RE(2)SPOND). a randomized clinical trial. Am J Respir Crit Care Med 2016;194:559–67.

31. Cazzola M, Calzetta L, Rogliani P, et al. Ensifentrine (RPL554): an investigational PDE3/4 inhibitor for the treatment of COPD. Expert Opin Investig Drugs 2019;28:827–33.

32. Albert RK, Connett J, Bailey WC, et al. Azithromycin for prevention of exacerbations of COPD. N Engl J Med 2011;365:689–98.

33. Uzun S, Djamin RS, Kluytmans JAJW, et al. Azithromycin maintenance treatment in patients with frequent exacerbations of chronic obstructive pulmonary disease (COLUMBUS): a randomised, double-blind, placebo-controlled trial. Lancet Respir Med 2014;2:361–8.

34. Seemungal TA, Wilkinson TM, Hurst JR, et al. Long-term erythromycin therapy is associated with decreased chronic obstructive pulmonary disease exacerbations. Am J Respir Crit Care Med 2008;178:1139–47.

35. Huckle AW, Fairclough LC, Todd I. Prophylactic antibiotic use in COPD and the potential anti-inflammatory activities of antibiotics. Respir Care 2018;63:609–19.

36. Cui Y, Luo L, Li C, et al. Long-term macrolide treatment for the prevention of acute exacerbations in

COPD: a systematic review and meta-analysis. Int J Chron Obstruct Pulmon Dis 2018;13:3813–29.

37. Suzuki T, Yanai M, Yamaya M, et al. Erythromycin and common cold in COPD. Chest 2001;120:730–3.

38. Han MK, Tayob N, Murray S, et al. Predictors of chronic obstructive pulmonary disease exacerbation reduction in response to daily azithromycin therapy. Am J Respir Crit Care Med 2014;189: 1503–8.

39. Sethi S, Jones PW, Theron MS, et al. Pulsed moxifloxacin for the prevention of exacerbations of chronic obstructive pulmonary disease: a randomized controlled trial. Respir Res 2010;11:10.

40. Decramer M, Janssens W. Mucoactive therapy in COPD. Eur Respir Rev 2010;19:134–40.

41. Cazzola M, Rogliani P, Calzetta L, et al. Impact of mucolytic agents on COPD exacerbations: a pairwise and network meta-analysis. COPD 2017;14: 552–63.

42. Manson SC, Brown RE, Cerulli A, et al. The cumulative burden of oral corticosteroid side effects and the economic implications of steroid use. Respir Med 2009;103:975–94.

43. Schols AM, Wesseling G, Kester AD, et al. Dose dependent increased mortality risk in COPD patients treated with oral glucocorticoids. Eur Respir J 2001;17(3):337–42.

44. Schols AM, Slangen J, Volovics L, et al. Weight loss is a reversible factor in the prognosis of chronic obstructive pulmonary disease. Am J Respir Crit Care Med 1998;157:1791–7.

45. Walters J, Walters E, Wood-Baker R. Oral corticosteroids for stable chronic obstructive pulmonary disease. Cochrane Database Syst Rev 2005;(3): CD005374.

46. Lee JH, Kim HJ, Kim YH. The effectiveness of antileukotriene agents in patients with COPD: a systemic review and meta-analysis. Lung 2015;193: 477–86.

47. Gottlieb SS, McCarter RJ, Vogel RA. Effect of betablockade on mortality among high-risk and low-risk patients after myocardial infarction. N Engl J Med 1998;339:489–97.

48. Dransfield MT, Voelker H, Bhatt SP, et al. Metoprolol for the prevention of acute exacerbations of COPD. N Engl J Med 2019;381:2304–14.

49. Criner GJ, Connett JE, Aaron SD, et al. Simvastatin for the prevention of exacerbations in moderate-to-severe COPD. N Engl J Med 2014;370:2201–10.

50. Parikh MA, Aaron CP, Hoffman EA, et al. Angiotensin-converting inhibitors and angiotensin II receptor blockers and longitudinal change in percent emphysema on computed tomography. The multiethnic study of atherosclerosis lung study. Ann Am Thorac Soc 2017;14:649–58.

51. Pavord ID. Biologics and chronic obstructive pulmonary disease. J Allergy Clin Immunol 2018;141: 1983–91.

52. Yousuf A, Brightling CE. Biologic drugs: a new target therapy in COPD? COPD 2018;15:99–107.

53. Woodruff PG, Agusti A, Roche N, et al. Current concepts in targeting chronic obstructive pulmonary disease pharmacotherapy: making progress towards personalised management. Lancet 2015; 385:1789–98.

54. Agusti A, Bel E, Thomas M, et al. Treatable traits: toward precision medicine of chronic airway diseases. Eur Respir J 2016;47:410–9.

55. Rennard SI, Flavin SK, Agarwal PK, et al. Long-term safety study of infliximab in moderate-to-severe chronic obstructive pulmonary disease. Respir Med 2013;107:424–32.

56. Dentener MA, Creutzberg EC, Pennings H-J, et al. Effect of infliximab on local and systemic inflammation in chronic obstructive pulmonary disease: a pilot study. Respiration 2008;76:275–82.

57. Pavord ID, Chanez P, Criner GJ, et al. Mepolizumab for eosinophilic chronic obstructive pulmonary disease. N Engl J Med 2017;377:1613–29.

58. Miravitlles M, Dirksen A, Ferrarotti I, et al. European Respiratory Society statement: diagnosis and treatment of pulmonary disease in α1-antitrypsin deficiency. Eur Respir J 2017;50. https://doi.org/10. 1183/13993003.00610-2017.

59. Ahmadi Z, Bernelid E, Currow DC, et al. Prescription of opioids for breathlessness in end-stage COPD: a national population-based study. Int J Chron Obstruct Pulmon Dis 2016;11:2651–7.

60. Barnes H, McDonald J, Smallwood N, et al. Opioids for the palliation of refractory breathlessness in adults with advanced disease and terminal illness. Cochrane Database Syst Rev 2016;2016. https:// doi.org/10.1002/14651858.CD011008.pub2.

Section V: Non-pharmacological Therapy in COPD

Smoking Cessation/ Vaccinations

Maria Montes de Oca, MD, PhD

KEYWORDS

- Chronic obstructive pulmonary disease • Smoking cessation • Counseling
- Nicotine replacement therapy • Bupropion • Varenicline • Influenza and pneumococcus vaccination

KEY POINTS

- A significant proportion of patients continue to smoke despite knowing they have chronic obstructive pulmonary disease (COPD).
- Smokers with COPD exhibit higher levels of nicotine dependence and have lower self-efficacy and self-esteem, which affects their ability to quit smoking.
- The combination of counseling plus pharmacotherapy is the most effective cessation treatment of smokers with COPD.
- Because of the high morbidity and mortality of influenza in patients with COPD, annual influenza vaccination has been recommended.
- Although the clinical efficacy of pneumococcal vaccination is uncertain in COPD, evidence suggests that it provides protection against CAP and reduces the likelihood of exacerbation. Therefore, several international health authorities routinely recommend this vaccination in patients with COPD.

SMOKING CESSATION IN CHRONIC OBSTRUCTIVE PULMONARY DISEASE

Cigarette smoking is the leading risk factor for chronic obstructive pulmonary disease (COPD) in developed countries and an important contributor to the burden in most societies around the world. Patients with COPD who continue to smoke have a higher prevalence of symptoms persistence, an accelerated decline in lung function, increased exacerbations, and higher mortality rate than non-smokers.[1–6] Therefore, smoking cessation has been identified as the single most cost-effective and effective strategy for slowing the progression of the disease.

SMOKING PREVALENCE IN CHRONIC OBSTRUCTIVE PULMONARY DISEASE

A significant proportion of patients with COPD continue to smoke despite knowing they have the disease, and as a consequence this behavior has a negative impact on the prognosis and progression of the disease.[7]

Several cross-sectional worldwide population-based studies have assessed the smoking status (never, former, and current smokers) in different COPD population. The IBERPOC study in Spain reported a prevalence of 15% and 12.8% for patients with COPD who are current and ex-smokers , respectively.[8] The Behavioral Risk Factor Surveillance System, a survey conducted in the United States, showed a frequency of current smoking in patients with COPD of 45.1%, higher than that observed among adults with other chronic disease (23%), asthma (20.3%), and no chronic disease (18.9%).[9] In Latin-America, the PLATINO study (Latin American Project for Investigation of Obstructive Lung Disease) reported that 31.5% of the patients with COPD were never smokers, 32.5% former smokers, and 36% current smokers.[10] In a more recent review from Latin-America, current smokers in COPD ranged from 13% in Bucaramanga (Colombia) to 38.5%

Servicio de Neumonología, Hospital Universitario de Caracas, Facultad de Medicina, Universidad Central de Venezuela, Centro Médico de Caracas, Av. Los Erasos, Edf. Anexo B, Piso 4, Consultorio 4B, San Bernardino, Caracas, Venezuela
E-mail address: montesdeoca.maria@gmail.com

Clin Chest Med 41 (2020) 495–512
https://doi.org/10.1016/j.ccm.2020.06.013
0272-5231/20/© 2020 Elsevier Inc. All rights reserved.

in Santiago de Chile (**Fig. 1**).[11] In a large survey from mainland China almost half of the patients with COPD were current smokers (47.7%), 15.8% former smokers, and 36.5% never smokers.[12] Results from the Health Survey for England showed that current smoking was higher among people with COPD (34.9%) than those without COPD (22.4%), and the smoking prevalence increased with disease severity (current smokers 29.5% in mild, 38.3% in moderate, and 40.5% in severe/very severe COPD).[13]

An analysis of individuals with COPD enrolled in the COPDGene cohort reported that 43.4% were current smokers,[14] and similar results have been reported by some recent COPD pharmacologic clinical trials (current smoker frequency between 35% and 47%) (**Table 1**).

CHARACTERISTICS OF SMOKERS WITH CHRONIC OBSTRUCTIVE PULMONARY DISEASE

There are differences in clinical characteristics between smoking patients with and without COPD. Smokers with COPD exhibit higher levels of nicotine dependence, smoke more cigarettes a day, have higher cotinine concentrations, and have less self-efficacy and self-esteem than those without the disease, all of which affect their ability to quit smoking.[13,23,24] This does not seem to be due to lack of motivation to quit, which was not different between smokers with and without COPD.[24] On the other hand, depression was more common among smokers with COPD, a fact that can influence the behavior of these patients.[25]

Smokers with COPD seem to have similar susceptibility to smoking cessation intervention than those without COPD. A study showed that 1-year quit rates in smokers with COPD was higher compared with those without the disease.[26] However, results of real-life studies and clinical trials found that the combination of brief or intensive counseling in smokers with COPD had comparable abstinence rates over 1 year to smokers in general.[27–30]

Data from the COPDGene study showed that current smokers were on average younger, had longer duration of cigarette smoking, and were more likely to be African American than former smokers.[31] The cigarette consumption in pack-years was similar between former and current smokers, as well as other functional parameters (forced expiratory volume in the first second of expiration [FEV_1]/forced vital capacity 0.54 vs 0.56 and FEV_1% 63.1% vs 63.3%, respectively).[31] In the visual analysis of CT, former smokers had an emphysema index 5.5% higher than current smokers, and the difference was evident in each GOLD categories.[31]

SMOKING DIAGNOSIS IN CHRONIC OBSTRUCTIVE PULMONARY DISEASE

The approach to the smoking patient in general should consider the mental situation in which the subject is at the time of consultation, paying attention to 2 aspects intimately linked with tobacco use: motivation and dependence.

Assessment of Motivation and Self-Efficacy in Smokers with Chronic Obstructive Pulmonary Disease

Self-efficacy in smokers with COPD is usually low and associated with low quit rates.[24] Therefore, increasing motivation and building self-efficacy are particularly important in these patients.

In general, the first approach to assess motivation is to classify the patient according to the phase model of Prochaska and Di Clemente. A correct phase motivational stage identification allows an adequate therapeutic intervention, timely treatment, appropriate use of resources, and increases the chances of success. It is not recommended to initiate pharmacotherapy for smoking cessation until the patient is in the preparation stage. **Fig. 2** shows a motivational phase diagnostic diagram.

Assessment of Tobacco Dependence in Smokers with Chronic Obstructive Pulmonary Disease

The assessment of the nicotine dependence in smokers involves the evaluation of the number of package-years, the degree of physical dependence to nicotine with the Fagerström test, the analysis of the previous attempts to quit, and determination of carbon monoxide (CO) levels in the exhaled air.

Number of package-years

The number of package-years can be obtained multiplying the amount of cigarette that the patient smokes per day by the number of years that the person has smoked, then divided by 20 (average number of cigarettes in a package). Patients with more than 5 package-years will have more difficulty quitting smoking than those with lower values.

Assessment of the degree of physical dependence to nicotine

The Fagerström test is the most used tool to measure nicotine dependence (**Table 2**). This test

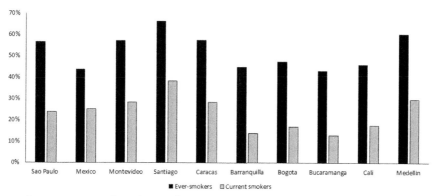

Fig. 1. Ever smokers versus current smokers review.

predicts the difficulty of quitting, severity of withdrawal symptoms, and need for pharmacologic treatment. The most distinctive indicators of nicotine dependence are as follows: How soon after you wake up do you smoke your first cigarette? and How many cigarettes do you smoke per day? Smokers who start within 30 min after waking and those who consume more than or equal to 20 cigarettes a day have a high degree of dependence.[32] Another indicator of high dependence is nocturnal smoking. A short version of the Fagerström test (Heaviness Smoking Index) that only include 2 questions has been developed.[33] Assessment of the Fagerström test and the Heaviness Smoking Index are shown in **Tables 2** and **3**, respectively.

Assessment of previous attempts to quit smoking

This assessment helps identify certain characteristics of the subject's smoking habit. Most smokers take 4 to 7 attempts to successfully quit and many have tried to quit before.[34,35] The characteristics of the attempts that led the subject to remain without

smoking for at least 24 hours should be considered, because they may help improve the chance of the next attempt. The following variables must be known: number of attempts made, duration of each abstinence, severity and timing of nicotine withdrawal symptoms, treatments used and its effects, and reasons for relapse.

The levels of carbon monoxide in the exhaled air

This test can be used to validate the withdrawal of the patient, to objectively measure the tobacco consumption, and as a motivating instrument to quit smoking. Levels of greater than or equal to 10 parts per million (ppm) of CO correspond to smoking subjects, between 5 and 10 ppm to sporadic smoking individuals or daily consumers of very small number of cigarettes, and less than 5 ppm for nonsmokers.

SMOKING CESSATION TREATMENTS

Several studies have shown that a combination of counseling plus pharmacotherapy is the most

Table 1
Smoking status among patients with COPD in some randomized pharmacologic clinical trials

Study	Subjects (n)	Age (y)	FEV$_1$ (%)	Former Smoker (%)	Current Smoker (%)
SUMMIT[15]	15,457	65.0	59.7	53.0	47.0
TRILOGY[16]	1367	63.5	36.6	53.1	46.9
TRINITY[17]	2691	63.1	36.6	52.2	47.8
DYNAGITO[18]	7880	66.4	44.5	63.0	37.0
TRIBUTE[19]	1532	64.5	36.4	55.4	44.6
IMPACT[20]	10,355	65.3	45.5	65.0	35.0
KRONOS[21]	1896	65.3	50.3	60.4	39.6
ETHOS[22]	8539	64.7	43.2	58.9	41.1

Data from Refs.[15–22]

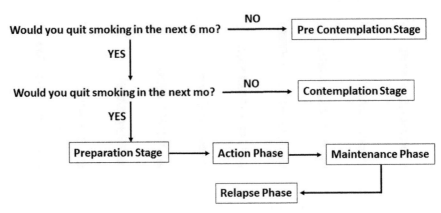

Fig. 2. Motivational phase diagnostic.

effective cessation intervention for smokers with COPD.[34–37]

Counseling and Behavioral Interventions

Smoking cessation counseling (SCC) can be offered individually, by group or by telephone.

In the general population of smokers, the effectiveness of simple advice from physicians has a small effect on cessation rates. Assuming an unassisted quit rate of 2% to 3%, a brief advice intervention can increase quitting by a further 1% to 3%.[38] Two meta-analysis in general smoker population reported that combining SCC and pharmacotherapy increase smoking cessation success compared with a minimal intervention or usual care.[39,40]

In patients with COPD a meta-analysis showed that SCC in combination with nicotine replacement therapy (NRT) had the greatest effect on prolonged abstinence rate: 5 times higher compared with no intervention or usual care (odds ratio [OR] 5.08, 95% confidence interval [CI] 4.32–

Table 2
The Fagerström test

Question	Response	Score
1. How soon after you wake up do you smoke your first cigarette?	After 60 min	0
	31–60 min	1
	6–30 min	2
	Within 5 min	3
2. Do you find it difficult to refrain from smoking in places where it is forbidden?	No	0
	Yes	1
3. Which cigarette would you hate most to give up?	The first in the morning	0
	Any other	1
4. How many cigarettes do you smoke per day?	10 or less	0
	11–20	1
	21–30	2
	31 or more	3
5. Do you smoke more frequently during the first hours after waking than during the rest of the day?	No	0
	Yes	1
6. Do you smoke even if you are so ill that you are in bed most of the day?	No	0
	Yes	1
Total		

Assessment:
  From 0–3: low dependence
  From 4–6: moderate dependence
  From 7–10: high dependence

Table 3
Heaviness smoking index

Question	Response	Score
1. How soon after you wake up do you smoke your first cigarette?	After 60 min	0
	31–60 min	1
	6–30 min	2
	Within 5 min	3
2. How many cigarettes do you smoke per day?	10 or less	0
	11–20	1
	21–30	2
	31 or more	3

Assessment:
  From 0–2: low dependence
  From 3–4: moderate dependence
  From 5–6: high dependence

5.97), 3 times higher compared with SCC alone (OR 2.80, 95% CI 1.49–5.26), and a nonsignificant statistical increase compared with SCC in combination with an antidepressant (OR 1.53, 95% CI 0.71–3.30).[34] A trend of SCC alone to be superior versus usual care (1.81, P = .07) was also observed.[34] In addition, another systematic review on smoking cessation in patients with COPD found an average 12-month continuous abstinence rates of 1.4% for usual care, 2.6% for minimal counseling, 6.0% for intensive counseling, and 12.3% for pharmacotherapy.[35]

Pharmacotherapy

Limited information exists regarding the use of pharmacotherapy for smoking cessation in patients with COPD. The main objectives of this pharmacotherapy are to control the long-term abstinence (nicotine patch, bupropion, and varenicline) and to provide rapid relief of acute cravings and withdrawal symptoms (rapidly acting nicotine replacement products).

A meta-analysis evaluated the effectiveness of SCC or pharmacologic smoking cessation interventions, or both, in smokers with COPD. NRT (risk ratio [RR] 2.60; 95% CI 1.29–5.24) and varenicline (RR 3.34; 95% CI 1.88–5.92) increased the quit rate over placebo. Pooled results also showed a positive effect of bupropion compared with placebo (RR 2.03; 95% CI 1.26–3.28).[36]

Table 4 shows the main results of some smoking cessation pharmacotherapy studies conducted in COPD.

Nicotine Replacement Therapy

Results from the Lung Health Study showed that after 12 months nicotine gum combined with an intensive behavioral program was more effective in helping smokers at risk for COPD to abstain from smoking than usual care.[41] Tønnesen and colleagues[27] found in smokers with COPD that the continuous abstinence rates from 2 to 12 months were superior in the NRT (14%) than the placebo group (5.4%) (OR 2.88; 95% CI, 1.34–6.15).

Bupropion Sustained Release

Bupropion sustained release (SR) is an antidepressant drug with an added effect on smoking cessation, particularly in patients with COPD.[29,42] Taskhin and colleagues[29] found a continuous abstinence rate at 6 months higher in the bupropion group (15.7%) versus placebo (9%) in patients with mild to moderate COPD. Another placebo-controlled randomized trial in smokers at risk for or with COPD showed that continuous abstinence rate at 6 months were 27.9%, 25%, and 14.6% for bupropion, nortriptyline, and placebo, respectively.[42] No significant difference was found between nortriptyline and placebo.[42]

Varenicline

Varenicline is a drug developed for smoking cessation that in "healthy" smokers has proven to over twice as effective as placebo and around 50% more effective than bupropion to promote long-term abstinence.

A study conducted in smokers with mild and moderate COPD showed a higher continuous abstinence rate at 1-year follow-up for varenicline (18.6%) versus placebo (5.6%) without differences in side effects.[43] Another study on smokers with severe-very severe COPD that received SCC plus pharmacotherapy showed an overall abstinence rate at 24-week of 48.5%.[44] The rates of continuous abstinence were 38.2% for NRT, 55.6% for bupropion and 58.3% for varenicline. Patients treated with varenicline for 24-week had

Table 4
Smoking cessation pharmacotherapy studies conducted in smoker patients with COPD

Study	Subjects (n)	FEV$_1$	Medication	Time Period	Sustained Quit Rates	OR (95% CI) or P Value
Anthonisen et al,[41] 1994	5887	78.3% pred	Nicotine gum	12 mo	Nicotine 35% Placebo 9%	Not available
Tønnesen et al,[27] 2006	370	56% pred	Nicotine sublingual tablets	2–12 mo	Nicotine 14% Placebo 5.4%	OR 2.88 (1.34–6.15)
Tashkin et al,[29] 2001	404	71.3% pred	Bupropion SR	7–26 wk	Bupropion 15.7% Placebo 9%	P = .040
Wagena et al,[42] 2005	144	Not available	Bupropion SR Nortriptyline	4–26 wk	Bupropion SR 27.3% Nortriptyline 21.2% Placebo 8.3%	% Difference Bupropion SR vs placebo 18.9 (3.6–34.2; P = .02) % Difference Nortriptyline vs placebo 12.9 (−0.8 to 26.4; P = .07)
Tashkin et al,[43] 2011	505	70% pred	Varenicline	9–52 wk	Varenicline 18.6% Placebo 5.6%	OR 4.04 (2.13–7.67)
Jiménez Ruiz et al,[44] 2012	472	Gold 3 (79%) Gold 4 (21%)	Nicotine patches Bupropion/ varenicline	9–24 wk	Nicotine patches 44% Bupropion alone 60% Varenicline alone 61%	Varenicline vs nicotine patches (OR: 1.98; 95% CI: 1.25–3.12; P = .003). Varenicline vs bupropion (OR: 1.43; 95% CI: 0.49–2.2)
Hernández Zenteno et al,[45] 2018	31 COPD 63 non-COPD	1.5 L 2.9 L	Varenicline	12 mo	COPD 61.2% Non-COPD 42.8%	P = .072

Data from Refs.[27,29,42–45]

higher abstinence rates than those treated for 12-week.[44] The onset of psychiatric symptoms due to medication was rare and evenly distributed across groups.[44] A recent study found no differences in the abstinence rate at 12-month between smokers with and without COPD (61.2% vs 42.8%, P = .072) receiving treatment with varenicline.[45]

Pharmacotherapies Approaches for Smoking Cessation in Chronic Obstructive Pulmonary Disorder

The doses and time of use of the different pharmacotherapies for smoking cessation are shown in **Table 5**. The treatment approach is based on the nicotine physical dependence severity. Smokers with mild to moderate degree of nicotine dependence can be treated with a controller drug (nicotine patch, bupropion, or varenicline) with or without a reliever medication (nicotine gum, lozenge, nasal spray, and oral inhaler). In those subjects with high degree of nicotine dependence, it is possible to combine controller drugs (bupropion and/or varenicline, or nicotine patch and/or bupropion, or combine the 3 controllers) with multiple relievers.[46]

Table 5
Dose and time of use of pharmacologic treatments for smoking cessation

Medication	Varenicline	Bupropion	Nicotine Replacement Therapy
Mechanism of action	Partial agonist for the $\alpha_4\beta_2$ nicotinic acetylcholine receptor (dopamine release in the nucleus accumbens)	Inhibit neuronal reuptake of dopamine and norepinephrine in the nucleus accumbens and locus ceruleus	Acts at the level of nicotinic central nervous system receptors

Dose	12 wk
	Days 1–3: 0.5 mg QD
	Days 4–7: 0.5 mg BD
	Days 8+: 1 mg BD
		12 wk.
		150 mg/12 h
		First week progressive dose
			16 h patches
			  25 mg/d 6 wk
			  15 mg/d 4 wk
			  10 mg/d 4 wk
			  5 mg/d 2 wk
			24 h patches
			  21 mg/d 6 wk
			  14 mg/d 4 wk
			  7 mg/d 4 wk
			Chewing gum 2–4 mg or *tablets* 1–2 mg if craving

Side effects	Nausea (most common), insomnia, vivid dreams, dyspepsia, constipation, flatulence, emesis	Insomnia (most common), dry mouth, anxiety, irritability, restlessness, headache, tinnitus, skin rash, seizures (rate)	Redness or itching of skin where patch applied Urticaria Headache Dizziness Nausea/vomiting Insomnia

SMOKING REDUCTION

Approved smoking cessation medications (NRT, bupropion, and varenicline) in combination with SCC have shown to double or triple quit rates under stringent settings of clinical trials. Nonetheless, relapse is common in the course of a smoking cessation; therefore, harm reduction has been considered as an alternative approach for resistant smokers with COPD or for those who are not ready to quit. This represents a dilemma for many pulmonary physicians and the results of the smoking reduction studies in patients with COPD have generated considerable controversy.[47–50]

Despite understanding that complete cessation is needed to minimize all the harmful effects of smoking, it is also known that reducing smoking increases the likelihood of quitting smoking in the future, so some smokers who are unable to quit abruptly may achieve it after a gradual reduction.[51,52] In all smoking reduction studies, several subjects who were unwilling or unable to stop smoking at baseline were abstinent at 4 months and 1 to 2 years, supporting the concept of smoking reduction as a step toward abstinence. However, one recent meta-analysis showed that neither reduction-to-quit nor abrupt quitting interventions result in superior long-term quit rates when compared with each other.[53] Evidence comparing the efficacy of reduction-to-quit interventions with no treatment was inconclusive and of low certainty.[53] There is also low-certainty evidence to suggest that reduction-to-quit interventions may be more effective when pharmacotherapy agents are used.[53]

E-CIGARETTES

Recently the use of novel tobacco products, particularly the electronic cigarette (EC) has increased probably due to the presumption that this is associated with less damage, as well as reducing the symptoms of anxiety and withdrawal from tobacco by sharing the same visual and sensory characteristics. Although the potential harm reduction due to switching from conventional cigarettes to EC in patients with COPD has not been studied, the perception exists that they are safer or are an effective NRT during the smoking cessation process.

The efficacy and safety of EC to help quit smoking is a subject of controversy. A meta-analysis that includes only randomized trials showed that EC with nicotine were more effective for smoking cessation (abstained for 6 month) than nicotine-free EC (RR 2.29, 95% CI 1.05–4.96), although there were concerns in the results due to the small number of trials and sample sizes.[54] Another meta-analysis that includes randomized trials, cohort, and cross-sectional studies showed that nicotine EC was more effective for cessation than those without nicotine (pooled RR 2.29, 95% CI 1.05–4.97).[55] Because of the lack of comparator groups in the studies included, the investigators were unable to comment on the efficacy of EC versus other interventions.[55] Another systematic review and meta-analysis of clinical trials and observational real-world studies showed that quitting cigarettes were 28% lower in those who used EC compared with those who did not use EC (OR 0.72, 95% CI 0.57–0.91).[56] However, the results from these meta-analyses did not assess the efficacy and safety of EC versus other effective interventions to quit smoking.[56]

More recently, the results of a trial aimed at evaluating the 1-year efficacy of EC, compared with NRT, as a smoking-cessation treatment showed that abstinence rate was 18% for EC group and 9.9% for the NRT group (RR 1.83, 95% CI 1.30–2.58).[57] An important finding to highlight in this study was that among participants with 1-year abstinence, 80% were using EC at 52 weeks in the EC group in comparison with 9% of those in the NRT.[57] This study was conducted in smokers who seek help; therefore, the results cannot be generalized to the entire population of smokers and to patients with COPD due to lack of information on the presence of this condition.

Health authorities and scientific societies have shown concern about issues surrounding safety of EC use.[58–63] The evidence of the modest effectiveness of nicotine EC in smoking cessation must be balanced against its short- and long-term health consequences. The efficacy and safety of EC for smoking cessation need also to be evaluated in high-risk populations (patients with pulmonary diseases), so based on the available evidence, its use cannot be recommended for smoking cessation in COPD patients with COPD.

VACCINATION IN PATIENTS WITH CHRONIC OBSTRUCTIVE PULMONARY DISEASE

Acute exacerbations are an important cause of morbidity and mortality in patients with COPD.

Although COPD exacerbations can be precipitated by factors, including environmental pollution, the most common causes seem to be respiratory tract infections by virus and bacteria (50%–70% of cases). Therefore, preventing exacerbations in patients with COPD is a major objective, and vaccination is accepted as an effective and simple preventive strategy to achieve this goal.[64] The most common vaccines given to patients with COPD are the influenza and pneumococcal vaccines.

VACCINATION RATES

Although immunization against influenza is recommended for all patients with COPD by several international health authorities and guidelines, the coverage rates of influenza vaccination for high-risk patients including those with chronic respiratory diseases, remain less than target levels in many countries.[65–70] In the United States coverage of high-risk adults was less than the target of 70% (47.6% for those between 18 and 64 years and 66.7% in adults ≥65 years) in 2014 to 2015 period, and the rate among adults aged 18 to 64 years with at least one high-risk condition (asthma, diabetes, or heart disease) was estimated to be 48%.[69] The European target for vaccine coverage among individuals with chronic medical conditions was 75% in 2012 to 2013 period, and the median influenza vaccine coverage for this population was 45.6% (ranging from 28% in Portugal to 80% in United Kingdom and Northern Ireland).[68]

In developed countries, the rates of vaccination in patients with COPD are heterogeneous and mostly describe suboptimal prevalence. Data from the Canadian Community Health Survey estimated that 47.9% of individuals with COPD were immunized for influenza within the year 2003.[71] Li and colleagues[72] reported an influenza vaccination rate of 47.7% in patients with COPD in Singapore. The prevalence of vaccination in Spain range between 52.2% and 87.2%, and the influenza vaccination decreased as the severity of COPD increased (65.3% for mild, 63.7% for moderate, 63% for severe, and 52% for very severe COPD).[73–75] Advanced age, increased exacerbation frequency, a history of pneumococcal vaccination, and the presence of comorbidities were associated with a higher percentage of influenza vaccination.[75] A study in patient with COPD from an outpatient clinic in Turkey found that 51.1% were vaccinated with influenza and pneumococcal vaccines,[64] and another study showed that 36.5% had influenza and 14.1% pneumococcal vaccination.[76] Both vaccination rates were significantly higher in patients with comorbidities in those with a white-collar occupation and higher education level.[76]

Data from 23 sites in 20 countries participating in the Burden of Obstructive Lung Disease study indicated that influenza vaccine was used significantly more in high-income countries than in low- to middle-income countries (mean rate 28.5% and 6.6%, respectively).[77] Rates of influenza vaccine ranged from 0% in Pune and Srinagar (India) to 57% in Sousse (Tunisia), whereas the probability of being vaccinated ranged from 0% in India to 70% in Sousse (Tunisia) among the same standard group. Influenza vaccination was more common in older participants (OR = 5.3, 95% CI 3.8–7.5), unemployed or retired (OR = 1.4, 95% CI 1.1–1.8), and in those with higher education (OR = 1.2, 95% CI 1.1–1.4).[77] It was also more common in those with respiratory symptoms (OR = 1.3, 95% CI 1.1–1.6), more severe COPD (OR = 1.5, 95% CI 1.0–2.3), comorbidities (OR = 1.4, 95%CI 1.1–1.6), and those who had a positive response to salbutamol (OR = 1.3, 95% CI 1.0–1.7).[77] Data from the PLATINO survey in Latin-American showed a variable and frequently suboptimal influenza vaccination (ranging from 5.1% in Caracas, Venezuela to 52% in Santiago de Chile).[78]

INFLUENZA DISEASE

Influenza are RNA viruses of the family orthomyxoviridae. Influenza A, B, and C are able to infect humans, with influenza A and B being the most common circulating types. Influenza A virus has been divided into subgroups based on the 2 core proteins hemagglutinin (H) and neuraminidase (N). There are at least 18 and 11 subtypes of hemagglutinin and neuraminidase, respectively; however only 3 H proteins (H1, H2, and H3) and 2 N proteins (N1 and N2) have been detected in human.

Influenza is an acute disease caused by the virus influenza A and B. Since 1977, influenza A (H1N1 and H3N2) viruses and influenza B (B/Victoria or B/Yamagata) viruses have circulated worldwide causing seasonal epidemics, and persistence of influenza has been attributed to the virus ability to evolve rapidly. Also common are antigenic variabilities that may partly result from a phenomenon called antigenic drift (amino acid changes that allow viral escape of neutralizing antibodies).[79]

The incidence rates of influenza infection vary according to the nature of the virus strains and the affected population. The rate of severe diseases is higher among older adults (>65 years), children younger than 2 years, and people with high-risk conditions such as COPD.

Influenza Vaccines Evidence of Efficacy and Recommendations in Patients with Chronic Obstructive Pulmonary Disease

Vaccination is the best intervention to prevent influenza virus infections. Nerveless, conventional vaccines are only active for a short period of time due to the propensity of influenza viruses to undergo antigenic changes; therefore, the antigenic content of influenza vaccines changes annually to reflect the virus strains in circulation. Strains used in licensed seasonal influenza vaccines are selected in February and September according to the influenza seasons in the northern and southern hemispheres, respectively. Three classes of licensed influenza vaccines are available and approved by the Food and Drug Administration: detergent-split inactivated influenza vaccine, recombinant influenza vaccine, and live attenuated influenza vaccine (**Table 6**).[80]

Current available seasonal influenza vaccines are either trivalent vaccines (TIVs) containing one strain of each of the 2 subtypes of influenza A virus (A/H1N1 and A/H3N2) and 1 of the 2 co-circulating B-virus lineages (B/Victoria or B/Yamagata) or quadrivalent vaccines (QIVs) containing both influenza A subtypes mentioned earlier and both influenza B co-circulating lineages. QIVs are expected to provide broader protection than TIVs and over the next years are expected to gradually replace TIVs globally.[81,82]

Bafadhel and colleagues[83] reported that of all exacerbations in COPD, 55%, 29%, and 28% were associated with bacteria, virus, or a sputum eosinophilia. Rhinovirus is the most frequent virus associated with these exacerbations and secondly influenza.

Because of the high morbidity and mortality of influenza in patients with COPD, annual influenza vaccination has been recommended by several guidelines.[65–70]

A Cochrane systematic review in patients with COPD showed that influenza vaccination significantly reduces the total number of exacerbations with an effectiveness of greater than 60% (mean difference −0.37, 95% CI −0.64 to −0.11), particularly in the first 4 weeks postvaccination.[84] No differences were found in the reduction of hospitalizations or all-cause mortality.[84] A systematic review that also included observational cohort studies found that influenza vaccination reduced all-cause mortality and deaths associated with a respiratory event in patients with COPD.[85] This finding was mainly driven by a study that showed that influenza vaccination was associated with a 41% reduction in risk of all-cause mortality (RR 0.59; 95% CI, 0.57–0.61).[86]

Table 6
Categories of influenza vaccines in United States, 2019–20 influenza season

Type of Vaccine	Virus Strain	Trade Name (Manufacturer)
IIV	Influenza A: H1N1 and H3N2 virus/influenza B: Victoria and/or Yamagata	IIV4—standard dose—egg based[a] Afluria Quadrivalent (Seqirus) Fluarix Quadrivalent (GlaxoSmithKline) FluLaval Quadrivalent (GlaxoSmithKline) Fluzone Quadrivalent (Sanofi Pasteur) IIV4—standard dose—cell culture–based (ccIIV4) Flucelvax Quadrivalent (Seqirus) IIV3—high dose—egg based[a] (HD-IIV3) Fluzone High-Dose (Sanofi Pasteur) IIV3—standard dose—egg based[a] with MF59 adjuvant (aIIV3) Fluad (Seqirus)
RIV	Contains the HA ectodomain amino acid sequence of cell-cultured vaccine prototype viruses suggested by WHO	RIV4—Recombinant HA Flublok Quadrivalent (Sanofi Pasteur)
LAIV	Subtypes of H1N1 and H3N2 (influenza A) and one influenza B	LAIV4—egg based[a] FluMist Quadrivalent (AstraZeneca)

Vaccination providers should consult FDA-approved prescribing information for 2019 to 2020 influenza vaccines for the most complete and updated information, including (but not limited to) indications, contraindications, warnings, and precautions. Package inserts for US-licensed vaccines are available at https://www.fda.gov/vaccines-blood-biologics/approved-products/vaccines-licensed-use-united-states.

Abbreviations: HA, hemagglutinin; IIV, inactivated influenza vaccine; LAIV, live attenuated influenza vaccine; RIV, recombinant influenza vaccine; WHO, World Health Organization.

[a] Persons with a history of egg allergy may receive any licensed, recommended influenza vaccine that is otherwise appropriate for their age and health status. Those who report having had reactions to egg involving symptoms other than urticaria (eg, angioedema or swelling, respiratory distress, lightheadedness, or recurrent emesis) or who required epinephrine or another emergency medical intervention should be vaccinated in an inpatient or outpatient medical setting (including, but not necessarily limited to, hospitals, clinics, health departments, and physician offices). Vaccine administration should be supervised by a health care provider who is able to recognize and manage severe allergic reactions.

A recent post-hoc analysis of a national multi-center prospective cohort study found that compared with hospitalized patients without influenza infection, patients with influenza were older (age >75 years; 50.8% vs 47.6%), more likely to be current smokers (34.4% vs 27.2%), to reside in long-term care (9.2% vs 7.0%), and less likely to be vaccinated during the season of hospitalization (58.9% vs 70.6%).[87] The adjusted analysis showed a 37.5% (95% CI, 27.3–46.2) reduction in influenza-related hospitalizations in vaccinated versus unvaccinated individuals.[87] Another retrospective study showed an association of influenza vaccination with decreased risk of respiratory failure (OR 0.87, 95% CI 0.79–0.96) in patients with COPD.[88]

PNEUMOCOCCAL DISEASES IN PATIENTS WITH CHRONIC OBSTRUCTIVE PULMONARY DISEASE

Streptococcus pneumoniae is an encapsulated gram-positive coccus and a major cause of community-acquired pneumonia (CAP) in adults worldwide, associated with considerable morbidity and mortality.[89–92]

Lower respiratory tract infections and COPD are the fourth and the third leading causes of death worldwide in 2016, respectively, and about half of all deaths from lower respiratory infections are attributable to pneumococcal pneumonia.[93]

A systematic review and meta-analysis reported an estimated proportion of CAP attributable to pneumococcus of 27.3% (95% CI: 23.9%–31.1%) and 24.8% (95% CI: 21.3%–28.9%) of bacteremic pneumococcal pneumonia.[91] A retrospective study cohort in the United States determined that in healthy adults, the risk of pneumococcal pneumonia was 5.2 times higher in persons aged 65 years or older compared with those aged 18 to 49 years and the incidence of pneumococcal pneumonia was 7.7-fold higher in adults aged 65 years or older with chronic respiratory diseases compared with those without comorbidity.[94]

COPD is one of the most common comorbidities in pneumonia, occurring in 30% of patients who require hospitalization and about half of the cases with severe pneumonia who require admission to the intensive care unit.[95,96] Patients with COPD are uniquely predisposed to develop CAP. In Europe the annual incidence of CAP in adults ranged between 1.07 and 1.2 per 1000 person-years,[97] whereas the rate in patients with COPD has been reported to be 22.4 (95% CI 21.7–23.2) per 1000 person-years (20-fold higher).[98] The presence of comorbidities (congestive heart failure, dementia, and severe COPD) and age greater than 65 years increased the risk of CAP in patients with COPD.[98] The risk of severe invasive pneumococcal disease has been reported to be 5-fold higher in patients with COPD than in general population.[99]

Patients with COPD may be more susceptible to respiratory infections, due to the impairment of mucociliary clearance mechanisms, and the increased production of specific cell adhesion molecules that mediate attachment of bacteria and viruses in the airways.[100,101] In addition, patients with COPD can experiment frequent exacerbations requiring inhaled corticosteroids that can further increase the risk of pneumonia.[102–104]

Although it has been debated whether pneumonia should be included as one of the causes of COPD exacerbation or if it is a differential diagnosis, the fact is that pneumonic exacerbation in COPD tends to be more severe than nonpneumonic exacerbation. Pneumonic exacerbation compared with nonpneumonic accounted for one-third of all first-time hospitalizations due to COPD exacerbation and are associated with more hospitalization in the ICU, longer hospitalization stays, and higher mortality.[105–107]

Pneumococcal Vaccines

Several efforts have been made to develop pneumococcal vaccines. Although more than 90 pneumococcus serotypes have been identified, only some of them cause infections.[108] Data from a Spanish group showed that the most prevalent serotypes in invasive CAP were 1, 3, 7F, 14, 19A, and 8, whereas 3, 7F, 19A, and 14 in noninvasive CAP.[109]

Two pneumococcal vaccines are recommended for adults in different guidelines: the 23-valent pneumococcal polysaccharide vaccine (PPSV-23), with antigens of serotypes 1, 3, 4, 5, 6B, 7F, 9V, 14, 18C, 19A, 19F, 23F, 2, 8, 9N, 10A, 11A, 12F, 15B, 17F, 20, 22F, and 33F42; and the 13-valent pneumococcal conjugate vaccine (PCV-13) containing antigens of serotypes 1, 3, 4, 5, 6A, 6B, 7F, 9V, 14, 18C, 19A, 19F, and 23F conjugated to nontoxic diphtheria CRM197 protein.[110,111]

For a long time, PPSV-23 has remained as the only antipneumococcal vaccine recommended for adults aged 65 years or older and other high-risk groups. More recently, this situation changed with the introduction of the PCV-13. A large study demonstrated the effectiveness of the PCV-13 in adults aged 65 years or older in preventing vaccine-type pneumococcal (45%), bacteremic, nonbacteremic CAP, and vaccine-type invasive pneumococcal disease, but no significant effect for all-cause CAP.[112] For this reason, the Advisory Committee on Immunization Practices (ACIP) recommended the adoption of PCV-13 use in adults aged 65 years or older who do not have an immunocompromising condition (based on shared clinical decision-making) but administered in series with PPSV-23.[113]

Results of different systematic reviews and meta-analysis indicated that although PPSV-23 is effective for invasive pneumococcal disease, there are inconclusive evidence of its effectiveness against pneumococcal or all-cause CAP.[114–117] Because of the uncertainty and variability of the clinical efficacy of PPSV-23, different public health agencies recognize that there is still an unmet medical need to protect older adults and high-risk groups against pneumococcal pneumonia.[118]

It is important to highlight that the type of immunity induced by PPSV-23 is mediated by a T-cell–independent B-cell response, and no immunologic memory is induced[119]; therefore, immunoresponses to PPSV-23 tend to decrease over time, and revaccination is recommended 5 years after the primary vaccination. On the other hand, PCV-

13 tends to be more consistently immunogenic than PPSV-23 and increases the duration and memory of antipneumococcal immunoresponses.[119] The PCV-13 vaccination contains pneumococcal polysaccharide antigens covalently linked to an immunogenic carrier protein that together induce T-cell–dependent humoral immunoresponses and stimulate T cells to help B cells produce antibodies to the vaccine and generate immune memory.[119]

Although the vaccination strategy for adults is still under debate and immunization guidelines vary among countries in terms of age and risk groups for vaccination, different guidelines worldwide recommend the use of both vaccines for primary vaccination in adults aged 65 years or older, administered always PCV-13 first.[113,120,121] The **Fig. 3** illustrated the common recommendation for pneumococcal vaccination guidelines for these individuals.

Pneumococcal Vaccines: Evidence of Efficacy and Recommendations in Chronic Obstructive Pulmonary Disease

The most recent GOLD document indicates that PPSV-23 has been shown to reduce the incidence of CAP in patients with COPD younger than 65 years with an FEV_1 less than 40% predicted and in those with comorbidities and that PCV-13 in general population of adults aged 65 years or older has demonstrated efficacy in reducing bacteremia and invasive pneumococcal disease.[70] However, the document does not propose a clear position on pneumococcal vaccination for patients with COPD.

A recently updated Cochrane meta-analysis showed that vaccination (primarily with PPSV-23) in patients with COPD provides significant protection against CAP compared with control (OR 0.62, 95% CI 0.43–0.89; GRADE: moderate), but findings did not indicate that vaccination reduced the risk of confirmed pneumococcal pneumonia (OR 0.26, 95% CI 0.05–1.31; GRADE: low).[122] The number needed to treat for an additional beneficial outcome (preventing one CAP episode) was 21 (95% CI 15–74). Pneumococcal vaccines had no significant effect on cardiorespiratory and all-cause mortality.[122] Pneumococcal vaccines also reduced the number of COPD exacerbations (NNT = 8; OR = 0.60; 95% CI, 0.39–0.93; moderate evidence) but did not reduce the number of hospitalizations.[122]

In another systematic review and meta-analysis of observational studies in persons with underlying risk factors, such as COPD, pneumococcal vaccine (PPSV-23) efficacy against any CAP varied widely among adults aged 65 years or older (−143% to 60%).[123] Among 4 studies the pneumococcal vaccine efficacy for pneumococcal CAP was 29% (95% CI −39 to 63) in those aged 50 years or older with chronic respiratory disease and for pneumococcal CAP hospitalization among those aged 65 years or older was 24% (95% CI −90 to 70) with chronic respiratory disease.[123]

A study in adult with chronic respiratory diseases found that exacerbation frequency was lower in the PPSV-23 plus influenza vaccination group than in the influenza vaccination–alone group ($P = .022$).[124] When these subjects were divided into subgroup an additive effect of PPSV-23 plus influenza vaccination in preventing

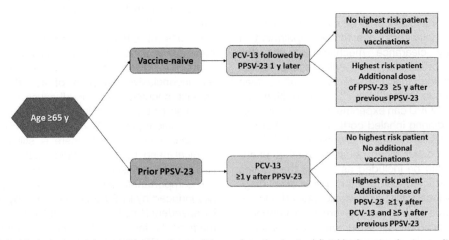

Fig. 3. High risk: includes patients with chronic conditions of cerebral spinal fluid leak, neurologic conditions that impair clearance of oral secretions, heart disease, lung disease, diabetes, kidney disease, and liver disease; cochlear implants; alcoholism; smoking; homelessness; and residing in long-term care.

infectious exacerbation was significant only in patients with COPD ($P = .037$).[124]

Although the clinical efficacy of PPSV-23 is uncertain and variable in patients with COPD, the benefit of vaccination could lie in the potential reduction of the cost and the annual burden of medical care related to avoiding (even in modest numbers) visits to emergency department. Therefore, the Centers for Disease Control and Prevention recommends that anyone with chronic pulmonary disease between 19 and 64 years of age should routinely receive the PCV-13 and the PPSV-23.[125] On the other hand, the ACIP in 2019 recommended 1 dose of PPSV-23 in immunocompetent persons with underlying medical condition such as chronic respiratory disease (includes chronic obstructive pulmonary disease, emphysema, and asthma) aged 19 to 64 years and 1 dose of PPSV-23 for persons aged 65 years or older; if PCV-13 has been given, then give PPSV-23 for more than or equal to 1 year after PCV-13 and more than or equal to 5 years after any PPSV-23 at age less than 65 years.[58]

SUMMARY

More than one-third of patients with COPD continue smoking despite knowing that they have the disease and that this behavior has a negative impact on the disease prognosis and progression. Smokers with COPD exhibit higher levels of nicotine dependence and lower self-efficacy and self-esteem, which affects their ability to quit smoking. A combination of counseling plus pharmacotherapy is the most effective cessation treatment of smokers with COPD. Varenicline seems to be the most effective pharmacologic intervention to promote long-term abstinence in these patients. There is a lack of information about the efficacy and safety of EC for smoking cessation in patients with COPD; therefore, its use cannot be recommended. Prevention of exacerbations in patients with COPD is a major objective, and vaccination (influenza and pneumococcal vaccination) is accepted to be an effective and simple preventive strategy to achieve this goal.

DISCLOSURE

M. Montes de Oca has stated that she has nothing to disclose.

REFERENCES

1. Godtfredsen NS, Lam TH, Hansel TT, et al. COPD-related morbidity and mortality after smoking cessation: status of the evidence. Eur Respir J 2008;32(4):844–53.

2. Kanner RE, Connett JE, Williams DE, et al. Effects of randomized assignment to a smoking cessation intervention and changes in smoking habits on respiratory symptoms in smokers with early chronic obstructive pulmonary disease: the Lung Health Study. Am J Med 1999;106(4): 410–6.

3. Au DH, Bryson CL, Chien JW, et al. The effects of smoking cessation on the risk of chronic obstructive pulmonary disease exacerbations. J Gen Intern Med 2009;24(4):457–63.

4. Kupiainen H, Kinnula VL, Lindqvist A, et al. Successful smoking cessation in COPD: association with comorbidities and mortality. Pulm Med 2012; 2012:725024.

5. Anthonisen NR, Skeans MA, Wise RA, et al. The effects of a smoking cessation intervention on 14.5-year mortality: a randomized clinical trial. Intern Med 2005;142(4):233–9.

6. Scanlon PD, Connett JE, Waller LA, et al. Smoking cessation and lung function in mild-to-moderate chronic obstructive pulmonary disease. The Lung Health Study. Am J Respir Crit Care Med 2000; 161(2 Pt 1):381–90.

7. Gritz ER, Vidrine DJ, Fingeret MC. Smoking cessation a critical component of medical management in chronic disease populations. Am J Prev Med 2007;33(6 Suppl):S414–22.

8. Peña VS, Miravitlles M, Gabriel R, et al. Geographic variations in prevalence and underdiagnosis of COPD: results of the IBERPOC multicentre epidemiological study. Chest 2000;118(4):981–9.

9. Schauer GL, Wheaton AG, Malarcher AM, et al. Smoking prevalence and cessation characteristics among U.S. adults with and without COPD: findings from the 2011 Behavioral Risk Factor Surveillance System. COPD 2014;11(6):697–704.

10. Menezes AM, Perez-Padilla R, Jardim JR, et al. Chronic obstructive pulmonary disease in five Latin American cities (the PLATINO study): a prevalence study. Lancet 2005;366(9500):1875–81.

11. Perez-Padilla R, Menezes AMB. Chronic obstructive pulmonary disease in Latin America. Ann Glob Health 2019;85(1) [pii:7].

12. Fang L, Gao P, Bao H, et al. Chronic obstructive pulmonary disease in China: a nationwide prevalence study. Lancet Respir Med 2018;6(6):421–30.

13. Shahab L, Jarvis MJ, Britton J, et al. Prevalence, diagnosis and relation to tobacco dependence of chronic obstructive pulmonary disease in a nationally representative population sample. Thorax 2006;61(12):1043–7.

14. Criner RN, Labaki WW, Regan EA, et al. Mortality and exacerbations by global initiative for chronic obstructive lung disease groups ABCD: 2011 versus 2017 in the COPDGene® cohort. Chronic Obstr Pulm Dis 2019;6(1):64–73.

15. Vestbo J, Anderson JA, Brook RD, et al. Fluticasone furoate and vilanterol and survival in chronic obstructive pulmonary disease with heightened cardiovascular risk (SUMMIT): a double-blind randomised controlled trial. Lancet 2016; 387(10030):1817–26.

16. Singh D, Papi A, Corradi M, et al. Single inhaler triple therapy versus inhaled corticosteroid plus long-acting β2-agonist therapy for chronic obstructive pulmonary disease (TRILOGY): a double-blind, parallel group, randomised controlled trial. Lancet 2016;388(10048):963–73.

17. Vestbo J, Papi A, Corradi M, et al. Single inhaler extrafine triple therapy versus long-acting muscarinic antagonist therapy for chronic obstructive pulmonary disease (TRINITY): a double-blind, parallel group, randomised controlled trial. Lancet 2017; 389(10082):1919–29.

18. Calverley PMA, Anzueto AR, Carter K, et al. Tiotropium and olodaterol in the prevention of chronic obstructive pulmonary disease exacerbations (DYNAGITO): a double-blind, randomised, parallel-group, active-controlled trial. Lancet Respir Med 2018;6(5):337–44.

19. Papi A, Vestbo J, Fabbri L, et al. Extrafine inhaled triple therapy versus dual bronchodilator therapy in chronic obstructive pulmonary disease (TRIBUTE): a double-blind, parallel group, randomised controlled trial. Lancet 2018;391(10125): 1076–84.

20. Lipson DA, Barnhart F, Brealey N, et al. Once-daily single-inhaler triple versus dual therapy in patients with COPD. N Engl J Med 2018; 378(18):1671–80.

21. Ferguson GT, Rabe KF, Martinez FJ, et al. Triple therapy with budesonide/glycopyrrolate/formoterol fumarate with co-suspension delivery technology versus dual therapies in chronic obstructive pulmonary disease (KRONOS): a double-blind, parallel-group, multicentre, phase 3 randomised controlled trial. Lancet Respir Med 2018;6(10):747–58.

22. Rabe KF, Martinez FJ, Ferguson GT, et al. A phase III study of triple therapy with budesonide/glycopyrrolate/formoterol fumarate metered dose inhaler 320/18/9.6 µg and 160/18/9.6 µg using co-suspension delivery technology in moderate-to-very severe COPD: the ETHOS study protocol. Respir Med 2019;158:59–66.

23. Jiménez-Ruiz CA, Masa F, Miravitlles M, et al. Smoking characteristics: differences in attitudes and dependence between healthy smokers and smokers with COPD. Chest 2001;119(5):1365–70.

24. Crowley TJ, Macdonald MJ, Walter MI. Behavioural anti-smoking trial in chronic obstructive pulmonary disease patients. Psychopharmacology (Berl) 1995;119(2):193–204.

25. Wagena EJ, Arrindell WA, Wouters EF, et al. Are patients with COPD psychologically distressed? Eur Respir J 2005;26(2):242–8.

26. Stratelis G, Mölstad S, Jakobsson P, et al. The impact of repeated spirometry and smoking cessation advice on smokers with mild COPD. Scand J Prim Health Care 2006;24(3):133–9.

27. Tønnesen P, Mikkelsen K, Bremann L. Nurse-conducted smoking cessation in patients with COPD using nicotine sublingual tablets and behavioral support. Chest 2006;130(2):334–42.

28. Tashkin DP, Rennard S, Hays JT, et al. Lung function and respiratory symptoms in a 1year randomized smoking cessation trial of varenicline in COPD patients. Respir Med 2011;105(11): 1682–90.

29. Tashkin D, Kanner R, Bailey W, et al. Smoking cessation in patients with chronic obstructive pulmonary disease: a double- blind, placebo-controlled, randomised trial. Lancet 2001; 357(9268):1571–5.

30. Gratziou Ch, Florou A, Ischaki E, et al. Smoking cessation effectiveness in smokers with COPD and asthma under real life conditions. Respir Med 2014;108(4):577–83.

31. Jou SS, Yagihashi K, Zach JA, et al. Relationship between current smoking, visual CT findings and emphysema index in cigarette smokers. Clin Imaging 2019;53:195–9.

32. Fagerström KO. Time to first cigarette: the best single indicator of tobacco dependence? Monaldi Arch Chest Dis 2003;59(1):91–4.

33. John U, Meyer C, Schumann A, et al. A short formof the Fagerström test for nicotine dependence and the heaviness of smokingindex in two adult population samples. Addict Behav 2004;29(6):1207–12.

34. Strassmann R, Bausch B, Spaar A, et al. Smoking cessation interventions in COPD: a network meta-analysis of randomised trials. Eur Respir J 2009; 34(3):634–40.

35. Hoogendoorn M, Feenstra TL, Hoogenveen RT, et al. Long-term effectiveness and cost-effectiveness of smoking cessation interventions in patients with COPD. Thorax 2010;65(8):711–8.

36. van Eerd EA, van der Meer RM, van Schayck OC, et al. Smoking cessation for people with chronic obstructive pulmonary disease. Cochrane Database Syst Rev 2016;(8):CD010744.

37. Thabane M, COPD Working Group. Smoking cessation for patients with chronic obstructive pulmonary disease (COPD): an evidence-based analysis. Ont Health Technol Assess Ser 2012;12(4): 1–50.

38. Stead LF, Buitrago D, Preciado N, et al. Physician advice for smoking cessation. Cochrane Database Syst Rev 2013;(5):CD000165.

39. Stead LF, Koilpillai P, Fanshawe TR, et al. Combined pharmacotherapy and behavioural interventions for smoking cessation. Cochrane Database Syst Rev 2016;(3):CD008286.

40. Hartmann-Boyce J, Hong B, Livingstone-Banks J, et al. Additional behavioural support as an adjunct to pharmacotherapy for smoking cessation. Cochrane Database Syst Rev 2019;(6):CD009670.

41. Anthonisen NR, Connett JE, Kiley JP, et al. Effects of smoking intervention and the use of an inhaled anticholinergic bronchodilator on the rate of decline of FEV1: the Lung Health Study. JAMA 1994;272(19):1497–505.

42. Wagena EJ, Knispchild PG, Huibers MJ, et al. Efficacy of bupropion and nortryptiline for smoking cessation among people at risk for or with COPD. Arch Intern Med 2005;165(19):2286–92.

43. Tashkin DP, Rennard S, Hays JT, et al. Effects of varenicline on smoking cessation in patients with mild to moderate COPD: a randomized controlled trial. Chest 2011;139(3):591–9.

44. Jiménez Ruiz CA, Ramos Pinedo A, Cicero Guerrero A, et al. Characteristics of COPD smokers and effectiveness and safety of smoking cessation medications. Nicotine Tob Res 2012;14(9):1035–9.

45. Hernández Zenteno RJ, Lara DF, Venegas AR, et al. Varenicline for long term smoking cessation in patients with COPD. Pulm Pharmacol Ther 2018;53:116–20.

46. Tashkin DP. Smoking cessation in chronic obstructive pulmonary disease. Semin Respir Crit Care Med 2015;36(4):491–507.

47. Simmons MS, Connett JE, NidesMA, et al. Smoking reduction and the rate of decline in FEV1: results from the Lung Health Study. Eur Respir J 2005; 25(6):1011–7.

48. Rennard SI, Daughton D, Fujita J, et al. Short-term smoking reduction is associated with reduction in measures of lower respiratory tract inflammation in heavy smokers. Eur Respir J 1990;3(7):752–9.

49. Jiménez-Ruiz C, Solano S, Viteri SA, et al. Harm reduction—a treatment approach for resistant smokers with tobacco-related symptoms. Respiration 2002;69(5):452–5.

50. Tønnesen P. Smoking reduction for smokers not able ormotivated to quit? Respiration 2002;69(6): 475–8.

51. Falba T, Jofre-Bonet M, Busch S, et al. Reduction of quantity smoked predicts future cessation among older smokers. Addiction 2004;99(1):93–102.

52. Hughes JR, Carpenter MJ. Does smoking reduction increase future cessation and decrease disease risk? A qualitative review. Nicotine Tob Res 2006;8(6):739–49.

53. Lindson N, Klemperer E, Hong B, et al. Smoking reduction interventions for smoking cessation. Cochrane Database Syst Rev 2019;(9):CD013183.

54. McRobbie H, Bullen C, Hartmann-Boyce J, et al. Electronic cigarettes for smoking cessation and reduction. Cochrane Database Syst Rev 2016;(9): CD010216.

55. Rahman MA, Hann N, Wilson A, et al. E-cigarettes and smoking cessation: evidence from a systematic review and meta-analysis. PLoS One 2015; 10(3):e0122544.

56. Kalkhoran S, Glantz SA. E-cigarettes and smoking cessation in real-world and clinical settings: a systematic review and meta-analysis. Lancet Respir Med 2016;4(2):116–28.

57. Hajek P, Phillips-Waller A, Przulj D, et al. A randomized trial of E-cigarettes versus nicotine-replacement therapy. N Engl J Med 2019;380(7): 629–37.

58. Davidson K, Brancato A, Heetderks P, et al. Outbreak of electronic-cigarette-associated acute lipoid pneumonia - North Carolina, July-August 2019. MMWR Morb Mortal Wkly Rep 2019;68(36): 784–6.

59. Hopkins Tanne J. Vaping: CDC investigates severe lung injuries. BMJ 2019;366:l5228.

60. Balmes JR. Vaping-induced acute lung injury: an epidemic that could have been prevented. Am J Respir Crit Care Med 2019;200(11):1342–4.

61. Kalininskiy A, Bach CT, Nacca NE, et al. E-cigarette, or vaping, product use associated lung injury (EVALI): case series and diagnostic approach. Lancet Respir Med 2019;7(12):1017–26.

62. Butt YM, Smith ML, Tazelaar HD, et al. Pathology of vaping-associated lung injury. N Engl J Med 2019; 381(18):1780–1.

63. Mukhopadhyay S, Mehrad M, Dammert P, et al. Lung biopsy findings in severe pulmonary illness associated with E-cigarette use (vaping). Am J Clin Pathol 2020;153(1):30–9.

64. Cimen P, Unlu M, Kirakli C, et al. Should patients with COPD be vaccinated? Respir Care 2015;60: 239–423.

65. Vaccines against influenza WHO position paper - November 2012. Wkly Epidemiol Rec 2012;87: 461–76.

66. Criner GJ, Bourbeau J, Diekemper RL, et al. Executive summary: prevention of acute exacerbation of COPD: American College of Chest Physicians and Canadian Thoracic Society Guideline. Chest 2015; 147(4):883–93.

67. Montes de Oca M, López Varela MV, Acuña A, et al. ALAT-2014 chronic obstructive pulmonary disease (COPD) clinical practice guidelines: questions and answers. Arch Bronconeumol 2015;51(8): 403–16.

68. European Centre for Disease Prevention and Control (ECDC). Seasonal influenza vaccination in Europe. Overview of vaccination recommendations and coverage rates in the EU member states for

the 2012–13 influenza season, Technical report. European Centre for Disease Prevention and Control; 2015.

69. Centers for Disease Control and Prevention (CDC). People at high risk of developing flu–related complications 2015. Available at: http://www.cdc.gov/flu/about/disease/high_risk.htm. Accessed February 24, 2016.

70. Global Initiative for Chronic Obstructive Lung Disease. Global strategy for the diagnosis, management and prevention of chronic obstructive pulmonary disease. Bethesda, GOLD. 2020. Available at: https://goldcopd.org/wp-content/uploads/2019/12/GOLD-2020-FINAL-ver1.2-03Dec19_WMV.pdf.

71. Vozoris NT, Lougheed MD. Influenza vaccination among Canadians with chronic respiratory disease. Respir Med 2009;103(1):50–8.

72. Li A, Chan YH, Liew MF, et al. Improving influenza vaccination coverage among patients with COPD: a pilot project. Int J Chron Obstruct Pulmon Dis 2019;14:2527–33.

73. Jiménez-García R, Ariñez-Fernandez MC, Garcia-Carballo M, et al. Influenza vaccination coverage and related factors among Spanish patients with chronic obstructive pulmonary disease. Vaccine 2005;23:3679–86.

74. Jiménez-García R, Ariñez-Fernandez MC, Hernández-Barrera V, et al. Compliance with influenza and pneumococcal vaccination among patients with chronic obstructive pulmonary disease consulting their medical practitioners in Catalonia, Spain. J Infect 2007;54(1):65–74.

75. Garrastazu R, García-Rivero JL, Ruiz M, et al. Prevalence of influenza vaccination in chronic obstructive pulmonary disease patients and impact on the risk of severe exacerbations. Arch Bronconeumol 2016;52(2):88–95.

76. Aka Aktürk Ü, Görek Dilektaşlı A, Şengül A, et al. Influenza and pneumonia vaccination rates and factors affecting vaccination among patients with chronic obstructive pulmonary disease. Balkan Med J 2017;34(3):206–11.

77. Gnatiuc L, Buist AS, Kato B, et al. Gaps in using bronchodilators, inhaled corticosteroids and influenza vaccine among 23 high- and low-income sites. Int J Tuberc Lung Dis 2015;19(1):21–30.

78. Lopez Varela MV, Muino A, Perez Padilla R, et al. Treatment of chronic obstructive pulmonary disease in 5 Latin American cities: the PLATINO study. Arch Bronconeumol 2008;44(2):58–64.

79. Kotey E, Lukosaityte D, Quaye O, et al. Current and novel approaches in influenza management. Vaccines (Basel) 2019;7(2) [pii:E53].

80. Jazayeri SD, Poh CL. Development of universal influenza vaccines targeting conserved viral proteins. Vaccines (Basel) 2019;7(4) [pii:E169].

81. Bekkat-Berkani R, Ray R, Jain VK, et al. Evidence update: GlaxoSmithKline's inactivated quadrivalent influenza vaccines. Expert Rev Vaccines 2016; 15(2):201–14.

82. Gresset-Bourgeois V, Leventhal PS, Pepin S, et al. Quadrivalent inactivated influenza vaccine (VaxigripTetra™). Expert Rev Vaccines 2018; 17(1):1–11.

83. Bafadhel M, McKenna S, Terry S, et al. Acute exacerbations of chronic obstructive pulmonary disease: identification of biologic clusters and their biomarkers. Am J Respir Crit Care Med 2011; 184(6):662–71.

84. Kopsaftis Z, Wood-Baker R, Poole P. Influenza vaccine for chronic obstructive pulmonary disease (COPD). Cochrane Database Syst Rev 2018;(6): CD002733.

85. Bekkat-Berkani R, Wilkinson T, Buchy P, et al. Seasonal influenza vaccination in patients with COPD: a systematic literature review. BMC Pulm Med 2017;17(1):79.

86. Schembri S, Morant S, Winter JH, et al. Influenza but not pneumococcal vaccination protects against all-cause mortality in patients with COPD. Thorax 2009;64(7):567–72.

87. Sunita M, Li L, Ye L, et al. Effectiveness of influenza vaccination on hospitalizations and risk factors for severe outcomes in hospitalized patients with COPD. Chest 2019;155(1):69–78.

88. Huang HH, Chen SJ, Chao TF, et al. Influenza vaccination and risk of respiratory failure in patients with chronic obstructive pulmonary disease: a nationwide population-based case-cohort study. J Microbiol Immunol Infect 2019;52(1):22–9.

89. Welte T, Torres A, Nathwani D. Clinical and economic burden of community acquired pneumonia among adults in Europe. Thorax 2012;67(1):71–9.

90. Rozenbaum MH, Pechlivanoglou P, van der Werf TS, et al. The role of Streptococcus pneumoniae in community-acquired pneumonia among adults in Europe: a meta-analysis. Eur J Clin Microbiol Infect Dis 2013;32(3):305–16.

91. Said MA, Johnson HL, Nonyane BA, et al. Estimating the burden of pneumococcal pneumonia among adults: a systematic review and meta-analysis of diagnostic techniques. PLoS One 2013;8(4):e60273.

92. Peto L, Nadjm B, Horby P, et al. The bacterial aetiology of adult community acquired pneumonia in Asia: a systematic review. Trans R Soc Trop Med Hyg 2014;108(6):326–37.

93. World Health Organization. The top 10 causes of death worldwide. Geneva (Switzerland): World Health Organization; 2018. Available at: www.who.int/mediacentre/factsheets/fs310/en/#. Accessed October 14, 2018.

94. Shea KM, Edelsberg J, Weycker D, et al. Rates of pneumococcal disease in adults with chronic medical conditions. Open Forum Infect Dis 2014;1(1): ofu024.

95. Menendez R, Ferrando D, Vallés JM, et al. Initial risk class and length of hospital stay in community-acquired pneumonia. Eur Respir J 2001;18(1):151–6.

96. Rello J, Rodríguez A, Torres A, et al. Implications of COPD in patients admitted to the intensive care unit by community-acquired pneumonia. Eur Respir J 2006;27(6):1210–6.

97. Torres A, Peetermans WE, Viegi G, et al. Risk factors for community-acquired pneumonia in adults in Europe: a literature review. Thorax 2013;68(11): 1057–65.

98. Mullerova H, Chigbo C, Hagan GW, et al. The natural history of community-acquired pneumonia in COPD patients: a population database analysis. Respir Med 2012;106(8):1124–33.

99. Inghammar M, Engström G, Kahlmeter G, et al. Invasive pneumococcal disease in patients with an underlying pulmonary disorder. Clin Microbiol Infect 2013;19(12):1148–54.

100. Shukla SD, Muller HK, Latham R, et al. Platelet-activating factor receptor (PAFr) is upregulated in small airways and alveoli of smokers and COPD patients. Respirology 2016;21(3):504–10.

101. Shukla SD, Mahmood MQ, Weston S, et al. The main rhinovirus respiratory tract adhesion site (ICAM-1) is upregulated in smokers and patients with chronic airflow limitation (CAL). Respir Res 2017;18(1):6.

102. Suissa S, Patenaude V, Lapi F, et al. Inhaled corticosteroids in COPD and the risk of serious pneumonia. Thorax 2013;68(11):1029–36.

103. Kew KM, Seniukovich A. Inhaled steroids and risk of pneumonia for chronic obstructive pulmonary disease. Cochrane Database Syst Rev 2014;(3): CD010115.

104. Suissa S, Coulombe J, Ernst P. Discontinuation of inhaled corticosteroids in COPD and the risk reduction of pneumonia. Chest 2015;148(5): 1177–83.

105. Andreassen SL, Liaaen ED, Stenfors N, et al. Impact of pneumonia on hospitalizations due to acute exacerbations of COPD. Clin Respir J 2014;8(1):93–9.

106. Søgaard M, Madsen M, Løkke A, et al. Incidence and outcomes of patients hospitalized with COPD exacerbation with and without pneumonia. Int J Chron Obstruct Pulmon Dis 2016;11:455–65.

107. Myint PK, Lowe D, Stone RA, et al. U.K. National COPD Resources and Outcomes Project 2008: patients with chronic obstructive pulmonary disease exacerbations who present with radiological pneumonia have worse outcome compared to those with non-pneumonic chronic obstructive pulmonary disease exacerbations. Respiration 2011;82(4): 320–7.

108. Hausdorff WP, Feikin DR, Klugman KP. Epidemiological differences among pneumococcal serotypes. Lancet Infect Dis 2005;5(2):83–93.

109. Menendez R, Espana PP, Perez-Trallero E, et al. The burden of PCV13 serotypes in accepted manuscript hospitalized pneumococcal pneumonia in Spain using a novel urinary antigen detection test. CAPA study. Vaccine 2017;35(39):5264–70.

110. Merck & Co. Pneumovax® 23 (pneumococcal vaccine polyvalent). Full prescribing information. Whitehouse Station (NJ): Merck & Co, Inc; 2015.

111. Pfizer, Inc. Prevnar 13® (pneumococcal 13-valent conjugate vaccine [diphtheria CRM197 protein]). Full prescribing information. Collegeville (PA): Pfizer, Inc; 2016.

112. Bonten MJ, Huijts SM, Bolkenbaas M, et al. Polysaccharide conjugate vaccine against pneumococcal pneumonia in adults. N Engl J Med 2015; 372(12):1114–25.

113. Matanock A, Lee G, Gierke R, et al. Use of 13-valent pneumococcal conjugate vaccine and 23-valent pneumococcal polysaccharide vaccine among adults aged ≥65 years: updated recommendations of the advisory committee on immunization practices. MMWR Morb Mortal Wkly Rep 2019;68(46):1069–75.

114. Kraicer-Melamed H, O'Donnell S, Quach C. The effectiveness of pneumococcal polysaccharide vaccine 23 (PPV23) in the general population of 50 years of age and older: a systematic review and meta-analysis. Vaccine 2016;34(13):1540–50.

115. Moberley S, Holden J, Tatham DP, et al. Vaccines for preventing pneumococcal infection in adults. Cochrane Database Syst Rev 2013;(1):CD000422.

116. Schiffner-Rohe J, Witt A, Hemmerling J, et al. Efficacy of PPV23 in preventing pneumococcal pneumonia in adults at increased risk—a systematic review and meta-analysis. PLoS One 2016;11(1): e0146338.

117. Diao WQ, Shen N, Yu PX, et al. Efficacy of 23-valent pneumococcal polysaccharide vaccine in preventing community-acquired pneumonia among immunocompetent adults: a systematic review and meta-analysis of randomized trials. Vaccine 2016; 34(13):1496–503.

118. Pneumococcal vaccines WHO position paper: 2012. Wkly Epidemiol Rec 2012;87(14):129–44.

119. van Werkhoven CH, Huijts SM. Vaccines to prevent pneumococcal community-acquired pneumonia. Clin Chest Med 2018;39(4):733–52.

120. Bonnave C, Mertens D, Peetermans W, et al. Adult vaccination for pneumococcal disease: a comparison of the national guidelines in Europe. Eur J Clin Microbiol Infect Dis 2019;38(4):785–91.

121. Kaplan A, Arsenault P, Aw B, et al. Vaccine strategies for prevention of community-acquired pneumonia in Canada: who would benefit most from pneumococcal immunization? Can Fam Physician 2019;65(9):625–33.

122. Walters JA, Tang JN, Poole P, et al. Pneumococcal vaccines for preventing pneumonia in chronic obstructive pulmonary disease. Cochrane Database Syst Rev 2017;(1):CD001390.

123. Htar MT, Stuurman AL, Ferreira G, et al. Effectiveness of pneumococcal vaccines in preventing pneumonia in adults, a systematic review and meta-analyses of observational studies. PLoS One 2017;12(5):e0177985.

124. Furumoto A, Ohkusa Y, Chen M, et al. Additive effect of pneumococcal vaccine and influenza vaccine on acute exacerbation in patients with chronic lung disease. Vaccine 2008;26(33): 4284–9.

125. Centers for Disease Control and Prevention, National Center for Immunization and Respiratory Diseases (NCIRD). Adult immunization schedule 2017. Atlanta (GA): 2017. Available at: https://www.cdc.gov/vaccines/schedules/easy-to-read/adult.html. Accessed June 5, 2017.

Pulmonary Rehabilitation

Jean Bourbeau, MD, MSC, FRCPC*, Sebastien Gagnon, MD,
Bryan Ross, MD, MSC, FRCPC

KEYWORDS

- COPD • Physical and rehabilitation medicine • Physical education and training • Exercise training
- Self-management • Exacerbation • Physical activity • Symptom flare up

KEY POINTS

- Pulmonary rehabilitation is an effective multidisciplinary nonpharmacological intervention that represents the standard of care in chronic obstructive pulmonary disease (COPD) management.
- Exercise training, education, and self-management behavior-modification are fundamental elements of a pulmonary rehabilitation program.
- Challenges encountered in program delivery (including exacerbations, advanced COPD, resource constraints, geographic constraints, and reductions in gains) can be effectively addressed (through exercise adjuncts, tailored prescriptions, community-based/tele-based/home-based delivery, and self-management intervention, respectively).

INTRODUCTION

With an aging population, the burden of chronic obstructive pulmonary disease (COPD) continues to rise, impacting patients, their families, the health care system, and the society. The clinical course of COPD follows a well-known vicious circle of dyspnea-inactivity often punctuated with acute exacerbations, resulting in a poor quality of life in affected patients.[1] This disease trajectory can be impacted by pulmonary rehabilitation (PR), considered now as an essential parts of COPD therapy.

There is robust evidence in the literature that PR leads to improvements in dyspnea, exercise capacity, health-related quality of life, and health care utilization in patients with COPD.[2,3] PR programs also emphasize self-management (SM) interventions to increase patient self-efficacy and healthy behaviors.[4] However, despite the documented benefits and strong recommendations for their use,[5,6] PR remains underprescribed and underused. In 2018, the reported rates of PR use in the United States were only 2.7% within 12 months of hospitalization in Medicare

beneficiaries, even though their hospitalization was within the 2 years since Medicare began reimbursement for PR.[7] Older age (≥75 years) and lower socioeconomic status were factors associated with nonusage. In Canada, the access remained limited to fewer than 1% of patients with COPD.[8] Increased awareness by health care providers, along with the development of strategies to facilitate access to PR, are needed.

This article provides a practical review of the elements of a PR program in addition to tackling relevant emerging topics, including alternate forms of organization and delivery, the role and training of the case manager, and specific challenges, such as patients with acute exacerbations of COPD (AECOPD) and those with advanced disease. Resources and online tools for health care professionals and patients are provided throughout the article.

DEFINITION, CONCEPT AND SOURCE DOCUMENTATIONS
Definition and Concept

PR is a comprehensive and multidisciplinary approach to the management of COPD. Given

Respiratory Epidemiology and Clinical Research Unit, Montréal Chest Institute, McGill University Health Centre, 5252 De Maisonneuve, Room 3D.62, Montréal, Québec H4A 3S5, Canada
* Corresponding author.
E-mail address: jean.bourbeau@mcgill.ca

Clin Chest Med 41 (2020) 513–528
https://doi.org/10.1016/j.ccm.2020.06.003

the robust evidence for benefit,[2,9–11] PR is an important component of the current standard of care in managing COPD, in addition to playing an ever-increasing role in the management of all chronic lung diseases. Society guidelines define PR as *"a comprehensive intervention based on a thorough patient assessment followed by patient-tailored therapies, which include, but are not limited to, exercise training, education, and behavior change, designed to improve the physical and psychological condition of people with chronic respiratory disease and to promote the long-term adherence of health-enhancing behaviors."*[9]

Although the setting and delivery of PR varies widely based on the fiscal, geographic, and personnel availabilities,[12] there is a general consensus on what constitutes the core components of a PR program. These include pre-rehabilitation assessment to individualize/optimize each individual's PR program experience; exercise training; body composition interventions; SM education; and psychological and social interventions.[9,13] Additional indicators of quality in a PR program include its duration, the frequency of supervised exercise, and the measurement of health outcomes before and after the program.[14] The multimodal approach also includes education on inhaler technique and adherence, energy utilization and conservation strategies, and how to recognize an exacerbation and the appropriate use of an Action Plan.[9]

In addition, the patients themselves must also actively engage and be equipped with the tools to manage their own disease. Education targeting self-management is an important component of PR promoting behavior change and allowing for the benefits of PR to persist after program completion.[15] SM reduces dyspnea, improves health-related quality of life, and reduces hospital admissions.[16] Its relative novelty and heterogeneity in delivery[16] prompted a standardized definition of SM in COPD management: *"structured but personalized and often multi-component, with the goals of motivating, engaging and supporting the patients to positively adapt their health behavior skills and develop skills to better manage their disease."*[17] The current SM model in modern PR programs emphasizes a collaborative approach; beyond didactic, passive instruction, the patient must also be motivated and confident to apply the knowledge they have learned following serial iterative interactions.[17] It is through this critical step that patients may become active agents in their own health and change their health and lifestyle behaviors in a sustainable manner, thereby promoting more enduring benefits following PR participation.[9]

Source Documentations

A comprehensive reference for PR is the "Rehabilitation" section of the Web site www.livingwellwithcopd.com, which includes resources for all of the elements of PR. In addition to many studies and clinical trials published to demonstrate its effectiveness, Living Well with COPD (LWWCOPD) is a high-quality resource referenced throughout this article, available to any health care provider following a simple account sign-up (https://www.livingwellwithcopd.com/en/become-member.html). Additional noteworthy resources include https://pulmonaryrehab.com.au, a Lung Foundation Australia open-access resource for high-yield PR materials, and http://www.livebetter.org, an American Thoracic Society/Gawlicki Family Foundation PR navigation tool geared toward patients with chronic lung disease.

EXERCISE TRAINING, TESTING AND PRESCRIPTION IN PULMONARY REHABILITATION

An important aim of PR is to stabilize or reverse the pathophysiological manifestations of the disease and to attempt to bring the patient to the highest possible functional capacity, achieved through SM intervention and exercise training.[9]

Exercise Training in Pulmonary Rehabilitation

Exercise training is the cornerstone of effective PR because it increases exercise capacity,[3] and improves activities of daily living (ADLs) and independent ADLs (IADLs).[18] Physical conditioning through exercise training is also an important way to achieve the personal goals identified by the patient at the outset of the program (participate in a sport or hobby that they were once able to do), which can provide the means to reconnect to social networks and enhance quality of life.

Exercise imparts a certain load onto the peripheral muscles, and this increases the oxygen needs of the body. The patient's respiratory system must exchange fuel (oxygen) for by-products (carbon dioxide) of metabolism, and transfer oxygen to the circulatory system; the heart and circulatory system must transport the oxygenated blood to the skeletal muscles used during exercise; and the mitochondria of these peripheral muscles must use oxygen efficiently in aerobic cellular respiration.[19] Any abnormality or breakdown along any of these organ systems can lead to a reduced exercise capacity. Depending on the underlying cause, symptoms in daily life are manifested as dyspnea and/or leg fatigue, the 2 principal components evaluated when using the Borg scale.[20] Adding to the complexity of exercise pathophysiology are layers of motivational and psychological aspects related to exercise, for example, the influence of previous traumatizing attacks of dyspnea,[21] on one's willingness to maximally exert one's self during exercise sessions.

Exercise Capacity Testing

The ability to determine the baseline exercise capacity, and the principal cause for exercise limitation, are pivotal in the ability to prescribe a tailored exercise plan for the patient with COPD. The gold standard remains the cardiopulmonary exercise test (CPET). In a CPET, valuable information is gained by the determination of peak workload and the collection of expired gases, pulse oximetry, electrocardiography, blood pressure, Borg scores, and in many cases serial spirometric maneuvers and dynamic operational lung volumes.[22] Through such data collection, not only can conventional measurements in performance athletics such as the ventilatory threshold and maximal (or peak) oxygen consumption be obtained, but additional critical respiratory limitations to exercise characteristics of COPD can be identified and quantified. In patients with COPD there are unique limitations, including ventilatory inefficiency and ventilation-perfusion mismatch, expiratory flow limitation and dynamic hyperinflation, a disproportionate work of breathing due to airway resistive and elastic abnormalities, and oxygen desaturation and hypercapnea.[19,22] Through incremental testing, the timing of these events in relation to peak workload, oxygen consumption, and Borg scores can help individualize the aerobic goals and limits for the exercise prescription.[22]

The accessibility to CPET varies greatly depending on the resources (expertise, personnel, equipment) and practice patterns within the milieu where the PR program operates. Alternative means of testing include the 6-minute walking test (6MWT)[23] or the incremental[24] shuttle walking tests (ISWT). Although the 6MWT encourages the patient to walk as far as possible at their own pace in 6 minutes, the ISWT progressively increases walking speed and is therefore felt to be more akin to an incremental CPET study.[25] Although less comprehensive from a physiologic and mechanistic perspective, useful information on exercise capacity can be collected from these alternative tests.[26]

Exercise Prescription, Type, and Intensity

A helpful framework for developing an exercise prescription is the "FITT'" paradigm: *Frequency,*

Intensity, Time, and *Type.*[27] Resources for upper and lower extremity aerobic and resistance prescriptions are available on the LWWCOPD Web site (https://www.livingwellwithcopd.com/286-exercisepr-program-overview-and-principles. html) as well as on the Lung Foundation Australia Web site (https://pulmonaryrehab.com.au/importance-of-exercise/exercise-prescription-table). Although endurance (aerobic) training has traditionally been the principal form of exercise in PR programs, many societies recommend that a combination of endurance and resistance types of training should be used.[14,28] Programs should initially allot time to introduce patients to the exercise equipment (treadmill, cycle ergometer, weights and resistance machines) such that they are familiarized with its safe use, particularly due to the known increased falls risk in patients with COPD.[29] Although the ideal exercise program duration in COPD remains controversial,[30] in general longer is better and at least 6 to 8 weeks is recommended.[9,28] Regarding aerobic exercise frequency, 3 to 5 sessions of 20 to 60 minutes each per week is recommended.[9,27]

Aerobic training is preferentially achieved through lower limb exercise[14]: in higher-resource settings this can be performed on a cycle ergometer or on a treadmill and in lower-resource settings by ground walking or by stair climbing. Aerobic training of the upper limbs is also possible, although less conventional.[14,31] **Table 1** provides an approach to setting the initial intensity for each modality of aerobic exercise. Regarding the resistance-type exercise prescription, the recommended frequency and timing is 1 (if higher repetitions) to 4 (if lower repetitions) sets of 8 to 12 repetitions on 2 to 3 days per week, and the recommended intensity is 60% to 70% of the patient's baseline 1-repetition maximum weight.[9,14] Resistance/weight machines, free weights, or elastic bands are commonly used, or even one's own body weight, a form of exercise referred to as calisthenics.

In both aerobic and resistance components of the training program, gradual increases in duration/repetitions and workload/resistance can be applied under the close supervision of trained PR personnel in a stepwise fashion. A printable exercise tracking sheet intended for point-of-care use is available on the LWWCOPD Web site (https://www.livingwellwithcopd.com/DATA/LIBRAIRIE/229_en~v~exercise-sheet.pdf). To continue to benefit from the program, it is important to iteratively titrate the exercise prescription in collaboration with the patient. Typically a "moving titration," targeting a Borg of 4 to 6, can allow for

Table 1
Modalities of training and recommended initial intensity of aerobic training

Aerobic Modality	Initial Intensity
Cycle ergometer	60% of peak workload on CPET
Treadmill	60%–80% of peak workload on CPET 80% of 6MWT speed[a] 75% of ISWT speed
Ground walking	80% of 6MWT speed[a]
Stair climbing	Borg 4–6
Upper extremity ergometer	75% of peak oxygen consumption (incremental upper extremity CPET)

Abbreviations: 6MWT, six-minute walk test; CPET, cardiopulmonary exercise testing; ISWT, incremental shuttle walk test.
  [a] 6MWT average speed = (6MWT distance × 10) ÷ 1000 km/h.
  Adapted from Living Well with COPD. McGill University Health Centre. Available at: https://www.livingwellwithcopd.com/286-exercisepr-program-overview-and-principles.html With permission. And Pulmonary Rehab. *Exercise Prescription Table. Lung Foundation Australia. Available at:* https://pulmonaryrehab.com.au/importance-of-exercise/exercise-prescription-table/ *With permission.*

progressively more demanding sessions as the program continues.[9,32]

PULMONARY REHABILITATION PATIENT SELECTION, SETTING, AND DELIVERY
Patient Selection

PR can benefit almost every patient with COPD irrespective of disease severity, sex, ethnicity, or age[33–35]; however, guidelines recognize that patients with a significant symptom burden despite optimal treatment or with an elevated risk of AECOPD would benefit the most from PR participation.[9,28,36] Comorbidities are not a contraindication to participation as long as they are not acute and uncontrolled and/or they do not interfere with the safe operation of the program; patients with comorbidities may in fact benefit the most from PR participation.[37,38] Initial selection and prioritization should not only focus on airflow obstruction severity but should additionally consider the patient's symptom burden and health status.

Pulmonary Rehabilitation Referral and Participation

Despite the robust evidence supporting PR efficacy, poor referral rates continue to contribute to limited participation.[39] Although PR referral should be considered by the physicians at any point in the chronic management of COPD, particular emphasis on referral should be placed during 3 key events: at diagnosis, before discharge following an AECOPD, and following progressive symptom deterioration.[36] The most common patient barriers prohibiting PR participation are significant travel distance, lack of perceived benefit, and being an active smoker.[40] To encourage participation in PR, the referring physician should first have a comprehensive discussion with the patient regarding the process and expected benefits of PR. Concerning the travel distance barrier, it has been proposed that PR delivery at peripheral community centers would increase both access and adherence. In support of this hypothesis, recent implementation studies have demonstrated that tele-health PR delivery to peripheral sites is feasible, safe, and effective.[41,42] Further studies are needed to better establish tele-rehabilitation strategies.

Setting and Delivery

PR can be conducted in a number of settings, from inpatient hospital-based, outpatient-based, and even home-based programs. The optimal setting for a specific program will vary according to community needs, available resources, and patient characteristics. Of note, patients with severe and advanced disease and those with multiple comorbidities often require hospital-based programs because of a greater need for supervision and multidisciplinary care.[43] Despite being the "gold standard," outpatient programs are limited by cost and availability constraints.[8,44] To overcome these limitations, home-based programs are under ongoing evaluation. Two studies demonstrated noninferiority of home-based versus hospital-based PR.[45,46] Short-term benefits on exercise capacity, breathlessness, and quality of life were observed, whereas adherence and completion rates were actually higher in home-based participants. Conflicting results in the literature[47] may be secondary to heterogeneity in design, intervention, and support structures. To be recognized as PR, a home-based program must be capable of preserving all core components that define PR, including exercise program supervision, a multidimensional approach, and education with SM interventions. Tele-health is a novel PR delivery method that incorporates rapidly growing technological advances in remote management.[48] Tele-health applications are numerous and can be incorporated in several clinical tasks including consultation, monitoring, and education. Tele-rehabilitation sessions can be delivered either within a health care institution or within the patient's home. When comparing an 8-week in-center tele-rehabilitation program with standard in-center PR, Stickland and colleagues[42] demonstrated that locally supervised group exercise sessions in combination with remote tele-casted education sessions resulted in similar benefits on quality of life and exercise capacity. At-home tele-rehabilitation is a further extension of remote PR. Although this has also demonstrated interesting results, larger studies are still needed.

Program Duration, Structure, and Staffing

Although the duration and number of PR sessions can vary by setting, minimal PR standards must still be met. Outpatient participants typically attend 2 to 3 sessions per week, whereas inpatient participants may attend up to 5 days per week. In the interest of program effectiveness, programs should contain at least 24 sessions. Although longer programs may produce greater gains,[9,30] physical capacity improvement tends to plateau after 12 weeks.[49] Therefore, in the interest of optimizing attendance, cost, and intervention efficacy, most programs last 8 to 12 weeks.[50] Typically, a PR team is interdisciplinary and the program is led by a medical director.[9,51]

A physiotherapist and/or kinesiologist with experience in clinical exercise training are essential for exercise prescription and supervision. Designation within the PR team of the patient's acting case manager (CM) should be considered; the CM can review the patient needs, coordinate individual and group education, and help the patient navigate the system.[52] All the health care professionals who are part of the PR team should be involved in an interdisciplinary approach. Based on resource availability, the team should be complemented by a social worker, nutritionist, occupational therapist, and psychologist.

Importance of the Case Manager

The CM stands to play an important role in SM intervention as the patient's principal health care system and chronic disease "navigator."[53] **Table 2** presents the many central roles of the CM in comprehensive patient care, in addition to CM training recommendations.[53] In those patients with recurrent AECOPD, the CM instructs and supports the patient on the timely completion of the written Action Plan. Recognition of symptom worsening ("problem learning"), deciding to adjust, change, or add medication ("decision making"), and contacting for assistance when needed are important tools acquired through the patient-CM relationship. Importantly, there is currently no evidence that an Action Plan without CM assistance is effective. A 2016 Cochrane review on Action plan[54] efficacy showed a reduction in hospital admission; however, the results were mainly driven by the trial of Rice and colleagues[55] that did include CM support. Training of the CM has not yet been studied and/or validated. In the absence of official guidelines, training in communication skills and in COPD care are recommended.[52] To optimize their effectiveness, the CM should also ideally be trained in the basic principles of behavior change and in motivational interviewing.

BEHAVIOR MODIFICATION, EXERCISE MAINTENANCE, AND INCREASED PHYSICAL ACTIVITY

The affected patient's adaptation, their associated comorbidities, and the social impact of the illness are important determinants that influence COPD morbidity. Adaptive behavior change using patient-centered communication strategies and SM training can help address these determinants and can ultimately stimulate intrinsically motivated actions.[9]

Self-Management Behavior Modification Intervention

Although education has always been an important part of the PR program, the paradigm shift from didactic to SM education was an important advancement that took place in the early 2000s. In 2003, Bourbeau and colleagues[56] demonstrated a reduction in admission for AECOPD by 39.8% following the combined interventions of exercise training with weekly home education sessions for 8 weeks as well as Action Plan teaching. Following this landmark study, multiple subsequent SM clinical trials duplicated these positive results A Cochrane meta-analysis

Table 2
Role of the case manager and training recommendations for self-management as part of the pulmonary rehabilitation program

Role of the case manager	1. Lead with the other team members the individual and group education sessions. 2. Guide/coach the patient in self-management behaviors that aid in achieving physical activity and other self-management goals (medication adherence, exacerbations), while improving daily COPD management. 3. Assess/record the patient's progress throughout the study using patient worksheets for measures of stage of change, motivation and self-efficacy tailored to the patient needs and make adaptations to the program as needed over time. 4. Use motivational enhanced communication strategies, goal setting, reinforcement. 5. Work with exercise staff to discuss patient goals and establish stage of change. 6. Provide direction to exercise staff for providing consistent message to the patient, evaluate barriers for a coordinated approach to the patient. 7. Reinforce skills during the exercise program such as the ability of the patient to use their inhaler properly, using oxygen appropriately, and discussing changes that should generate or consider using the Action Plan.
Training[a] of the case manager	1. Training can be based on a self-management program such as "Living Well with COPD," which is designed to help patients with COPD and their families cope with their disease on a daily basis. 2. Reference guides "Living Well with COPD" should be provided to assist the case manager/health coach in engaging with their patients and facilitating improved disease self-management. 3. Basic training in motivational communication skills should be provided as an important component of the training and includes the following: • Using open questions and building motivation to engage patients in more physical activity and other behaviors • Using reflective listening to manage and overcome resistance • Providing information by offering, sharing. and asking patients for feedback

Abbreviation: COPD, chronic obstructive pulmonary disease.
   [a] This training should be delivered to the other members of the pulmonary rehabilitation team as well.
   Adapted from Clini E HA, Pitta F, Troosters T (Eds). Textbook of Pulmonary Rehabilitation. Springer International Publishing AG; 2018. p. 224; with permission. (Table 3 in original)

comprising 22 studies and 3854 participants demonstrated that SM resulted in an overall improvement in health-related quality of life and a reduction in respiratory-related hospital admissions.[57] Although the heterogeneity of each SM intervention studied makes it difficult to determine the optimal form and content of an effective SM intervention, it is prudent and important to continue to apply the benefits of SM intervention toward PR program design.

Educational Components

The American Thoracic Society and European Respiratory Society[9] emphasize the need to promote adaptive behavior change and SM in particular. The precise content of an SM educational intervention will depend on individual needs, the comorbidity profile, and the patient's own capacity to manage his or her disease (self-efficacy, literacy, numeracy). **Table 3** presents the common skills that require mastery and the healthy behaviors to be adopted and maintained through PR education.[4] Content tailoring and small-group educational delivery (4–8 patients) are effective PR program approaches that encourage mutual enrichment through peer learning.

Table 3
Self-management skills and healthy behaviors for COPD self-management

Healthy Behavior	Self-Management Skill (Strategy)
Live in a smoke-free environment	Quit smoking, remain nonsmoker, and avoid second-hand smoke
Comply with your medication	Take medication as prescribed on a regular basis and use proper inhalation techniques
Manage to maintain comfortable breathing	Use according to directives: • The pursed-lip breathing technique • The forward body position
Conserve your energy Manage your stress and anxiety	Prioritize your activities, plan your schedule, and pace yourself Use your relaxation and breathing techniques, try to solve one problem at a time, talk about your problems and do not hesitate to ask for help, and maintain a positive attitude
Prevent and seek early treatment of COPD exacerbations	Get your flu shot every year and your vaccine for pneumonia Identify and avoid factors that can make your symptoms worse Use your plan of action according to the directives (recognition of symptom deterioration and actions to perform) Contact your resource person when needed
Maintain an active lifestyle	Maintain physical activities (eg, activities of daily living, walking, climbing stairs) Exercise regularly (according to a prescribed home exercise program)
Keep a healthy diet	Maintain a healthy weight, eat food high in protein and eat smaller meals more often (5–6 meals per day)
Have good sleep habits	Maintain a routine, avoid heavy meals and stimulants, and relax before bedtime
Maintain a satisfying sex life	Use positions that require less energy Share your feelings with your partner Do not limit yourself to intercourse, create a romantic atmosphere Use your breathing, relaxation, and coughing techniques
Get involved in leisure activities	Choose leisure activities that you enjoy Choose environments in which your symptoms will not be aggravated Pace yourself through the activities while using your breathing techniques Respect your strengths and limitations

Abbreviation: COPD, chronic obstructive pulmonary disease.

Adapted from Bourbeau J, Nault D. Self-management strategies in chronic obstructive pulmonary disease. Clin Chest Med. 2007;28(3):617-628, vii; with permission.

Pulmonary Rehabilitation Maintenance and Increased Physical Activity

After PR completion, the gains made risk being lost if the patient does not continue to be active.[58] Therefore, a major goal of PR is to ensure the implementation of a maintenance exercise program and/or a sustainable increase in physical activity. The challenge is considerable, but worth it: physically active patients with COPD demonstrate a lower hospital utilization and a better survival than their inactive counterparts.[59–61]

When patients have to exercise on their own following PR completion, regular exercise participation can drop more than 50% by 12 months.[62,63] Three distinct patterns of patient evolution have been described in one PR study in which patients were followed,[63] 2 of which display difficulty in maintaining exercise activity in the 12 months following PR completion. A systematic review of qualitative studies identified common barriers to maintaining exercise included symptoms during exercise, restricted social support, lack of positive feedback, and absence of maintenance sessions following PR.[64] Collectively, these results suggest that by implementing appropriate interventions during and after the PR program, it may be possible to promote better long-term adherence to home exercise and/or physical activity.

Maintenance Considerations

After PR completion, supervised exercise maintenance may be the most appropriate option for certain patients. In a recently published meta-analysis, continued supervised exercise maintenance following PR resulted in a reduction in the risk of experiencing at least 1 respiratory-related hospitalization compared with usual care.[65] This result was mainly driven by the recent study by Güell and colleagues,[66] which reported a 3-year follow-up to an 8-week PR program followed by a weekly home-based supervised exercise maintenance program using cycle ergometers. Over the first 2 years, the BODE index[67] and 6MWD were preserved, but progressively declined thereafter. Following previous disappointing results regarding supervised exercise maintenance,[50] this study challenged previous beliefs and put forth the possibility of maintaining the benefits of a short-term PR program over 2 years. Because it is more economic and practical to perform maintenance programs from home, this is an interesting concept in need of further research. Two prior studies using maintenance unsupervised training reported preservation of exercise capacity at 18 months. It should be noted that both trials used a long initial program (3 and 6 months, respectively), which may explain the observed benefits and is therefore likely not applicable to most real-world practice settings.

To increase access to maintenance programs, home-based tele-rehabilitation offers a promising solution. Following an 8-week PR program, Vasilopoulou and colleagues[68] randomized 147 patients to either home-based maintenance, outpatient maintenance or usual care. Although the home-based tele-rehabilitation program was as effective as the hospital-based program in reducing the risk of AECOPD and hospitalization, emergency department visits were lower in the tele-rehabilitation program. Future research on maintenance modalities should focus on overcoming common barriers experienced by patients linked with mechanisms that strengthen the link between the hospital and the community.

Role of Self-Management on Physical Activity

Without self-efficacy and SM skills learned from motivational and self-management behavior-modification (SMBM) interventions, there is a risk that the benefits gained from PR may not translate into a sustainable change in physical activity and in behaviors after PR completion.[15] This is classically described as the inability to translate from "can do" to "do do."[69]

The PHYSACTO study evaluated the fundamental role of SM to promote an increase in physical activity.[70] This randomized controlled trial (RCT) prospectively assessed whether the addition of dual bronchodilation to an SMBM program (based on the LWWCOPD program [www.livingwellwithcopd.com]), with or without exercise training, would improve exercise endurance time and physical activity over a 12-week period. Patients were randomized to 1 of 4 groups: SMBM alone, SMBM with tiotropium, SMBM with tiotropium/olodaterol, and SMBM with dual bronchodilation and exercise training. Unsurprisingly, the group with exercise training and combined bronchodilators had the greatest improvement in exercise capacity. However, when looking at physical activity at 12 weeks, SMBM alone significantly increased the daily step-count to a similar magnitude as the increase observed in the other groups. This striking finding supports SMBM (when of a highly standardized caliber as is observed in this RCT) as a major determinant of change in physical activity. Furthermore, a study embedded within the PHYSACTO study demonstrated that SMBM intervention delivered using a motivational counseling approach increases physical activity mediated by an improvement of 3 key hypothesized mechanisms of change: readiness to change, autonomous motivation, and confidence. For the first time, this study shows that an SMBM program can be successful in changing the mechanisms of change targeted by the intervention.

PULMONARY REHABILITATION, ACUTE EXACERBATIONS, AND ADVANCED DISEASE

COPD Exacerbation

COPD exacerbations represent a unique challenge to PR intervention as PR is conventionally delivered through standard multi-week programs. Also, the participation in PR can be challenging in very advanced disease even in the absence of AECOPD. The present section discusses the role of peri-exacerbation PR, as well as strategies and adjuncts in the delivery of PR in advanced and severe COPD.

Acute Exacerbations of Chronic Obstructive Pulmonary Disease

AECOPDs represent important events in the natural history and trajectory of disease. An AECOPD is defined as an acute worsening of respiratory symptoms requiring additional therapy and is classified as mild, moderate, and severe based on the pharmacologic treatment and/or health care setting required in its management.[71] Severe AECOPDs are independently associated with an increase in overall mortality.[72] AECOPDs affect not only respiratory function but are also associated with systemic inflammation,[73] nutritional deficiency,[74] and marked deconditioning, atrophy, and physical activity decline.[75,76]

Pulmonary Rehabilitation Delivery Following an Acute Exacerbation of Chronic Obstructive Pulmonary Disease

There is overwhelming evidence that participation in PR following an AECOPD improves exercise capacity, health-related quality of life and hospitalizations,[10,77] and prevents future exacerbations.[78] Although PR participation following AECOPD has also been found to reduce mortality,[77] due to heterogeneity in the literature,[10] further evidence is required to confirm this effect. Applying the positive results seen in postexacerbation PR, it was hypothesized that even *very early* physical activity (ie, in the midst of an actual exacerbation) would outperform traditional/conventional bed rest in improving the negative consequences of an AECOPD. This was tested in a prospective RCT and to the surprise of the investigators, not only was the readmission rate not affected but there was also an observed *increase* in mortality.[79] This was in contrast to other inpatient rehabilitation trials that had demonstrated benefit.[80,81] The surprising result was felt in part to reflect a low observed length of hospital stay (for the inpatient intervention) and a low adherence to the unsupervised outpatient program in that trial.[82] In this sense, major guidelines recommend PR participation within 3[9] to 4[28,71,78] weeks of an AECOPD hospitalization, as this does clearly improve patient outcomes.[83–85]

Despite its proven benefit, timely referral and participation in PR following AECOPD is unacceptably low.[86] Public, political, and health care professional awareness, as well as program access and capacity in relation to the proportion of eligible patients, are principal system issues.[8,87] From the perspective of the average health care provider, a gap in knowledge of what PR is, its benefits in COPD, and referral process details have been identified.[39] From the perspective of the patient, despite the wealth of evidence supporting the practice of participating in PR shortly after their AECOPD, this is often in direct contrast to how unwell they feel during this critical period. Interventions that improve patient knowledge and readiness to participate, including introductory/educational sessions and materials during their inpatient AECOPD, remain a research priority[88] and are under ongoing development.[89]

Guiding Patients Who Have Stopped Exercising

Patients often terminate exercise training for a number of reasons including AECOPD. For patients who have previously completed a PR program and experience an AECOPD, and for those whose program is interrupted by an exacerbation, the health care professional must be able to ease them back toward a gradual return to their program. **Table 4** provides a resource for health care professionals to assist them in guiding their patients who fall into this category. Helpful resources specific to patients who stop their maintenance exercise training can be found on the LWWCOPD Web site (www.livingwellwithcopd.com) under the tab "Rehabilitation - Exercise maintenance at home" under "Healthy Lifestyle, a Guide for the gradual return to exercise."

Advanced chronic obstructive pulmonary disease and adjunct therapies

A primary challenge of exercise training in COPD is to overcome the respiratory limitations of these patients. The traditional scheme described by Wasserman,[19] the coupling of external to cellular respiration by organ systems in series, provides an excellent analogy to the strategic application of PR adjunct therapies in advanced COPD. Conceptually, the use of adjuncts allows the patient and PR team to bypass or overcome the obvious rate-limiting *"Lungs"* step, to better supply oxygen and remove carbon dioxide from the *"Heart"*/*"Blood"* and *"Muscle"*/*"Mitochondria"* steps.

Bronchodilators, Oxygen Supplementation, Helium, and Noninvasive Ventilation

The incorporation of bronchodilators and supplemental oxygen, into PR can be thought as program "adjuncts." Poiseuille's law describes that small increases in airway radius can lead to large reductions (to the fourth power) in airway resistance. At rest, bronchodilators not only dilate the airways and reduce airway resistance, but also consequently reduce lung volumes in patients with

Table 4
Guiding patients who have stopped exercising, including those who have stopped due to an AECOPD

Define the Cause of Exercise Cessation		
Lack of motivation, vacation, changes in habits, etc. Define the duration of exercise cessation	*Exercise, worsening of the respiratory condition*	*Guide for a gradual return to the exercise program*
1–4 wk • Tell your patient to resume his or her exercise program as soon as possible 1–3 mo • Tell your patient to follow the guide for a gradual return to the exercise program (right column) >3 mo • See your patient for an evaluation and if not possible in the short term, tell your patient to follow the guide for a gradual return to the exercise program (on the right column) until he or she can see you For every duration • If the cause is a lack of motivation, help your patient to identify the barriers to motivation and give some advice, such as changing the type of activity, doing group exercises, or using fitness technology If the cause of exercise cessation is from a new symptom such as chest pain, joint pain, or dizziness: tell your patient to contact his or her physician	At home with additional medication • See your patient for an evaluation and tell him or her to resume activities as soon as possible with, temporarily, a lower intensity. • Tell your patient to follow the guide for a gradual return to the exercise program (on the right) At the hospital • Tell your patient to move and walk as tolerated while at the hospital, unless told otherwise by the physician • At the hospital, does your patient have access to a professional to advise him or her on how to resume activities at home after discharge? • If NO instruction: after discharge, your patient must do as tolerated for 3 wk (no training), then, start the exercises of the first week of the guide for a gradual return to the exercise program (on the right column) • If the exercises are not tolerated after 3 wk, see your patient for an evaluation	Week 1 Strengthening: • 1 series of each exercise with lighter weights Cardiovascular exercises: • Resume progressively, with a low intensity, duration as tolerated Week 2 Strengthening: • 1–2 series of each exercise with lighter weights Cardiovascular exercise: • Increase duration Week 3 Strengthening: • 1–2 series of each exercise with regular weights Cardiovascular exercises • Increase intensity (3–5 on the Borg scale: the patient must be able to talk while exercising) Week 4 Back to the regular program

Adapted from Canadian Pulmonary Rehabilitation Program. Guide for a Gradual Return to the Exercise Program. Living Well with COPD. Available at: https://www.livingwellwithcopd.com/DATA/LIBRAIRIE/289_en~v~guide-for-a-gradual-return-to-the-exercise.pdf; with permission.

hyperinflation.[90] Through these same mechanisms during exercise training, bronchodilators reduce the severity of expiratory flow limitation and dynamic hyperinflation,[91] thereby reducing resistive and elastic work of breathing, improving exercise capacity, and reducing dyspnea scores.[92] Long-acting bronchodilator with PR outperforms short-acting bronchodilator therapy with PR in exercise tolerance in COPD.[93]

The use of supplemental oxygen therapy, even in patients with severe COPD who are not hypoxemic and do not desaturate with exercise,[94] has been shown to normalize breathing patterns and delay dynamic hyperinflation and improve exercise tolerance and dyspnea in a dose-dependent manner.[94] Furthermore, providing supplemental oxygen longitudinally over many exercise sessions allows for more intense training sessions,[95] which could help to maximize overall PR program gains in exercise capacity. However, in addition to mixed results in the literature there is a traditional concern regarding hyperoxia in COPD (particularly in "carbon dioxide retainers"). This is unlikely to occur in clinical practice.

The addition of helium to oxygen promotes laminar flow, which greatly reduces the overall work of breathing. Although the physiologic rationale for helium-oxygen mixtures is sound, and there is evidence of improved 6MWD in COPD with this gas mixture,[96] PR trials using helium-oxygen adjuncts have not consistently improved exercise capacity.[97] Therefore, from a pragmatic perspective, patients with COPD selected for supplemental oxygen and helium-oxygen adjuncts must be done so carefully.[9]

Supplemental oxygen improves alveolar oxygenation by increasing the fraction of inspired oxygen (FiO_2). Alternatively, noninvasive ventilation (NIV) can increase the driving pressure, effectively increasing the "atmospheric pressure" (P_{ATM}) part of the alveolar gas equation; to varying degrees (depending on the modality), NIV can also improve alveolar ventilation (and reduce the partial pressure of carbon dioxide part of the equation). NIV unloads the respiratory muscles, reduces the work of breathing during exercise, and improves gas exchange; if also prescribed at night, this may allow for further rest and recovery of the respiratory muscles.[98] Devices and modes ranging from continuous positive airway pressure,[99] heated and high-flow nasal cannula,[100] and assisted pressure-controlled ventilation[101] have all been tested in severe COPD, each with positive results. Cumulatively, there is literature[98] and guidelines support for NIV as a useful adjunct in augmenting exercise capacity gains during a PR program. Such an adjunct requires a highly specialized center with appropriate resources and personnel.

Opioid Adjuncts to Alleviate Dyspnea

The many mechanisms of respiratory limitation in COPD cumulatively lead to neuromechanical uncoupling, a phenomenon that is felt to be central in the unpleasant and pervasive sensation of dyspnea.[102] This sensation amplifies during stressful stimuli such as exercise, which can directly interfere with exercise capacity. To maximize the gains from exercise sessions during PR, methods to help alleviate dyspnea can be powerful adjuncts. Opioids such as morphine are effective in treating dyspnea in COPD and are recommended in clinical guidelines.[21,71,103] Although the safety and efficacy of low-dose opioids are well-established in COPD,[104] in the setting of PR only 1 randomized trial demonstrated that immediate-release morphine can reduce dyspnea and increase exercise endurance.[105] Other forms of opioids continue to be studied for their effectiveness and safety as exercise adjuncts in COPD.[106]

Alternative Training Types as Exercise Adjuncts

Although endurance and resistance training are recommended in PR programs,[28] interval training is an alternative "adjunct." Interval training involves interposing phases of high-intensity exercise between periods of rest or lower exercise intensity. In high-performance athletics, interval training is one of the most effective modalities to increase cardiorespiratory fitness.[107] Applied to the patient with advanced COPD, critical respiratory and metabolic limits are avoided while at the same time providing a very intense exercise stimulus to the musculature.[108] The intensity and duration of the exercise phase can be tailored to the individual patient, and can reduce breathlessness while increasing the training load.[109,110]

One-legged exercise is based on a similar rationale: by isolating a smaller muscle mass during exercise, the leg being exercised can be exposed to a higher exercise intensity without being inhibited by the compromised ventilatory system.[111] This approach has been demonstrated with good effect in COPD[112] and appears to be an adjunct that is easy to incorporate into PR programs.[113]

Endurance cycle training using eccentric muscle actions (whereby the muscle lengthens while simultaneously producing force) is a potentially effective training strategy for patients with exercise intolerance. Eccentric exercise results in greater gains in muscle power with a lower metabolic and cardiorespiratory demand (by 4-fold to 5-fold) than conventional concentric exercise (whereby the muscle shortens while simultaneously producing force).[114–116] A randomized trial in patients with severe COPD demonstrated that eccentric cycle exercise training achieves a similar increase in exercise capacity, with an acceptable safety profile and greater improvements in isometric quadriceps strength than with conventional concentric cycle exercise training.[117] These findings provide a strong scientific rationale for eccentric exercise training as an alternative and/or adjunct exercise training modality for patients with advanced COPD.

Finally, pursed-lip breathing is a fundamental technique taught in PR educational sessions. This technique itself can be thought of as an exercise "adjunct" in severe COPD. Pursed-lip breathing alters the adaptive pattern of respiratory muscle recruitment during exercise,[118] and furthermore has also been shown to normalize breathing during exercise in COPD (ie, increasing tidal breathing and reducing respiratory rate for a given minute ventilation).[119]

SUMMARY

PR is supported by a strong evidence demonstrating its effectiveness in patients with COPD over a large spectrum of acuity and severity. And yet, only a fraction of patients with COPD worldwide access PR. The key to an effective PR program for COPD is exercise, primarily of the lower extremities. However, a fundamental and now well-recognized component is SMBM, which increases the likelihood of exercise maintenance post PR, increases physical activity, and improves the daily outpatient self-management of COPD. Adaptive behavior change using patient-centered communication strategies and SM training can ultimately stimulate intrinsically motivated actions. Among the challenges to deliver PR we must consider the patient's disease severity, and resource and geographic constraints. Progress has been made to overcome these challenges through exercise adjuncts, tailored prescriptions, community-based/tele-based/home-based delivery, and SM intervention, respectively. Finally, particular attention must be given to patients around the critical period of an AECOPD. We must support the expansion and evolution of PR, an intervention that is critical for the quality of life of our patients.

DISCLOSURE

J. Bourbeau reports no funding pertaining to this article. He reports grants from CIHR and Canadian Respiratory Research Network (CRRN), Foundation of the McGill University Health Center, Aerocrine, AstraZeneca, Boehringer Ingelheim, Grifols, GlaxoSmithKline, Novartis, and Trudell; personal conference and advisory board fees from Canadian Thoracic Society, CHEST, Astra Zeneca, Boehringer Ingelheim, Grifols, GlaxoSmithKline, Novartis, and Trudell. S. Gagnon and B. Ross do not report any commercial, financial, or other conflicts of interest.

REFERENCES

1. Ramon MA, Ter Riet G, Carsin AE, et al. The dyspnoea-inactivity vicious circle in COPD: development and external validation of a conceptual model. Eur Respir J 2018;52(3):1800079.
2. McCarthy B, Casey D, Devane D, et al. Pulmonary rehabilitation for chronic obstructive pulmonary disease. Cochrane Database Syst Rev 2015;(2): CD003793.
3. Lacasse Y, Cates CJ, McCarthy B, et al. This Cochrane Review is closed: deciding what constitutes enough research and where next for pulmonary rehabilitation in COPD. Cochrane Database Syst Rev 2015;(11):CD000107.
4. Bourbeau J, Nault D. Self-management strategies in chronic obstructive pulmonary disease. Clin Chest Med 2007;28(3):617–28, vii.
5. Vogelmeier CF, Criner GJ, Martinez FJ, et al. Global strategy for the diagnosis, management, and prevention of chronic obstructive lung disease 2017 Report: GOLD executive summary. Am J Respir Crit Care Med 2017;53(3):128–49.
6. Vogelmeier CF, Criner GJ, Martinez FJ, et al. Global strategy for the diagnosis, management, and prevention of chronic obstructive lung disease 2017 report: GOLD executive summary. Eur Respir J 2017;49(3):1700214.
7. Spitzer KA, Stefan MS, Priya A, et al. Participation in pulmonary rehabilitation after hospitalization for chronic obstructive pulmonary disease among Medicare beneficiaries. Ann Am Thorac Soc 2019;16(1):99–106.
8. Camp PG, Hernandez P, Bourbeau J, et al. Pulmonary rehabilitation in Canada: a report from the Canadian Thoracic Society COPD Clinical Assembly. Can Respir J 2015;22(3):147–52.
9. Spruit MA, Singh SJ, Garvey C, et al. An official American Thoracic Society/European Respiratory Society statement: key concepts and advances in pulmonary rehabilitation. Am J Respir Crit Care Med 2013;188(8):e13–64.
10. Puhan MA, Gimeno-Santos E, Cates CJ, et al. Pulmonary rehabilitation following exacerbations of chronic obstructive pulmonary disease. Cochrane Database Syst Rev 2016;(12):CD005305.
11. Puhan MA, Lareau SC. Evidence-based outcomes from pulmonary rehabilitation in the chronic obstructive pulmonary disease patient. Clin Chest Med 2014;35(2):295–301.
12. Spruit MA, Pitta F, Garvey C, et al. Differences in content and organisational aspects of pulmonary rehabilitation programmes. Eur Respir J 2014; 43(5):1326–37.
13. Nici L, Donner C, Wouters E, et al. American Thoracic Society/European Respiratory Society statement on pulmonary rehabilitation. Am J Respir Crit Care Med 2006;173(12):1390–413.
14. Dechman G, Cheung W, Ryerson CJ, et al. Quality indicators for pulmonary rehabilitation programs in Canada: a Canadian Thoracic Society expert working group report. Can J Resp Crit Care Sleep 2019; 3(4):199–209.
15. Blackstock FC, Lareau SC, Nici L, et al. Chronic obstructive pulmonary disease education in pulmonary rehabilitation. An official American Thoracic Society/Thoracic Society of Australia and New Zealand/Canadian Thoracic Society/British Thoracic Society workshop report. Ann Am Thorac Soc 2018;15(7):769–84.

16. Zwerink M, Brusse-Keizer M, van der Valk P, et al. Self-management for patients with chronic obstructive pulmonary disease. Cochrane Database Syst Rev 2014;(3):CD002990.

17. Effing TW, Vercoulen JH, Bourbeau J, et al. Definition of a COPD self-management intervention: international expert group consensus. Eur Respir J 2016;48(1):46–54.

18. Casaburi R, ZuWallack R. Pulmonary rehabilitation for management of chronic obstructive pulmonary disease. N Engl J Med 2009;360(13):1329–35.

19. Wasserman K. Diagnosing cardiovascular and lung pathophysiology from exercise gas exchange. Chest 1997;112(4):1091–101.

20. Borg G. Psychosocial bases of perceived exertion. Med Sci Sports Exerc 1982;14:377–81.

21. Marciniuk DD, Goodridge D, Hernandez P, et al. Managing dyspnea in patients with advanced chronic obstructive pulmonary disease: a Canadian Thoracic Society clinical practice guideline. Can Respir J 2011;18(2):69–78.

22. American Thoracic Society, American College of Chest Physicians. ATS/ACCP statement on cardiopulmonary exercise testing. Am J Respir Crit Care Med 2003;167(2):211–77.

23. ATS Committee on Proficiency Standards for Clinical Pulmonary Function Laboratories. ATS statement: guidelines for the six-minute walk test. Am J Respir Crit Care Med 2002;166(1):111–7.

24. Revill SM, Morgan MD, Singh SJ, et al. The endurance shuttle walk: a new field test for the assessment of endurance capacity in chronic obstructive pulmonary disease. Thorax 1999; 54(3):213–22.

25. Singh SJ, Morgan MD, Scott S, et al. Development of a shuttle walking test of disability in patients with chronic airways obstruction. Thorax 1992;47(12):1019–24.

26. Celli B, Tetzlaff K, Criner G, et al. The 6-minute-walk distance test as a chronic obstructive pulmonary disease stratification tool. insights from the COPD biomarker qualification consortium. Am J Respir Crit Care Med 2016;194(12):1483–93.

27. Garber CE, Blissmer B, Deschenes MR, et al. Quantity and quality of exercise for developing and maintaining cardiorespiratory, musculoskeletal, and neuromotor fitness in apparently healthy adults: guidance for prescribing exercise. Med Sci Sports Exerc 2011;43(7):1334–59.

28. Marciniuk D, Brooks D, Butcher S, et al. Optimizing pulmonary rehabilitation in chronic obstructive pulmonary disease–practical issues: a Canadian Thoracic Society Clinical Practice Guideline. Can Respir J 2010;17(4):159–68.

29. Beauchamp MK, Janaudis-Ferreira T, Parreira V, et al. A randomized controlled trial of balance training during pulmonary rehabilitation for individuals with COPD. CHEST 2013;144(6):1803–10.

30. Beauchamp MK, Janaudis-Ferreira T, Goldstein RS, et al. Optimal duration of pulmonary rehabilitation for individuals with chronic obstructive pulmonary disease - a systematic review. Chron Respir Dis 2011;8(2):129–40.

31. Epstein SK, Celli BR, Martinez FJ, et al. Arm training reduces the VO2 and VE cost of unsupported arm exercise and elevation in chronic obstructive pulmonary disease. J Cardiopulm Rehabil 1997;17(3):171–7.

32. Horowitz MB, Littenberg B, Mahler DA. Dyspnea ratings for prescribing exercise intensity in patients with COPD. Chest 1996;109(5):1169–75.

33. Berry MJ, Rejeski WJ, Adair NE, et al. Exercise rehabilitation and chronic obstructive pulmonary disease stage. Am J Respir Crit Care Med 1999; 160(4):1248–53.

34. Baltzan MA, Kamel H, Alter A, et al. Pulmonary rehabilitation improves functional capacity in patients 80 years of age or older. Can Respir J 2004;11(6):407–13.

35. Verrill D, Barton C, Beasley W, et al. The effects of short-term and long-term pulmonary rehabilitation on functional capacity, perceived dyspnea, and quality of life. Chest 2005;128(2):673–83.

36. Singh D, Agusti A, Anzueto A, et al. Global strategy for the diagnosis, management, and prevention of chronic obstructive lung disease: the GOLD science committee report 2019. Eur Respir J 2019; 53(5):1900164.

37. Tunsupon P, Lal A, Abo Khamis M, et al. Comorbidities in patients with chronic obstructive pulmonary disease and pulmonary rehabilitation outcomes. J Cardiopulm Rehabil Prev 2017;37(4):283–9.

38. Mesquita R, Vanfleteren LE, Franssen FM, et al. Objectively identified comorbidities in COPD: impact on pulmonary rehabilitation outcomes. Eur Respir J 2015;46(2):545–8.

39. Milner SC, Boruff JT, Beaurepaire C, et al. Rate of, and barriers and enablers to, pulmonary rehabilitation referral in COPD: a systematic scoping review. Respir Med 2018;137:103–14.

40. Keating A, Lee A, Holland AE. What prevents people with chronic obstructive pulmonary disease from attending pulmonary rehabilitation? A systematic review. Chron Respir Dis 2011;8(2): 89–99.

41. Knox L, Dunning M, Davies CA, et al. Safety, feasibility, and effectiveness of virtual pulmonary rehabilitation in the real world. Int J Chron Obstruct Pulmon Dis 2019;14:775–80.

42. Stickland M, Jourdain T, Wong EY, et al. Using telehealth technology to deliver pulmonary rehabilitation in chronic obstructive pulmonary disease patients. Can Respir J 2011;18(4):216–20.

43. Spruit MA, Wouters EFM. Organizational aspects of pulmonary rehabilitation in chronic respiratory diseases. Respirology 2019;24(9):838–43.

44. Desveaux L, Janaudis-Ferreira T, Goldstein R, et al. An international comparison of pulmonary rehabilitation: a systematic review. Copd 2015;12(2):144–53.

45. Holland AE, Mahal A, Hill CJ, et al. Home-based rehabilitation for COPD using minimal resources: a randomised, controlled equivalence trial. Thorax 2017;72(1):57–65.

46. Maltais F, Bourbeau J, Shapiro S, et al. Effects of home-based pulmonary rehabilitation in patients with chronic obstructive pulmonary disease: a randomized trial. Ann Intern Med 2008;149(12):869–78.

47. Nolan CM, Kaliaraju D, Jones SE, et al. Home versus outpatient pulmonary rehabilitation in COPD: a propensity-matched cohort study. Thorax 2019;74(10):996–8.

48. Field MJ. Telemedicine: a guide to assessing telecommunications in healthcare. J Digit Imaging 1997;10(3 Suppl 1):28.

49. Rejbi IB, Trabelsi Y, Chouchene A, et al. Changes in six-minute walking distance during pulmonary rehabilitation in patients with COPD and in healthy subjects. Int J Chron Obstruct Pulmon Dis 2010;5:209–15.

50. Alison JA, McKeough ZJ, Johnston K, et al. Australian and New Zealand pulmonary rehabilitation guidelines. Respirology 2017;22(4):800–19.

51. Garvey C, Carlin B, Raskin J. Program organization in pulmonary rehabilitation. Clin Chest Med 2014;35(2):423–8.

52. Bourbeau J, Lavoie KL, Sedeno M. Comprehensive self-management strategies. Semin Respir Crit Care Med 2015;36(4):630–8.

53. Bourbeau J, Alsowayan W, Wald J. Self-management in pulmonary rehabilitation. In: Clini EH, Holland A, Pitta F, et al, editors. Textbook of pulmonary rehabilitation. 1st edition. Springer; 2018. p. 27–232.

54. Howcroft M, Walters EH, Wood-Baker R, et al. Action plans with brief patient education for exacerbations in chronic obstructive pulmonary disease. Cochrane Database Syst Rev 2016;(12): CD005074.

55. Rice KL, Dewan N, Bloomfield HE, et al. Disease management program for chronic obstructive pulmonary disease: a randomized controlled trial. Am J Respir Crit Care Med 2010;182(7):890–6.

56. Bourbeau J, Julien M, Maltais F, et al. Reduction of hospital utilization in patients with chronic obstructive pulmonary disease: a disease-specific self-management intervention. Arch Intern Med 2003; 163(5):585–91.

57. Lenferink A, Brusse-Keizer M, van der Valk PD, et al. Self-management interventions including action plans for exacerbations versus usual care in patients with chronic obstructive pulmonary disease. Cochrane Database Syst Rev 2017;(8): CD011682.

58. Carr SJ, Goldstein RS, Brooks D. Acute exacerbations of COPD in subjects completing pulmonary rehabilitation. Chest 2007;132(1):127–34.

59. Garcia-Aymerich J, Lange P, Benet M, et al. Regular physical activity reduces hospital admission and mortality in chronic obstructive pulmonary disease: a population based cohort study. Thorax 2006;61(9):772–8.

60. Waschki B, Kirsten A, Holz O, et al. Physical activity is the strongest predictor of all-cause mortality in patients with COPD: a prospective cohort study. Chest 2011;140(2):331–42.

61. Cote CG, Celli BR. Pulmonary rehabilitation and the BODE index in COPD. Eur Respir J 2005;26(4):630–6.

62. Brooks D, Krip B, Mangovski-Alzamora S, et al. The effect of postrehabilitation programmes among individuals with chronic obstructive pulmonary disease. Eur Respir J 2002;20(1):20–9.

63. Soicher JE, Mayo NE, Gauvin L, et al. Trajectories of endurance activity following pulmonary rehabilitation in COPD patients. Eur Respir J 2012;39(2):272–8.

64. Robinson H, Williams V, Curtis F, et al. Facilitators and barriers to physical activity following pulmonary rehabilitation in COPD: a systematic review of qualitative studies. NPJ Prim Care Respir Med 2018;28(1):19.

65. Jenkins AR, Gowler H, Curtis F, et al. Efficacy of supervised maintenance exercise following pulmonary rehabilitation on health care use: a systematic review and meta-analysis. Int J Chron Obstruct Pulmon Dis 2018;13:257–73.

66. Güell MR, Cejudo P, Ortega F, et al. Benefits of long-term pulmonary rehabilitation maintenance program in patients with severe chronic obstructive pulmonary disease. three-year follow-up. Am J Respir Crit Care Med 2017;195(5):622–9.

67. Celli BR, Cote CG, Marin JM, et al. The body-mass index, airflow obstruction, dyspnea, and exercise capacity index in chronic obstructive pulmonary disease. N Engl J Med 2004;350(10):1005–12.

68. Vasilopoulou M, Papaioannou AI, Kaltsakas G, et al. Home-based maintenance tele-rehabilitation reduces the risk for acute exacerbations of COPD, hospitalisations and emergency department visits. Eur Respir J 2017;49(5):1602129.

69. Koolen EH, van Hees HW, van Lummel RC, et al. "Can do" versus "do do": a novel concept to better understand physical functioning in patients with chronic obstructive pulmonary disease. J Clin Med 2019;8(3):340.

70. Troosters T, Maltais F, Leidy N, et al. Effect of bronchodilation, exercise training, and behavior

modification on symptoms and physical activity in chronic obstructive pulmonary disease. Am J Respir Crit Care Med 2018;198(8):1021–32.

71. From the global strategy for the diagnosis, management, and prevention of COPD: global initiative for chronic obstructive lung disease (GOLD). 2020. Available at: https://goldcopd.org/gold-reports/.

72. Soler-Cataluña JJ, Martínez-García MÁ, Román Sánchez P, et al. Severe acute exacerbations and mortality in patients with chronic obstructive pulmonary disease. Thorax 2005;60(11):925–31.

73. Agusti A, Edwards LD, Rennard SI, et al. Persistent systemic inflammation is associated with poor clinical outcomes in COPD: a novel phenotype. PLoS One 2012;7(5):e37483.

74. Vermeeren MA, Wouters EF, Geraerts-Keeris AJ, et al. Nutritional support in patients with chronic obstructive pulmonary disease during hospitalization for an acute exacerbation; a randomized controlled feasibility trial. Clin Nutr 2004;23(5): 1184–92.

75. Pitta F, Troosters T, Probst VS, et al. Physical activity and hospitalization for exacerbation of COPD. Chest 2006;129(3):536–44.

76. Cote CG, Dordelly LJ, Celli BR. Impact of COPD exacerbations on patient-centered outcomes. Chest 2007;131(3):696–704.

77. Puhan MA, Gimeno-Santos E, Scharplatz M, et al. Pulmonary rehabilitation following exacerbations of chronic obstructive pulmonary disease. Cochrane Database Syst Rev 2011;(10): CD005305.

78. Criner GJ, Bourbeau J, Diekemper RL, et al. Executive summary: prevention of acute exacerbation of COPD: American College of Chest Physicians and Canadian Thoracic Society guideline. Chest 2015; 147(4):883–93.

79. Greening NJ, Williams JEA, Hussain SF, et al. An early rehabilitation intervention to enhance recovery during hospital admission for an exacerbation of chronic respiratory disease: randomised controlled trial. BMJ 2014;349:g4315.

80. Troosters T, Probst VS, Crul T, et al. Resistance training prevents deterioration in quadriceps muscle function during acute exacerbations of chronic obstructive pulmonary disease. Am J Respir Crit Care Med 2010;181(10):1072–7.

81. He M, Yu S, Wang L, et al. Efficiency and safety of pulmonary rehabilitation in acute exacerbation of chronic obstructive pulmonary disease. Med Sci Monit 2015;21:806–12.

82. Ibrahim W, Harvey-Dunstan TC, Greening NJ. Rehabilitation in chronic respiratory diseases: in-hospital and post-exacerbation pulmonary rehabilitation. Respirology 2019;24(9):889–98.

83. Man WDC, Polkey MI, Donaldson N, et al. Community pulmonary rehabilitation after hospitalisation for acute exacerbations of chronic obstructive pulmonary disease: randomised controlled study. BMJ 2004;329(7476):1209.

84. Seymour JM, Moore L, Jolley CJ, et al. Outpatient pulmonary rehabilitation following acute exacerbations of COPD. Thorax 2010;65(5):423–8.

85. Ko FWS, Cheung NK, Rainer TH, et al. Comprehensive care programme for patients with chronic obstructive pulmonary disease: a randomised controlled trial. Thorax 2017;72(2):122–8.

86. Jones SE, Green SA, Clark AL, et al. Pulmonary rehabilitation following hospitalisation for acute exacerbation of COPD: referrals, uptake and adherence. Thorax 2014;69(2):181–2.

87. Rochester CL, Vogiatzis I, Holland AE, et al. An official American Thoracic Society/European Respiratory Society policy statement: enhancing implementation, use, and delivery of pulmonary rehabilitation. Am J Respir Crit Care Med 2015; 192(11):1373–86.

88. Jones AW, Taylor A, Gowler H, et al. Systematic review of interventions to improve patient uptake and completion of pulmonary rehabilitation in COPD. ERJ Open Res 2017;3(1). 00089-2016.

89. Milner SC, Bourbeau J, Ahmed S, et al. Improving acceptance and uptake of pulmonary rehabilitation after acute exacerbation of COPD: acceptability, feasibility, and safety of a PR "taster" session delivered before hospital discharge. Chron Respir Dis 2019;16. 1479973119872517.

90. Newton MF, O'Donnell DE, Forkert L. Response of lung volumes to inhaled salbutamol in a large population of patients with severe hyperinflation. Chest 2002;121(4):1042–50.

91. Belman MJ, Botnick WC, Shin JW. Inhaled bronchodilators reduce dynamic hyperinflation during exercise in patients with chronic obstructive pulmonary disease. Am J Respir Crit Care Med 1996; 153(3):967–75.

92. O'Donnell DE, Lam MIU, Webb KA. Measurement of symptoms, lung hyperinflation, and endurance during exercise in chronic obstructive pulmonary disease. Am J Respir Crit Care Med 1998;158(5): 1557–65.

93. Casaburi R, Kukafka D, Cooper CB, et al. Improvement in exercise tolerance with the combination of tiotropium and pulmonary rehabilitation in patients with COPD. Chest 2005;127(3):809–17.

94. Somfay A, Porszasz J, Lee SM, et al. Dose-response effect of oxygen on hyperinflation and exercise endurance in nonhypoxaemic COPD patients. Eur Respir J 2001;18(1):77–84.

95. Emtner M, Porszasz J, Burns M, et al. Benefits of supplemental oxygen in exercise training in

nonhypoxemic chronic obstructive pulmonary disease patients. Am J Respir Crit Care Med 2003; 168(9):1034–42.

96. Marciniuk DD, Butcher SJ, Reid JK, et al. The effects of helium-hyperoxia on 6-min walking distance in COPD: a randomized, controlled trial. Chest 2007;131(6):1659–65.

97. Scorsone D, Bartolini S, Saporiti R, et al. Does a low-density gas mixture or oxygen supplementation improve exercise training in COPD? Chest 2010;138(5):1133–9.

98. Corner E, Garrod R. Does the addition of non-invasive ventilation during pulmonary rehabilitation in patients with chronic obstructive pulmonary disease augment patient outcome in exercise tolerance? A literature review. Physiother Res Int 2010;15(1):5–15.

99. Petrof BJ, Calderini E, Gottfried SB. Effect of CPAP on respiratory effort and dyspnea during exercise in severe COPD. J Appl Physiol (1985) 1990; 69(1):179–88.

100. Cirio S, Piran M, Vitacca M, et al. Effects of heated and humidified high flow gases during high-intensity constant-load exercise on severe COPD patients with ventilatory limitation. Respir Med 2016;118:128–32.

101. Gloeckl R, Andrianopoulos V, Stegemann A, et al. High-pressure non-invasive ventilation during exercise in COPD patients with chronic hypercapnic respiratory failure: a randomized, controlled, cross-over trial. Respirology 2019;24(3):254–61.

102. O'Donnell DE, Banzett RB, Carrieri-Kohlman V, et al. Pathophysiology of dyspnea in chronic obstructive pulmonary disease. Proc Am Thorac Soc 2007;4(2):145–68.

103. Mahler DA, Selecky PA, Harrod CG, et al. American College of Chest Physicians consensus statement on the management of dyspnea in patients with advanced lung or heart disease. Chest 2010; 137(3):674–91.

104. Ekstrom M, Nilsson F, Abernethy AA, et al. Effects of opioids on breathlessness and exercise capacity in chronic obstructive pulmonary disease. A systematic review. Ann Am Thorac Soc 2015; 12(7):1079–92.

105. Abdallah SJ, Wilkinson-Maitland C, Saad N, et al. Effect of morphine on breathlessness and exercise endurance in advanced COPD: a randomised crossover trial. Eur Respir J 2017;50(4):1701235.

106. Verberkt CA, van den Beuken-van Everdingen MH, Franssen FM, et al. A randomized controlled trial on the benefits and respiratory adverse effects of morphine for refractory dyspnea in patients with COPD: protocol of the MORDYC study. Contemp Clin trials 2016;47:228–34.

107. Buchheit M, Laursen PB. High-intensity interval training, solutions to the programming puzzle: Part I: cardiopulmonary emphasis. Sports Med 2013;43(5):313–38.

108. Kortianou EA, Nasis IG, Spetsioti ST, et al. Effectiveness of interval exercise training in patients with COPD. Cardiopulm Phys Ther J 2010;21(3): 12–9.

109. Bravo DM, Gimenes AC, Amorim BC, et al. Excess ventilation in COPD: implications for dyspnoea and tolerance to interval exercise. Respir Physiol Neurobiol 2018;250:7–13.

110. Vogiatzis I, Nanas S, Roussos C. Interval training as an alternative modality to continuous exercise in patients with COPD. Eur Respir J 2002;20(1): 12–9.

111. Dolmage TE, Goldstein RS. Response to one-legged cycling in patients with COPD. Chest 2006;129(2):325–32.

112. Dolmage TE, Goldstein RS. Effects of one-legged exercise training of patients with COPD. Chest 2008;133(2):370–6.

113. Evans RA, Dolmage TE, Mangovski-Alzamora S, et al. One-legged cycle training for chronic obstructive pulmonary disease. A pragmatic study of implementation to pulmonary rehabilitation. Ann Am Thorac Soc 2015;12(10):1490–7.

114. Isner-Horobeti M-E, Dufour SP, Vautravers P, et al. Eccentric exercise training: modalities, applications and perspectives. Sports Med 2013;43(6): 483–512.

115. Roig M, O'Brien K, Kirk G, et al. The effects of eccentric versus concentric resistance training on muscle strength and mass in healthy adults: a systematic review with meta-analysis. Br J Sports Med 2009;43(8):556–68.

116. Roig M, Shadgan B, Reid WD. Eccentric exercise in patients with chronic health conditions: a systematic review. Physiother Can 2008;60(2):146–60.

117. Bourbeau J, De Sousa Sena R, Taivassalo T, et al. Eccentric versus conventional cycle training to improve muscle strength in advanced COPD: a randomized clinical trial. Respir Physiol Neurobiol 2020;276:103414.

118. Breslin EH. The pattern of respiratory muscle recruitment during pursed-lip breathing. Chest 1992;101(1):75–8.

119. Spahija J, de Marchie M, Grassino A. Effects of imposed pursed-lips breathing on respiratory mechanics and dyspnea at rest and during exercise in COPD. Chest 2005;128(2):640–50.

Oxygen Therapy and Noninvasive Ventilation in Chronic Obstructive Pulmonary Disease

Ayham Daher, MD, Michael Dreher, MD*

KEYWORDS

- Chronic obstructive pulmonary disease • Respiratory failure • Oxygen therapy
- Noninvasive ventilation

KEY POINTS

- Supplemental oxygen therapy is recommended in patients with severe hypoxemia, and also those with moderate hypoxemia if there is concomitant pulmonary hypertension, heart failure or polycythemia.
- Noninvasive ventilation (NIV) improves the prognosis in patients with hypercapnic chronic obstructive pulmonary disease (COPD) exacerbation and may allow invasive ventilation to be avoided.
- Data for long-term NIV in chronic hypercapnic respiratory failure are not conclusive, but the body of evidence for benefit is growing.
- After COPD exacerbation, long-term NIV should be prescribed only to patients with persistent hypercapnia.
- In this setting, it is important to target NIV to achieve a significant reduction in carbon dioxide levels.

INTRODUCTION

Progressive chronic obstructive pulmonary disease (COPD) is associated with the development of respiratory failure, which worsens disease prognosis and predicts high mortality. The main feature of respiratory failure is inadequate blood oxygenation and/or decarboxylation by the lungs. Supplemental oxygen therapy (SOT) and mechanical ventilation are important components of therapeutic strategies for respiratory failure, and can improve oxygenation and decarboxylation. However, although these are simple therapeutic concepts, currently available evidence to support their usage in COPD is complex. Furthermore, the heterogenicity of COPD and the variety of associated respiratory failure phenotypes make definitive unified clinical judgments about these therapies very difficult.

This review provides an overview of the best published evidence relating to the use of SOT and noninvasive ventilation (NIV) in the management of COPD. The most recent recommendations are also presented, although it is important to note that these are not always consistent. However, we have tried to unify the recommendation when possible or represent the most obvious recommendation with the strongest evidence when there are inconsistencies in current guidelines.

SUPPLEMENTAL OXYGEN THERAPY IN CHRONIC OBSTRUCTIVE PULMONARY DISEASE

The general indications, technical details and different application systems are outside the scope of this article. The focus here is on use of SOT in COPD.

Department of Pneumology and Intensive Care Medicine, University Hospital Aachen, Pauwelsstrasse 30, Aachen 52074, Germany
* Corresponding author.
E-mail address: mdreher@ukaachen.de

Clin Chest Med 41 (2020) 529–545
https://doi.org/10.1016/j.ccm.2020.06.014

Pathophysiology and Burden of Hypoxemia in Chronic Obstructive Pulmonary Disease

The pathophysiology of hypoxemia in COPD is complex and multifactorial (**Box 1**); however, uncorrected chronic hypoxemia is associated with the development of adverse sequelae of COPD, including secondary pulmonary hypertension (PH), secondary polycythemia, systemic inflammation, neurocognitive dysfunction, and skeletal and respiratory muscle dysfunction.[1,2] A combination of these factors leads to reduced exercise tolerance and quality of life (QoL), and increased cardiovascular morbidity and death.[2]

Positive Effects of Supplemental Oxygen Therapy in Chronic Obstructive Pulmonary Disease

From a physiologic point of view, SOT affects not only blood oxygenation but also tissue/cellular oxygenation. Arterial lactate levels are elevated in hypoxemic patients with COPD,[4] which reflects a greater reliance on anaerobic metabolism[1] and is a strong mortality predictor.[5] SOT reduces lactate levels,[6] which indirectly indicates improved tissue oxygenation. Consequently, SOT leads to improvements of multiple physiologic functions (**Table 1**).[6–16]

From a clinical point of view, 2 clinical trials conducted in the early 1980s investigated the effect of long-term oxygen therapy (LTOT) on survival and established its use in COPD: the Nocturnal Oxygen Therapy Trial (NOTT)[11] and the Medical Research Council (MRC) Long-Term Domiciliary Oxygen Therapy Trial[14] (**Table 2**).

These were the only trials for decades showing positive effects of LTOT in a very selected group of patients with COPD (with cardiac comorbidity), and with the most positive effects in patients with mild hypercapnia.[11,14] Other trials assessing LTOT in patients with moderate hypoxemia (moderate resting, isolated moderate exercise-induced or isolated sleep-related hypoxemia) were not able to reproduce LTOT beneficial effects on survival,[17–20] or on pulmonary hemodynamics.[19,20] In a recent randomized controlled trial (RCT) (The Long-Term Oxygen Treatment Trial [LOTT]),[18] LTOT was not associated with a reduction in the combined endpoint (death and first hospitalization) event rate in patients with moderate resting or exercise-induced moderate hypoxemia. However, this trial has some serious limitations, making it difficult to form clear conclusions about the value of LTOT in moderate hypoxemia.[21]

To the best of our knowledge, the populations with moderate hypoxemia and polycythemia and/or PH that were included in the NOTT and MRC

trials were arbitrarily defined, and the reduction in mortality in patients with COPD with these characteristics is still not clearly established. Nevertheless, according to expert opinion, LTOT is indicated in these situations.

Other clinical benefits of LTOT include improved QoL (but with some concerns regarding the negative aspects of cylinder gas use, such as social stigma, social isolation, lack of self-confidence,

---

Box 1
Pathophysiological causes of hypoxemia in chronic obstructive pulmonary disease

1. V/Q mismatch[1,2]:
   - The most important cause!
   - Due to 2 mechanisms:
      a. Airflow limitation.
      b. Emphysematous destruction of the pulmonary capillary bed.

2. Alveolar hypoventilation/diminished ventilatory response to hypoxemia[2]:
   - Due to 2 disorders:
      a. Defective neural control mechanisms.
      b. Malfunctioning inspiratory muscle/dynamics and hyperinflation (more importantly!).

3. Pulmonary vascular remodeling/secondary PH[1,2]

4. Obesity[2,3]:
   - Increasingly prevalent among patients with COPD.
   - Leads to absolute and relative hypoxemia in many mechanisms:
      a. Small airway dysfunction
      b. Worsening chest wall compliance
      c. Worsening V/Q mismatch
      d. Increasing peripheral oxygen consumption
      e. Associated sleep-disordered breathing (nocturnal hypoxemia).

5. Nocturnal hypoxemia[2]:
   - Complex mechanisms, but mainly due to:
      a. Alveolar hypoventilation (multifactorial)
      b. Commonly coexisting OSA (ie, overlap syndrome)

Abbreviations: COPD, chronic obstructive pulmonary disease; OSA, obstructive sleep apnea; PH, pulmonary hypertension; V/Q, ventilation/perfusion.
Data from Refs.[1–3]

Table 1
Physiologic effects of oxygen therapy on different organ functions

Lung[6–9]	• Reduces exercise minute ventilation. • Reduces ventilatory requirements at submaximal work and therefore improves exercise endurance and reduces dynamic hyperinflation. • No stable effect on resting minute ventilation.
Cardiovascular system[1,7,10–12]	• Reduces pulmonary artery pressure and increases cardiac output (through eliminating hypoxic vasoconstriction). • Reduces the resting heart rate, without affecting the ejection fraction.
Kidney[13]	• Improves renal blood flow with resulting diuresis.
Bone marrow[14,15]	• Reverses secondary polycythemia. • May improve platelet survival time.
Central nervous system[16]	• Neuropsychiatric improvement.

Data from Refs.[1,6–16]

depression and fear of dependence),[1,22–24] and reduced breathlessness[9,25] (partially due to a placebo effect).[26]

Negative Effects of Supplemental Oxygen Therapy and Hyperoxia in Chronic Obstructive Pulmonary Disease

The adverse consequences of SOT and higher than normal oxygen levels need to be taken into account when prescribing LTOT. In his book *Evidence-Based Critical Care*,[27] Paul E. Marik wrote the following under the heading "*Too much oxygen kills*": "*It is essentially impossible to get a Pao_2 of much about 100 mm Hg if you only have 21% oxygen to breathe, which is all we had for millennia. There's no evolutionary response to deal with hyperoxia.*"

Oxygen toxicity has been the subject of many studies, and it is now well known that hyperoxia leads to the formation of reactive oxygen species.[1] Although these have positive roles in mediating cell signaling and enhancing phagocytic antimicrobial action and inflammatory response,[1] high concentrations cause cellular damage and degrade bioactive nitric oxide, triggering cellular necrosis and apoptosis.[1] Breathing supplemental oxygen in high concentrations for a long time may be associated with toxic side effects (**Table 3**). These side effects, especially the pulmonary toxicities, are obviously very counterproductive in patients with COPD.

Oxygen inhalation might precipitate or worsen hypercapnic ventilatory failure via several mechanisms.[1] First, some patients with COPD (those with chronic hypercapnia) are largely dependent

Table 2
Study populations and key findings of the NOTT and MRC trials

	NOTT[11]	MRC[14]
Inclusion criteria	• Pao_2 ≤55 mm Hg (≤7.3 kPa), or • Pao_2 ≤59 mm Hg (≤7.87 kPa) accompanied by either edema, P-pulmonale (electrocardiogram) or raised hematocrit (≥55%)	• Pao_2 40–60 mm Hg (5.3–8 kPa) and at least 1 recorded episode of heart failure with ankle edema
Results	The 24-mo mortality rate was significantly lower in patients randomized to continuous oxygen therapy (mean usage ~18 h/d) than in those randomized to 12 h/d of nocturnal oxygen therapy (22.4% vs 40.8%, respectively; *P*<.01)	The 5-y mortality rate was significantly lower in the LTOT group (usage ≥15 h/d) than in control subjects who did not receive LTOT (risk of death 12%/y vs 29%/y, respectively; *P* = .04)

Abbreviations: LTOT, long-term oxygen therapy; MRC, Medical Research Council long-term domiciliary oxygen therapy trial; NOTT, nocturnal oxygen therapy trial; Pao_2, arterial partial pressure of oxygen.
Data from Refs.[11,14]

on hypoxemia for stimulating breathing via peripheral chemoreceptor activity (carotid bodies). Removal of the hypoxemia stimulus reduces the work of breathing (WOB) despite worsening Pa_{CO_2} (arterial partial pressure of carbon dioxide) values.[1,28] As hypercapnia worsens, this stimulus loses its natural ability to increase ventilatory drive via central chemoreceptors in upper brainstem in most patients with COPD.[1,28] Second, oxygen reduces airway resistance and improves respiratory system impedance, which itself can contribute to reduced ventilatory drive.[1] Other mechanisms may also have roles in oxygen-induced hypercapnia in COPD, including the Haldane effect, which refers to oxygen displacing CO_2 from hemoglobin, and (more importantly) impaired hypoxic pulmonary vasoconstriction (Euler-Liljestrand mechanism) with a resulting increase in ventilation/perfusion (V/Q) mismatch and an increase in CO_2 content in shunted blood.[1,8,28]

P. Marik mentioned the term "permissive hypoxemia" in the following context[27]: "hyperoxia appears to be more harmful to the host than hypoxemia. The human has developed elaborate mechanisms to compensate for hypoxemia and may tolerate permissive hypoxemia with minimal adverse effects. However, the human has not evolved to deal with hyperoxia which appears to be associated with significant adverse effects." He also mentioned that "there appears to be a dose-dependent association between supranormal oxygen tension and risk of adverse outcomes."

Long-Term Oxygen Therapy Indications in Chronic Obstructive Pulmonary Disease

It is first important to note that oxygen is a treatment for hypoxemia, not breathlessness.[29] Thus, although improvements in dyspnea and exercise tolerance could be important benefits of LTOT,[29] LTOT remains an expensive treatment modality and, like other medical treatments, has potential side effects.[23] On the other hand, determining the "safe degree of hypoxemia" for an individual subject is exceedingly difficult.[27] Interestingly, Magnet and colleagues[23] noted that the NOTT and MRC trials were performed in the late 1970s, when patients with COPD had fewer comorbidities than they do currently and therapeutic approaches were different, meaning that the findings of these studies might not necessarily be applicable today.

When prescribing LTOT it is important to consider current guidelines and to make a careful risk-benefit evaluation. Guidelines are useful in some areas, but lacking in others. Furthermore, some need to be updated with the latest evidence. However, the current recommendations regarding LTOT indications are summarized in **Tables 4, 5** and **Fig. 1**.

Although respiratory failure is usually defined as an arterial partial pressure of oxygen (Pa_{O_2}) less than 60 mm Hg, in reality it is the arterial oxygen

Table 3
Toxic effects of hyperoxia and hyperoxia-generated oxygen-derived radicals

Neurologic toxicity[1,27,80–82]	Visual disturbance Ear problems Dizziness Confusion Nausea Convulsions Unconsciousness Retina damage Myopia Decreased cerebral blood flow Ischemia-induced brain damage
Pulmonary toxicity[1,27,83–85]	Tracheobronchial irritation with impaired mucociliary clearance Decline in lung function Resorptive atelectasis Alveolar protein leakage Enhanced expression of leukotrienes by alveolar macrophages Increases in alveolar neutrophils Diffuse alveolar damage Acute respiratory distress syndrome Chronic pulmonary fibrosis and emphysema
Systemic toxicity[86,87]	Increased vascular resistance and decreased cardiac output Impaired innate immune responses resulting in increased susceptibility to infection

Data from Refs.[1,27,80–87]

saturation (SaO_2) that should be used to make clinical decisions and to titrate SOT.[27] As shown by the arterial oxygen content equation (**Box 2**), oxygen delivery is almost entirely dependent on SaO_2 and cardiac output rather than PaO_2 (which contributes to the small amount of oxygen dissolved in serum).[27]

Further details about the diagnostic approach before prescribing LTOT, and about titration of therapeutic oxygen flow rates are presented in **Tables 6** and **7**.

Hours of Use

Based on evidence from NOTT and MRC trials,[11,14] current guidelines recommend use of LTOT for a minimum of 15 to 16 hours per day.[29–31] In general, up to 24 hours of use is recommended based on presumed additional benefit, although some evidence suggests that survival is not improved when oxygen is prescribed for more than 16 hours per day.[32]

Long-Term Oxygen Therapy for Patients Who Still Smoke

This is a complex issue, which has been somewhat sidestepped, and there is no obvious evidence about this subject.[30] Magnet and colleagues[23] suggested that LTOT should neither be wholly denied nor recommended to active smokers, and the decision of whether or not to prescribe LTOT

Table 4
Indications for LTOT in COPD from different published guidelines/recommendations

Recommending Society	1st Indication: Severe Resting Hypoxemia (Classical Criteria)	2nd Indication: Milder Hypoxemia
BTS[29]	$PaO_2 \leq 55$ mm Hg (≤ 7.3 kPa)	$PaO_2 > 55–60$ mm Hg ($> 7.3–8.0$ kPa) plus: • peripheral edema • secondary polycythemia (HCT $\geq 55\%$), or • evidence of PH
DGP[30]		
ACCP[88]	$PaO_2 \leq 55$ mm Hg (≤ 7.3 kPa)	PaO_2 55–59 mm Hg (7.3–7.8 kPa) plus: • dependent edema • P-pulmonale on ECG (>3 mm in standard lead II, III, or aVF), or • HCT >56%
ATS[37]		PaO_2 55–59 mm Hg or $SaO_2 < 89\%$ plus: • Congestive heart failure, • ECG evidence of right atrial enlargement, or • HCT $\geq 55\%$
TSANZ[34]		PaO_2 56–59 mm Hg (7.4–7.8 kPa) plus evidence of hypoxic organ damage, including • Clinical, electrocardiographic, or echocardiographic evidence of PH, or • Episodes of right heart failure, or • HCT >55%
GOLD[31]	$PaO_2 \leq 55$ mm Hg (≤ 7.3 kPa) or $SaO_2 \leq 88\%$	PaO_2 55–60 mm Hg (7.3–8.0 kPa) or SaO_2 88% plus • Peripheral edema • Evidence of PH, or • HCT >55%
ACP[89]	$PaO_2 \leq 55$ mm Hg (≤ 7.3 kPa) or $SaO_2 \leq 88\%$	PaO_2 55–59 mm Hg plus • Cor pulmonale, or • Polycythemia

Abbreviations: ACCP, American College of Chest Physicians; ACP, American College of Physicians; ATS, American Thoracic Society; BTS, British Thoracic Society; DGP, Deutsche Gesellschaft für Pneumologie und Beatmungsmedizin; ECG, electrocardiogram; GOLD, Global Initiative for Chronic Obstructive Lung Disease; HCT, hematocrit; PaO_2, arterial partial pressure of oxygen; PH, pulmonary hypertension; SaO_2, arterial oxygen saturation; TSANZ, Thoracic Society of Australia and New Zealand.
Data from Refs.[29–31,34,37,88,89]

Table 5
Indications of AOT and NOT

AOT	• AOT should only be offered to patients already on LTOT if they are[29]
	  ○ Mobile outdoors (so they can achieve the required duration of daily usage), or
	  ○ Too symptomatic to leave home without AOT.
	• Two of 3 of the following criteria should be met to prescribe AOT (expert consensus, no solid evidence):[29]
	  ○ SpO2 can be kept constantly >90% during exercise with oxygen
	  ○ Improvement of 6MWT by ≥10%
	  ○ Improvement of dyspnea (≥1 point improvement on the Borg scale)
	• Regarding patients with COPD with exercise-induced desaturation who do not have the classic criteria at rest:
	  ○ They probably do not benefit from AOT regarding mortality, exercise capacity or dyspnea during exercise[18,90,91]
	  ○ Because AOT transiently improves their exercise capacity,[92] they should get AOT as part of a rehabilitation program.[23,29,30]

NOT	• Regarding patients who do not meet the classic LTOT criteria at rest,
	  ○ NOT is not recommended in most guidelines
	  ○ In many trials, NOT did not improve pulmonary hemodynamics, survival, QoL, or sleep quality[11,19,93]
	  ○ An ongoing trial (INOX; NCT01044628) is evaluating the effects of NOT in patients with COPD; results are expected soon
	  ○ NOT can be considered for hypoxemic patients receiving LT-NIV for treatment of hypercapnic respiratory failure, but the evidence and practical details are lacking.[23]

Abbreviations: 6MWT, six-minute walk test; AOT, ambulatory oxygen therapy; COPD, chronic obstructive pulmonary disease; LT-NIV, long-term noninvasive ventilation; LTOT, long-term oxygen therapy; NOT, nocturnal oxygen therapy; QoL, quality of life; SpO$_2$, oxygen saturation on pulse oximeter.
  Data from Refs.[11,18,19,23,29,30,90–93]

should be assessed on an individual basis, taking into account the advantages and disadvantages.[30] Patients do need to be informed about the risk of burns/deflagration when using open fire sources near oxygen.[33]

Box 2
Arterial oxygen content and arterial oxygen delivery equations

$$CaO_2 \text{ [mL/L]} = (Hb \text{ [g/dL]} \times 1.34 \text{ [mL]} \times SaO_2 \text{ [\%]}) + (Pao_2 \text{ [mm Hg]} \times 0.031)$$

$$DaO_2 \text{ [mL/min]} = CaO_2 \text{ [mL/L]} \times \text{cardiac output [L/min]}$$

1.34 = oxygen combining capacity of hemoglobin.

0.031 = solubility coefficient of oxygen in human plasma.

Abbreviations: CaO$_2$, oxygen content of arterial blood; DaO$_2$, arterial oxygen delivery; Hb, hemoglobin level; Pao$_2$, arterial partial pressure of oxygen; SaO2, arterial oxygen saturation.

Supplemental Oxygen Therapy During Air Travel

As a general rule, SOT is unlikely to be required if resting peripheral oxygen saturation on pulse oximeter [SpO$_2$] is ≥95% (or arterial partial pressure of oxygen [Pao$_2$] >72 mm Hg) and 6-minute walk test–SaO$_2$ is greater than 84% at sea level, but is recommended when there is an indication for home LTOT.[31,34–36] However, these criteria do not completely exclude the possibility of a patient developing severe hypoxemia during air travel, and careful consideration should be given to any comorbidity that may impair oxygen delivery to tissues (eg, cardiac impairment or anemia).[31] In patients with a sea level saturation between the preceding values, Pao$_2$ at altitude can be predicted (however inaccurately) from baseline data using the following calculation (**Box 3**):[37]

Furthermore, it is recommended to advise against air travel when there is a usual oxygen requirement at sea level at flow rate exceeding 4 L/min[35]; however, a laboratory-based altitude simulation provides more accurate estimates of real oxygenation at altitude,[34] and Pao$_2$ should be maintained at greater than 50 mm Hg (≥6.6 kPa) or SpO$_2$ ≥85% during flight.[31,34,38] Titrating SOT

Table 6
Timing of LTOT initiation and first-line diagnostics

When to Initiate LTOT?	
Timing of LTOT initiation in stable patients	• Patients should undergo 2 blood gas analyses at least 3 wk apart during a period of apparent clinical stability and while receiving adequate COPD therapy[29–31] (expert opinion based on MRC protocol,[14] no data from controlled trials)[30]
LTOT in post-exacerbation COPD patients	• After an exacerbation, patients should not be discharged from hospital with LTOT unless they are breathless, cannot manage without oxygen, and have an SpO_2 <92% while breathing room air[29] • Even then, the LTOT indication should be reassessed after ≥8 wk of stability (patients who become hypoxemic during COPD exacerbation could have improvements in gas exchange after 8 wk)[3,23,94,95]
What is the best first-line diagnostic tool?	
ABG	• Recommended as first-line diagnostic tool for hypoxemia[23,29,31] • Not always practical, especially in an ambulatory setting[29,30]
CBG	• Underestimates Pao_2[96] (patients could receive LTOT inappropriately)[94] • A combination of CBG and oximetry can be used, even as primary approach[29,30]
Pulse oximetry	• Pulse oximeters have a bias of 0.2%–1% and a standard deviation (precision) of <2% when SaO_2 is >80%[27,97] • SpO_2 of ≤92% can be safely used for screening patients (SpO_2 ≤94% with clinical evidence of peripheral edema, polycythemia or PH)[29] • Oximetry cannot be used alone for formal assessment without at least a CBG analysis[29,30]

Abbreviations: ABG, arterial blood gas analysis; CBG, capillary blood gas analysis; COPD, chronic obstructive pulmonary disease; LTOT, long-term oxygen therapy; Pao_2, arterial partial pressure of oxygen; PH, pulmonary hypertension; SaO_2, arterial oxygen saturation; SpO_2, oxygen saturation on pulse oximeter.
Data from Refs.[3,14,23,27,29–31,94–97]

flow rate to the value needed while flying requires a simulation test in most cases (see **Table 7**).[37]

Long-Term Oxygen Therapy in Patients with Compensatory Hyperventilation

In some situations, oxygenation can be falsely increased/normal due to hyperventilation, which can be recognized if there is hypocapnia in patients with COPD. In these situations, the real Pao_2 (namely standard Pao_2) could be calculated (**Box 4**).[39]

This calculation allows an accurate estimation of the respiratory failure degree if there is accompanying hypocapnia. It simply shows the value of Pao_2 if the patient was not able to hyperventilate to compensate for hypoxemia. Nevertheless, it is not obvious how to use LTOT in these patients, who could have different scenarios such as

hypoxemia with hypocapnia or borderline oxygenation with hypocapnia.

Supplemental Oxygen Therapy Using Nasal High-Flow Cannula

Nasal high-flow cannula (NHFC) represents a promising option for the treatment of patients with type-1 acute respiratory failure. The most important NHFC benefits in COPD are listed in **Box 5**.[40]

Follow-Up Visits and Termination of Long-Term Oxygen Therapy

After prescribing LTOT, reevaluation should be done within 2 to 3 months, both while the patient is breathing room air and using the therapeutic oxygen flow rate, to determine whether LTOT is still indicated

Table 7
Titration of oxygen flow rates at rest, under exercise, during sleep, and during air travel

At rest	• SpO2 titration is recommended as follows:[29,30] 　○ Start with 1 L/min. 　○ Increasing by 1 L/min every 20 min until SpO_2 reaches >90%. 　○ Afterward, an ABG test should confirm $Pao_2 \geq 60$ mm Hg (≥ 8 kPa)[29,30] (based on NOTT protocol).[11] • A combination of CBG and SpO_2 can be used instead of ABG.[29,30] • In patients who do not achieve $Pao_2 \geq 60$ mm Hg under high flow rates, an increase of >10 mm Hg (1.33 kPa) could also be acceptable[30] (in this case, investigations should be performed to identify comorbidities with high volumes of right-left shunt).[30]
LTOT in patients with elevation in $Paco_2$ under titration test	• Symptomatic hypercapnia before initiating LTOT is not a contraindication to LTOT.[30] • Patients who develop a >7.5 mm Hg (>1 kPa) increase in $Paco_2$ and/or respiratory acidosis under titration test should be considered as unstable and undergo further medical optimization.[29] In this situation, a reassessment is indicated and, if the problem persists while the patient is clinically stable, then LTOT should be ordered in combination with nocturnal NIV.[29]
Under exercise (6MWT)	• Estimation of the required flow rate based on the lowest SpO_2 during 6MWT on room air can be made:[29,38] 　○ 86%–89% → 3 L/min 　○ 80%–85% → 4 L/min 　○ 74%–79% → 5 L/min 　○ ≤73% → 6 L/min • Next, the test should be repeated using the estimated flow rate (after a resting preoxygenation period of at least 20 min).[29] • Titration should be performed using pulse oximetry (SpO_2) while carrying or wheeling the oxygen device to mimic everyday life requirements.[29] • The previously described 3 criteria for AOT should be considered.
During sleep	• Oxygen flow rates during sleep should be increased by 1 L/min comparing with daytime flow rates in the absence of any contraindications (eg, chronic hypercapnia).[29]
During air travel	• Titrating the SOT flow rate to the value needed while flying requires a simulation test in most cases.[37] • Rule of thumb: 2 L/min for patients without home LTOT, and double usual flow rates in LTOT patients.[38]

Abbreviations: 6MWT, six-minute walk test; ABG, arterial blood gas analysis; AOT, ambulatory oxygen therapy; CBG, capillary blood gas analysis; LTOT, long-term oxygen therapy; NIV, noninvasive ventilation; NOTT, nocturnal oxygen therapy trial; $Paco_2$, arterial partial pressure of carbon dioxide; Pao_2, arterial partial pressure of oxygen; SOT, supplemental oxygen therapy; SpO_2, oxygen saturation on pulse oximeter.
Data from Refs.[29,30,37,38]

Box 3
Calculation of predicted Pao_2 at altitude

$$Pao_{2\ [at\ 8000\ ft]} = [0.238 \times (Pao_{2\ [sea\ level]})] + [20.098 \times (FEV_1/FVC)] + 22.258$$

Abbreviations: FEV_1, forced expiratory volume in 1 second; FVC, forced vital capacity; Pao_2, arterial partial pressure of oxygen.

Box 4
Standard Pao_2 equation

$$Pao_{2\ Standard\ [mm\ Hg]} = Pao_{2\ Measured\ [mm\ Hg]} - \{1.66 \times (40\_Paco_{2\ Measured\ [mm\ Hg]})\}$$

Abbreviations: $Paco_2$ arterial partial pressure of carbon dioxide; Pao_2, arterial partial pressure of oxygen.

and still providing therapeutic benefit.[29–31] Further follow-ups should be performed at 6 to 12 months, or sooner if the clinical condition changes.[23,29] Home visits after 4 weeks are also recommended and appear to be more effective than hospital follow-up visits.[41] LTOT should be withdrawn if the patient no longer requires it or if he or she is noncompliant (ie, usage <15 h/d, inconsistent ambulatory oxygen therapy [AOT] usage).[23,29]

NONINVASIVE VENTILATION IN CHRONIC OBSTRUCTIVE PULMONARY DISEASE

This section focuses specifically on the use of NIV in patients with COPD; the general indications, contraindications, side effects, and technical details of NIV are not part of the scope of this article.

Pathophysiology of Hypercapnic Respiratory Failure in Chronic Obstructive Pulmonary Disease

The "respiratory pump" consists of anatomic and functional units that allow normal lung ventilation.[42] It includes interactions of the respiratory center, nerves, muscles, skeletal system, and airways.[43] Although functional limitations of the lung tissue and circulation induce primary hypoxemia, limitations of the "respiratory pump" result in an inability to maintain an alveolar ventilation level sufficient to eliminate CO_2, resulting in so called "ventilatory failure" with primary hypercapnia.[43,44]

Ventilatory failure in COPD appears to result from an imbalance between load and capacity of the respiratory pump in a variety of ways. From a

---

Box 5
Benefits of nasal high-flow cannula oxygen therapy

Warming and humidification of inspired air

Enhancement of ciliary action and secretion removal

More reliable delivery of a targeted inspired oxygen fraction

Washout of dead space in the upper respiratory tract due to high flow rates, which improve ventilation efficacy and reduce $Paco_2$

Reduced work of breathing

Buildup of a small amount of extrinsic PEEP, which leads to partial antagonization of the increased intrinsic PEEP

Abbreviations: $Paco_2$, arterial partial pressure of carbon dioxide; PEEP, positive end-expiratory pressure. *Data from* De Troyer A, Leeper JB, McKenzie DK, et al. Neural drive to the diaphragm in patients with severe COPD. Am J Respir Crit Care Med 1997;155(4):1335-40; with permission.

---

mechanical point of view, inspiratory muscles in patients with COPD are usually in a very unsuitable configuration, primarily due to lung hyperinflation, which worsens the dynamic thoracic relationship and represents an extra load on the inspiratory muscles.[44–46] Furthermore, respiratory muscles have to overcome the increased resistance of obstructive airways.[46] The combination of these factors increases WOB[46] and increases respiratory muscle energy requirements, creating higher metabolic demand and a potential metabolic imbalance between supply and demand.[46,47] Other systemic factors, such as inflammation, oxidative stress, nutritional depletion, and the effect of certain drugs, further weaken the respiratory muscles.[46] Another important component of ventilatory failure in COPD is reduced alveolar ventilation due to reduced neurologic drive. Generally, when COPD progresses, the respiratory center (which is primarily sensitive to changes in $Paco_2$), increases respiratory neural drive to adapt ventilation so that $Paco_2$ does not increase significantly[28,48]; however, cost of this compensation is increased WOB and higher metabolic demands.[28] In some patients, the respiratory center will keep making this increased effort ("pink puffer" patients), whereas in others it will drive a breathing pattern that minimizes WOB at the expense of reduced ventilation and increasing $Paco_2$ ("blue bloater" patients).[28,48] It is believed that increased mechanical loads on the respiratory muscles in COPD leads to reduced ventilatory responsiveness to elevations in $Paco_2$ due to a reduction in the neural center chemosensitivity to changes in $Paco_2$, prioritizing peripheral chemoreceptors that are primarily responsive to Pao_2.[28] The consequences of ventilatory failure are chronic hypercapnia and (compensated) respiratory acidosis,[49] which seem to be inversely associated with overall prognosis and mortality.[49,50]

Physiologic Benefits of Noninvasive Ventilation in Chronic Obstructive Pulmonary Disease

The most important physiologic benefits of properly applied, synchronous NIV in COPD are summarized in **Table 8**.

Overall, reduced lung hyperinflation and increased ventilatory chemosensitivity to CO_2 appear to be the main mechanisms underlying the effectiveness of NIV in COPD.[51] From a clinical point of view, NIV is indicated in patients with COPD for the treatment of acute, chronic, and acute-on-chronic hypercapnic respiratory failure (**Fig. 1**, **Table 9**).

Table 8
Potential physiologic benefits of properly applied, synchronous NIV in COPD

Effect of NIV	Main Effecting Factor/Mechanism
Augments minute ventilation and increases alveolar ventilation, which improves decarboxylation.[98]	IPAP, controlled breaths
Unloads ventilatory muscles facing respiratory system elastic recoil and airway resistance, with indirect positive effects[98]: • Facilitating respiratory muscle recovery and improving its endurance and strength even during NIV-free periods.[98] • Redirecting blood flow from respiratory muscles to limbs, improving perfusion of extremities and contributing to improved exercise tolerance.[99]	IPAP, controlled breaths
Improves and stabilizes alveolar recruitment, with indirect positive effects:[98] • Improving V/Q-match and oxygenation • Improving ventilation and decarboxylation • Preventing surfactant breakdown and improving lung compliance	Mainly through applied PEEP.
Opens airways and prevents small airway collapse,[100] with indirect positive effects: • Reduction of distal airway resistance and amelioration of distal airway collapse during use of PEEP leads to better emptying of the lungs during expiration, which in turn reduces air trapping and lung hyperinflation.[69,100,101] This improves respiratory dynamics and reduces WOB.[98] • Increased respiratory system compliance, reducing the elastic resistance to inspiration.[98] • Positive effects on the pathophysiological changes in the airway wall and lumen, and may lead to a stable improvement in lung function.[71]	Mainly through applied PEEP. Reductions in hypercapnia during NIV could decrease fluid retention in airway walls caused by hypercapnia-triggered activation of the renin–angiotensin–aldosterone system.[71]
Resets the ventilatory control system and increases respiratory center chemosensitivity to CO_2[98,102]	Indirect result of improved gas exchange, reduced muscle loads, and reduced dyspnea.
Maintains upper-airway patency[98,103]	Applied PEEP

Abbreviations: COPD, chronic obstructive pulmonary disease; IPAP, inspiratory positive airway pressure; NIV, noninvasive ventilation; PEEP, positive end-expiratory pressure; V/Q, ventilation/perfusion; WOB, work of breathing.
Data from Refs.[69,71,98–103]

Noninvasive Ventilation for Acute Hypercapnic Respiratory Failure Due to Chronic Obstructive Pulmonary Disease

Use of NIV in this setting has been shown to reduce $Paco_2$ and increase pH.[52] More significantly, in addition to standard therapy, NIV improves dyspnea during COPD exacerbation, reduces mortality, decreases the need for endotracheal intubation, and shortens the length of the hospital stay.[52,53] Therefore, NIV is usually the first-line treatment option in patients with acute hypercapnic respiratory failure due to COPD who need mechanical ventilation; use of NIV avoids the side effects of invasive ventilation.

However, NIV does not improve the situation during COPD exacerbation in 20% to 30% of cases (**Box 6**).[54]

NIV can be discontinued when acidosis and hypercapnia have resolved. This should be done in a stepwise manner to avoid relapse of hypercapnic failure,[57] although some new data suggest that immediate withdrawal of NIV is safe. More evidence is needed to define how to wean patients from acute NIV therapy.

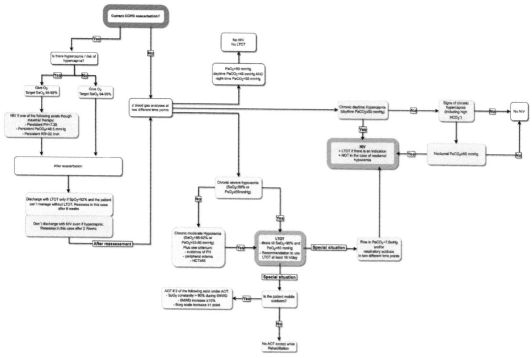

Fig. 1. A suggested algorithm for the nonmedical management of respiratory/ventilatory failure. HCT, hematocrit; NOT, nocturnal oxygen therapy; RR, respiratory rate.

Table 9
Indications for NIV in COPD (current recommendations from BTS/ICS and German national guidelines for long-term NIV)

Clinical Situation	Recommendation
Hypercapnic COPD exacerbation	NIV is recommended if one of the following criteria exists despite optimal pharmacologic and controlled oxygen therapy[57]: • Persistent acidosis (pH <7.35) • Persistent hypercapnia (Paco$_2$ >48.5 mm Hg (>6.5 kPa) • Persistent tachypnea (respiratory rate >22 breaths/min)
Following an acute exacerbation	Wait and reassess hypercapnia at least 2 wk after terminating acute mechanical ventilatory support Start NIV if Paco$_2$ is >53 mm Hg (based on the German guideline[75])
Chronic hypercapnic respiratory failure	Start NIV in the chronic setting when 1 of the following criteria exists (based on the German guideline[75]): • Chronic daytime hypercapnia with Paco$_2$ ≥50 mm Hg • Nocturnal hypercapnia with Paco$_2$ ≥55 mm Hg • Mild daytime hypercapnia with Paco$_2$ 46–50 mm Hg and an increase in PtcCO$_2$ of ≥10 mm Hg during sleep • After prolonged weaning, if a decannulation of tracheostomy is only possible with the help of NIV, and when NIV is necessary to control symptoms and avoid hypercapnia over the long term after hospital discharge

Abbreviations: BTS/ICS, British Thoracic Society/Intensive Care Society; COPD, chronic obstructive pulmonary disease; NIV, noninvasive ventilation; Paco$_2$, arterial partial pressure of carbon dioxide; PtcCO$_2$, percutaneous carbon dioxide pressure.
Data from Refs.[57,75]

Young age[55]

APACHE-II score greater than 20.5 at presentation[54,55]

Persistent tachycardia (>100 beats/min) 1 to 2 hours after initiation of NIV[56]

Persistent tachypnea (>30 breaths/min) 1 to 2 hours after initiation of NIV[54,56]

Persistent acidosis (pH <7.35) 1 to 2 hours after initiation of NIV[54,56]

Decreased consciousness (GCS <15) 1 to 2 hours after initiation of NIV[54,56]

Bad oxygenation (Pao_2/Fio_2 <150) 1 to 2 hours after initiation of NIV[56]

Abbreviations: APACHE-II, acute physiology and chronic health evaluation II score; COPD, chronic obstructive pulmonary disease; Fio_2, fraction of inspired oxygen; GCS, Glasgow coma scale; NIV, noninvasive ventilation; Pao_2, arterial partial pressure of oxygen.
Data from Refs.[54–56]

Noninvasive Ventilation for Chronic Hypercapnic Respiratory Failure due to Chronic Obstructive Pulmonary Disease

The clinical benefit of long-term-NIV in patients with stable hypercapnic respiratory failure due to COPD has been a controversial subject,[58,59] and despite a growing body of evidence, there is still the need for more clinical trial data to inform a solid evidence-based approach.[60] Although it has become standard in Europe, long-term-NIV in COPD remains underused in the United States.[60]

Patients with COPD with chronic hypercapnia require more frequent hospital admissions, have worse outcomes during and after an exacerbation,[61] and have higher mortality rates compared with normocapnic patients.[50,62] There are some data that chronic hypercapnia suppresses innate immunity and that reducing levels of CO_2 might ameliorate this issue, leading to a reduction in exacerbations.[50]

Available data suggest that long-term NIV is associated with improvements in exercise capacity,[49,63] exercise-related dyspnea,[63] diurnal sleepiness,[64] pulmonary cachexia,[65] QoL,[49,63,66] and probably sleep quality.[67] Furthermore, long-term NIV has been shown to slow the rate of clinical worsening, and decrease outpatient visits, frequency of hospital admissions, and length of hospital stay, thus reducing overall treatment costs.[64,68]

The results of one randomized, controlled study by McEvoy and colleagues[66] concluded that only small improvements in survival in patients with stable hypercapnic COPD came at the expense of reductions in QoL. However, this conclusion is counterintuitive given the known pathophysiological burdens of hypercapnic respiratory failure and the physiologic benefits of NIV. Perhaps the most important limitation of this trial was that ventilator settings were not titrated to normalize $Paco_2$ levels (the inspiratory positive airway pressure [IPAP], difference between IPAP and positive end-expiratory pressure [PEEP], and frequency were all too low) and there was no significant improvement in pulmonary function tests (PFTs); that is, there was no resolution of ventilatory failure and respiratory dynamics were apparently not improved, leading some experts to describe the intervention as inadequate.[58] Subsequently, additional trials,[69,70] including one RCT,[49] used NIV with higher inspiratory pressures and high backup frequencies, which significantly improved or even normalized hypercapnia. Improvements were also seen in other physiologic parameters (gas exchange, PFTs, exercise endurance, and respiratory muscle function), with comparable, if not better, compliance and sleep quality in the NIV group.[71] The results of the RCT showed a significant 1-year survival benefit in patients randomized to long-term NIV compared with control, along with an improvement in QoL.[49]

In summary, current evidence for the positive effects of domiciliary long-term NIV for chronic stable COPD is not conclusive, but continues to grow. Based on existing data, the overall aim during NIV therapy should be to significantly decrease elevated $Paco_2$ (eg, by using adequately high inspiratory pressure).

Current European recommendations for the use of long-term NIV are conditional, based on some evidence for improvements in QoL, dyspnea, and exercise tolerance, and reductions in mortality and hospitalizations, with the suggestion that the lack of mortality benefit in some trials was likely due to inadequacy of pressure support.[58,60] The benefits of long-term NIV are thought to outweigh the potential harms, including minor adverse events, especially because NIV has been shown to be cost-effective, especially in patients with COPD with frequent exacerbations and hospital admissions.[58]

Noninvasive Ventilation for Acute-On-Chronic Hypercapnic Respiratory Failure due to Chronic Obstructive Pulmonary Disease

It is well known that patients with COPD needing mechanical ventilation during an episode of acute

Table 10
Study populations and key findings of the RESCUE and HOT-HMV trials

	RESCUE[73]	HOT-HMV[74]
Inclusion criteria	Hypercapnia shortly after termination of ventilatory support during an episode of acute hypercapnic failure "Hypercapnia directly after exacerbation"	Hypercapnia at a longer period (2–4 wk) after termination of ventilatory support during an episode of acute hypercapnic failure "Prolonged hypercapnia after exacerbation"
Randomization	NIV + LTOT vs LTOT alone shortly after exacerbation (before discharge)	NIV + LTOT vs LTOT alone 2–4 wk after exacerbation
Results	At 1 y, there was no significant between-group difference in the rate of the primary outcome (combination of mortality and readmission)	Treatment with NIV + LTOT significantly increased the time to readmission or death over 1 y of follow-up (4.3 vs 1.4 mo; adjusted HR 0.49, 95% confidence interval 0.31–0.77; $P = .002$)

Abbreviations: HOT-HMV, Home Oxygen Therapy–Home Mechanical Ventilation; HR, hazard ratio; LTOT, long-term oxygen therapy; NIV, noninvasive ventilation; RESCUE, REspiratory Support in COPD after acUte Exacerbation.
Data from Refs.[73,74]

respiratory failure are at very high risk of readmission and mortality after discharge.[72] Two large RCTs have evaluated the use of NIV in this setting: the RESCUE-Trial[73] and the HOT-HMV-Trial[74] (**Table 10**).

One criticism of the RESCUE-Trial was that patients were recruited too soon after the acute exacerbation meaning that some could have been randomized during a period of potentially reversible acute hypercapnic failure and probably would not have needed NIV if they had been evaluated later. These 2 trials helped formation of a consensus regarding the importance of carefully selecting post-acute exacerbation patients with hypercapnic COPD who would be most likely to benefit from long-term NIV. Therefore, patients need to be assessed to determine which have transient acute hypercapnia that will spontaneously resolve over time (ie, unlikely to benefit from long-term NIV) and which have a real "mostly acute-on-chronic" hypercapnic failure that would respond to treatment with long-term NIV.

Noninvasive Ventilation Settings

Current recommendations state that NIV should be titrated in a "targeted way" to normalize or significantly reduce $Paco_2$ levels with the best possible patient acceptance.[58,75] Stepwise increases in IPAP and measurement of blood gases to determine whether a significant reduction in $Paco_2$ has occurred seems to be a practical approach and has been shown to be effective.[69,70,76] Combining effective IPAP titration with a pressure-controlled mode of ventilation and a high backup respiratory rate, just below the patient's spontaneous breathing frequency, is one technique that has been used to maximally support respiratory work,[69] and was shown to improve relevant physiologic and clinical variables, with very good compliance.[58] A combination of high-pressure support levels and low backup rate might be a good alternative strategy with comparable outcomes, but has not yet been widely studied.[77] Generally, the potential for negative cardiopulmonary interactions needs to be taken into account when a very high IPAP is used.[78] On the other hand, there is not enough evidence on this topic, and effective NIV was shown to be associated with a significant reduction in N-terminal pro-B-type natriuretic peptide levels, indicating improved cardiac function.[71,79]

SUMMARY

Current guidelines recommend the use of SOT in patients with COPD with severe hypoxemic respiratory failure and moderate hypoxemic failure in the presence of concomitant PH, congestive heart failure, or polycythemia; however, the benefits should be weighed against the burden and possible side effects of LTOT. Treatment with NIV is known to improve prognosis in patients with a hypercapnic COPD exacerbation and may prevent the need for invasive mechanical ventilation. A growing body of evidence also suggests that long-term NIV targeted to significantly reduce $Paco_2$ has significant and important clinical benefits in patients with COPD with confirmed, prolonged chronic hypercapnia at least 2 to 4 weeks after an acute exacerbation. Current European guidelines reflect the latest data, but there is a gap between available evidence and clinical practice in other settings, especially the United States.

ACKNOWLEDGMENTS

English language editing assistance was provided by Nicola Ryan, independent medical writer.

DISCLOSURE

The authors report no commercial or financial conflicts of interest or outside funding sources.

REFERENCES

1. Barjaktarevic I, Cooper CB. Supplemental oxygen therapy for patients with chronic obstructive pulmonary disease. Semin Respir Crit Care Med 2015; 36(4):552–66.

2. Kent BD, Mitchell PD, Mcnicholas WT. Hypoxemia in patients with COPD: cause, effects, and disease progression. Int J Chron Obstruct Pulmon Dis 2011;6:199–208.

3. Young T, Palta M, Dempsey J, et al. The occurrence of sleep-disordered breathing among middle-aged adults. N Engl J Med 1993;328(17): 1230–5.

4. Engelen MPKJ, Schols AMWJ, Does JD, et al. Exercise-induced lactate increase in relation to muscle substrates in patients with chronic obstructive pulmonary disease. Am J Respir Crit Care Med 2000; 162(5):1697–704.

5. Shapiro NI, Howell MD, Talmor D, et al. Serum lactate as a predictor of mortality in emergency department patients with infection. Ann Emerg Med 2005;45(5):524–8.

6. Stein DA, Bradley BL, Miller WC. Mechanisms of oxygen effects on exercise in patients with chronic obstructive pulmonary disease. Chest 1982;81(1): 6–10.

7. Cotes JE, Pisa Z, Thomas AJ. Effect of breathing oxygen upon cardiac output, heart rate, ventilation, systemic and pulmonary blood pressure in patients with chronic lung disease. Clin Sci 1963;25: 305–21.

8. Aubier M, Murciano D, Milic-Emili J. Effects of administration of O2 on ventilation and blood gases in patients with chronic obstructive pulmonary disease during acute respiratory failure. Am Rev Respir Dis 1980;122(5):747–54.

9. Davidson AC, Leach R, George RJD, et al. Supplemental oxygen and exercise ability in chronic obstructive airways disease. Thorax 1988;43(12): 965–71.

10. Hunt JM, Copland J, McDonald CF, et al. Cardiopulmonary response to oxygen therapy in hypoxaemic chronic airflow obstruction. Thorax 1989;44(11):930–6.

11. Kvale PA, Conway WA, Coates EO. Continuous or nocturnal oxygen therapy in hypoxemic chronic obstructive lung disease. A clinical trial. Ann Intern Med 1980;93(3):391–8.

12. Abraham AS, Hedworth-Whitty RB, Bishop JM. Effects of acute hypoxia and hypervolaemia singly and together, upon the pulmonary circulation in patients with chronic bronchitis. Clin Sci 1967;33(2): 371–80.

13. Baudouin SV, Bott J, Ward A, et al. Short term effect of oxygen on renal haemodynamics in patients with hypoxaemic chronic obstructive airways disease. Thorax 1992;47(7):550–4.

14. Stuart-Harris C, Bishop JM, Cark TJH, et al. Long term domiciliary oxygen therapy in chronic hypoxic cor pulmonale complicating chronic bronchitis and emphysema. Report of the Medical Research Council Working Party. Lancet 1981;1(8222):681–6.

15. Johnson TS, Ellis JH, Steele PP. Improvement of platelet survival time with oxygen in patients with chronic obstructive airway disease. Am Rev Respir Dis 1978;117(2):255–7.

16. Heaton RK, Grant I, McSweeny AJ, et al. Psychologic effects of continuous and nocturnal oxygen therapy in hypoxemic chronic obstructive pulmonary disease. Arch Intern Med 1983;143(10): 1941–7.

17. Górecka D, Gorzelak K, Śliwiński P, et al. Effect of long term oxygen therapy on survival in patients with chronic obstructive pulmonary disease with moderate hypoxaemia. Thorax 1997;52(8):674–9.

18. Albert RK, Au DH, Blackford AL, et al. A randomized trial of long-term oxygen for COPD with moderate desaturation. N Engl J Med 2016; 375(17):1617–27.

19. Chaouat A, Weitzenblum F, Kessler R, et al. A randomized trial of nocturnal oxygen therapy in chronic obstructive pulmonary disease patients. Eur Respir J 1999;14(5):1002–8.

20. Ekström M, Ringbaek T. Which patients with moderate hypoxemia benefit from long-term oxygen therapy? Ways forward. Int J Chron Obstruct Pulmon Dis 2018;13:231–5.

21. Yusen RD, Criner GJ, Sternberg AL, et al. The long-term oxygen treatment trial for chronic obstructive pulmonary disease: rationale, design, and lessons learned. Ann Am Thorac Soc 2018;15(1):89–101.

22. Fleetham J, West P, Mezon B, et al. Sleep, arousals, and oxygen desaturation in chronic obstructive pulmonary disease. The effect of oxygen therapy. Am Rev Respir Dis 1982;126(3):429–33.

23. Magnet FS, Schwarz SB, Callegari J, et al. Long-term oxygen therapy: comparison of the German and British guidelines. Respiration 2017;93(4): 253–63.

24. Cullen DL. Long term oxygen therapy adherence and COPD: what we don't know. Chron Respir Dis 2006;3(4):217–22.

25. Woodcock AA, Gross ER, Geddes DM. Oxygen relieves breathlessness in "pink puffers". Lancet 1981;317(8226):907–9.

26. Lilker ES, Karnick A, Lerner L. Portable oxygen in chronic obstructive lung disease with hypoxemia and cor pulmonale. A controlled double blind crossover study. Chest 1975;68(2):236–41.

27. Marik PE. Evidence-based critical care. 3rd edition. Cham: Springer; 2015.

28. Jacono FJ. Control of ventilation in COPD and lung injury. Respir Physiol Neurobiol 2013;189(2):371–6.

29. Hardinge M, Annandale J, Bourne S, et al. British Thoracic Society guidelines for home oxygen use in adults. Thorax 2015;70(Suppl 1):i1–43.

30. Magnussen H, Kirsten AM, Köhler D, et al. Leitlinien zur langzeit-sauerstofftherapie: Deutsche gesellschaft für pneumologie und beatmungsmedizin e. V. Pneumologie 2008;62:748–56.

31. Global Initiative for Chronic Obstructive Lung Disease. Global strategy for the diagnosis, management, and prevention of chronic obstructive pulmonary disease: 2019 report. Available at: https://goldcopd.org/wp-content/uploads/2018/11/GOLD-2019-v1.7-FINAL-14Nov2018-WMS.pdf. Accessed January 13,2020.

32. Ahmadi Z, Sundh J, Bornefalk-Hermansson A, et al. Long-term oxygen therapy 24 vs 15 h/day and mortality in chronic obstructive pulmonary disease. PLoS One 2016;11(9):e0163293.

33. Galligan C, Markkanen P, Fantasia L, et al. A growing fire hazard concern in communities: home oxygen therapy and continued smoking habits. New Solut 2015;24(4):535–54.

34. McDonald CF, Whyte K, Jenkins S, et al. Clinical practice guideline on adult domiciliary oxygen therapy: executive summary from the Thoracic Society of Australia and New Zealand. Respirology 2016;21(1):76–8.

35. Shrikrishna D, Coker RK. Managing passengers with stable respiratory disease planning air travel: British Thoracic Society recommendations. Thorax 2011;66(9):831–3.

36. Edvardsen A, Akerø A, Christensen CC, et al. Air travel and chronic obstructive pulmonary disease: a new algorithm for pre-flight evaluation. Thorax 2012;67(11):964–9.

37. Kim V, Benditt JO, Wise RA, et al. Oxygen therapy in chronic obstructive pulmonary disease. Proc Am Thorac Soc 2008;5(4):513–8.

38. Cornish L, Dyer F, Cheema K, et al. P38 Is it possible to predict ambulatory oxygen (AO) requirements? Thorax 2013;68(Suppl 3):A92.

39. Frost N, Rosseau S. Standard-pO2 zur Unterscheidung von primärer und sekundärer Hypoxämie. Med Klin Intensivmed Notfmed 2014;109(1):62–5.

40. Hill NS. High flow nasal cannula, is there a role in COPD? Tanaffos 2017;16(Suppl 1):S12.

41. Pépin JL, Barjhoux CE, Deschaux C, et al. Long-term oxygen therapy at home: compliance with medical prescription and effective use of therapy. ANTADIR Working Group on Oxygen Therapy. Association Nationale de Traitement à Domicile des Insuffisants Respiratories. Chest 1996;109(5):1144–50.

42. Pfeifer M. Respiratory pump failure. Clinical symptoms, diagnostics and therapy | Versagen der atempumpe klinik, diagnostik und therapie. Internist 2012;53(5):534–44.

43. Qaseem A. Diagnosis and management of stable chronic obstructive pulmonary disease: a clinical practice guideline update from the American College of Physicians, American College of Chest Physicians, American Thoracic Society, and European Respiratory Society. Ann Intern Med 2011;155(3):179–91.

44. Calverley PMA. Respiratory failure in chronic obstructive pulmonary disease. Eur Respir J Suppl 2003;47:26s–30s.

45. Similowski T, Yan S, Gauthier AP, et al. Contractile properties of the human diaphragm during chronic hyperinflation. N Engl J Med 1991;325(13):917–23.

46. Gea J, Pascual S, Casadevall C, et al. Muscle dysfunction in chronic obstructive pulmonary disease: update on causes and biological findings. J Thorac Dis 2015;7(10):E418–38.

47. Barreiro E, Gea J. Respiratory and limb muscle dysfunction in COPD. COPD 2015;12(4):413–26.

48. De Troyer A, Leeper JB, McKenzie DK, et al. Neural drive to the diaphragm in patients with severe COPD. Am J Respir Crit Care Med 1997;155(4):1335–40.

49. Köhnlein T, Windisch W, Köhler D, et al. Non-invasive positive pressure ventilation for the treatment of severe stable chronic obstructive pulmonary disease: a prospective, multicentre, randomised, controlled clinical trial. Lancet Respir Med 2014;2(9):698–705.

50. Foucher P, Baudouin N, Merati M, et al. Relative survival analysis of 252 patients with COPD receiving long- term oxygen therapy. Chest 1998;113(6):1580–7.

51. Turkington PM, Elliott MW. Rationale for the use of non-invasive ventilation in chronic ventilatory failure. Thorax 2000;55(5):417–23.

52. Bott J, Keilty SEJ, Elliott MW, et al. Randomised controlled trial of nasal ventilation in acute ventilatory failure due to chronic obstructive airways disease. Lancet 1993;341(8860):1555–7.

53. Brochard L, Mancebo J, Wysocki M, et al. Noninvasive ventilation for acute exacerbations of chronic obstructive pulmonary disease. N Engl J Med 1995;341(8860):1555–7.

54. Confalonieri M, Garuti G, Cattaruzza MS, et al. A chart of failure risk for noninvasive ventilation in

patients with COPD exacerbation. Eur Respir J 2005;25(2):348–55.

55. Corrêa TD, Sanches PR, de Morais LC, et al. Performance of noninvasive ventilation in acute respiratory failure in critically ill patients: a prospective, observational, cohort study. BMC Pulm Med 2015;15:144.

56. Duan J, Wang S, Liu P, et al. Early prediction of noninvasive ventilation failure in COPD patients: derivation, internal validation, and external validation of a simple risk score. Ann Intensive Care 2019;9(1):108.

57. Davidson AC, Banham S, Elliott M, et al. BTS/ICS guideline for the ventilatory management of acute hypercapnic respiratory failure in adults. Thorax 2016;71(Suppl 2):ii1–35.

58. Ergan B, Oczkowski S, Rochwerg B, et al. Early View Task Force Report. European Respiratory Society guideline on long-term home non-invasive ventilation for management of chronic obstructive pulmonary disease. 2019. Available at: https://www.ers-education.org/lrmedia/2019/pdf/418656.pdf. Accessed January 13,2020.

59. Rochwerg B, Brochard L, Elliott MW, et al. Official ERS/ATS clinical practice guidelines: noninvasive ventilation for acute respiratory failure. Eur Respir J 2017;50(2) [pii:1602426].

60. Coleman JM, Wolfe LF, Kalhan R. Noninvasive ventilation in chronic obstructive pulmonary disease. Ann Am Thorac Soc 2019;16(9):1091–8.

61. Ahmadi Z, Bornefalk-Hermansson A, Franklin KA, et al. Hypo- and hypercapnia predict mortality in oxygen-dependent chronic obstructive pulmonary disease: a population-based prospective study. Respir Res 2014;15:30.

62. Connors AF, Dawson NV, Thomas C, et al. Outcomes following acute exacerbation of severe chronic obstructive lung disease. The SUPPORT investigators (Study to Understand Prognoses and Preferences for Outcomes and Risks of Treatments). Am J Respir Crit Care Med 1996;154(4 Pt 1):959–67.

63. Duiverman ML, Wempe JB, Bladder G, et al. Nocturnal non-invasive ventilation in addition to rehabilitation in hypercapnic patients with COPD. Thorax 2008;63(12):1052–7.

64. Tsolaki V, Pastaka C, Karetsi E, et al. One-year noninvasive ventilation in chronic hypercapnic COPD: effect on quality of life. Respir Med 2008;102(6):904–11.

65. Budweiser S, Heinemann F, Meyer K, et al. Weight gain in cachectic COPD patients receiving noninvasive positive-pressure ventilation. Respir Care 2006;51(2):126–32.

66. McEvoy RD, Pierce RJ, Hillman D, et al. Nocturnal non-invasive nasal ventilation in stable hypercapnic COPD: a randomised controlled trial. Thorax 2009;64(7):561–6.

67. Meecham Jones DJ, Paul EA, Jones PW, et al. Nasal pressure support ventilation plus oxygen compared with oxygen therapy alone in hypercapnic COPD. Am J Respir Crit Care Med 1995;152(2):538–44.

68. Tuggey JM, Plant PK, Elliott MW. Domiciliary noninvasive ventilation for recurrent acidotic exacerbations of COPD: an economic analysis. Thorax 2003;58(10):867–71.

69. Dreher M, Storre JH, Schmoor C, et al. High-intensity versus low-intensity non-invasive ventilation in patients with stable hypercapnic COPD: a randomised crossover trial. Thorax 2010;65(4):303–8.

70. Windisch W, Kostić S, Dreher M, et al. Outcome of patients with stable COPD receiving controlled noninvasive positive pressure ventilation aimed at a maximal reduction of PaCO2. Chest 2005;128(2):657–62.

71. Duiverman ML. Noninvasive ventilation in stable hypercapnic COPD: what is the evidence? ERJ Open Res 2018;4(2) [pii:00012-02018].

72. Chu CM, Chan VL, Lin AWN, et al. Readmission rates and life threatening events in COPD survivors treated with non-invasive ventilation for acute hypercapnic respiratory failure. Thorax 2004;59(12):1020–5.

73. Struik FM, Sprooten RTM, Kerstjens HAM, et al. Nocturnal non-invasive ventilation in copd patients with prolonged hypercapnia after ventilatory support for acute respiratory failure: a randomised, controlled, parallel-group study. Thorax 2014;69(9):826–34.

74. Murphy PB, Rehal S, Arbane G, et al. Effect of home noninvasive ventilation with oxygen therapy vs oxygen therapy alone on hospital readmission or death after an acute COPD exacerbation: a randomized clinical trial. JAMA 2017;317(21):2177–86.

75. Windisch W, Dreher M, Geiseler J, et al. S2k-Leitlinie: nichtinvasive und invasive Beatmung als Therapie der chronischen respiratorischen Insuffizienz – revision 2017. Pneumologie 2017;71(11):722–95.

76. Windisch W, Haenel M, Storre JH, et al. High-intensity non-invasive positive pressure ventilation for stable hypercapnic COPD. Int J Med Sci 2009;6(2):72–6.

77. Murphy PB, Brignall K, Moxham J, et al. High pressure versus high intensity noninvasive ventilation in stable hypercapnic chronic obstructive pulmonary disease: a randomized crossover trial. Int J Chron Obstruct Pulmon Dis 2012;7:811–8.

78. Lukácsovits J, Carlucci A, Hill N, et al. Physiological changes during low- and high-intensity noninvasive ventilation. Eur Respir J 2012;39(4):869–75.

79. Dreher M, Schulte L, Müller T, et al. Influence of effective noninvasive positive pressure ventilation on inflammatory and cardiovascular biomarkers in

stable hypercapnic COPD patients. Respir Med 2015;109(10):1300–4.

80. Hampson N, Atik D. Central nervous system oxygen toxicity during routine hyperbaric oxygen therapy. Undersea Hyperb Med 2003;30(2):147–53.

81. Floyd TF, Clark JM, Gelfand R, et al. Independent cerebral vasoconstrictive effects of hyperoxia and accompanying arterial hypocapnia at 1 ATA. J Appl Physiol (1985) 2003;95(6):2453–61.

82. Mickel HS, Vaishnav YN, Kempski O, et al. Breathing 100% oxygen after global brain ischemia in Mongolian gerbils results in increased lipid peroxidation and increased mortality. Stroke 1987;18(2):426–30.

83. Dripps RD, Comroe JH. The effect of the inhalation of high and low oxygen concentrations on respiration, pulse rate, ballistocardiogram and arterial oxygen saturation (oximeter) of normal individuals. Am J Physiol 1947;149(2):277–91.

84. Jackson RM. Pulmonary oxygen toxicity. Chest 1985;88(6):900–5.

85. De Jonge E, Peelen L, Keijzers PJ, et al. Association between administered oxygen, arterial partial oxygen pressure and mortality in mechanically ventilated intensive care unit patients. Crit Care 2008;12(6):R156.

86. Anderson KJ, Harten JM, Booth MG, et al. The cardiovascular effects of normobaric hyperoxia in patients with heart rate fixed by permanent pacemaker. Anaesthesia 2010;65(2):167–71.

87. Baleeiro CEO, Wilcoxen SE, Morris SB, et al. Sublethal hyperoxia impairs pulmonary innate immunity. J Immunol 2003;171(2):955–63.

88. Stoller JK, Panos RJ, Krachman S, et al. Oxygen therapy for patients with COPD: current evidence and the long-term oxygen treatment trial. Chest 2010;138(1):179–87.

89. Qaseem A. Diagnosis and management of stable chronic obstructive pulmonary disease: a clinical practice guideline update from the American College of Physicians, American College of Chest Physicians, American Thoracic Society, and European Respiratory Society. Ann Intern Med 2011;155(3):179–91.

90. Eaton T, Garrett JE, Young P, et al. Ambulatory oxygen improves quality of life of COPD patients: a randomised controlled study. Eur Respir J 2002;20(2):306–12.

91. Ejiofor SI, Bayliss S, Gassamma A, et al. Ambulatory oxygen for exercise-induced desaturation and dyspnea in chronic obstructive pulmonary disease (COPD): systematic review and meta-analysis. Chronic Obstr Pulm Dis 2016;3(1):419–34.

92. Bradley JM, Lasserson T, Elborn S, et al. A systematic review of randomized controlled trials examining the short-term benefit of ambulatory oxygen in COPD. Chest 2007;131(1):278–85.

93. Fletcher EC, Donner CF, Midgren B, et al. Survival in COPD patients with a daytime PaO2 >60 mm Hg with and without nocturnal oxyhemoglobin desaturation. Chest 1992;101(3):649–55.

94. Eaton T, Rudkin S, Garrett JE. The clinical utility of arterialized earlobe capillary blood in the assessment of patients for long-term oxygen therapy. Respir Med 2001;95(8):655–60.

95. Chaney JC, Jones K, Grathwohl K, et al. Implementation of an oxygen therapy clinic to manage users of long-term oxygen therapy. Chest 2002;122(5):1661–7.

96. Zavorsky GS, Cao J, Mayo NE, et al. Arterial versus capillary blood gases: a meta-analysis. Respir Physiol Neurobiol 2007;155(3):268–79.

97. Louw A, Cracco C, Cerf C, et al. Accuracy of pulse oximetry in the intensive care unit. Intensive Care Med 2001;27(10):1606–13.

98. MacIntyre NR. Physiologic effects of noninvasive ventilation. Respir Care 2019;64(6):617–28.

99. Ambrosino N, Cigni P. Non invasive ventilation as an additional tool for exercise training. Multidiscip Respir Med 2015;10:14.

100. Hajian B, De Backer J, Sneyers C, et al. Pathophysiological mechanism of long-term noninvasive ventilation in stable hypercapnic patients with COPD using functional respiratory imaging. Int J Chron Obstruct Pulmon Dis 2017;12:2197–205.

101. Schönhofer B, Polkey MI, Suchi S, et al. Effect of home mechanical ventilation on inspiratory muscle strength in COPD. Chest 2006;130(6):1834–8.

102. Nickol AH, Hart N, Hopkinson NS, et al. Mechanisms of improvement of respiratory failure in patients with restrictive thoracic disease treated with non-invasive ventilation. Thorax 2005;60(9):754–60.

103. McNicholas WT. Chronic obstructive pulmonary disease and obstructive sleep apnoea-the overlap syndrome. J Thorac Dis 2016;8(2):236–42.

Interventional Bronchoscopic Therapies for Chronic Obstructive Pulmonary Disease

Nathaniel Marchetti, DO*, Sean Duffy, MD, Gerard J. Criner, MD

KEYWORDS

- Bronchoscopic lung volume reduction • Targeted lung denervation • Chronic bronchitis

KEY POINTS

- Endobronchial valves improve lung function, exercise performance, and quality of life in patients with severely hyperinflated emphysema with heterogeneous and homogeneous emphysema.
- Determining fissure integrity is key to successful bronchoscopic lung volume reduction and endobronchial valves should not be deployed if collateral ventilation between lobes exists.
- Bronchoscopic targeted lung denervation using radiofrequency ablation to alter the parasympathetic innervation of the airways is currently under investigation as a viable option for further decreasing acute exacerbations of chronic obstructive pulmonary disease.
- Bronchoscopic techniques to treat mucus hypersecretion and chronic bronchitis using liquid nitrogen cryospray and bronchial rheoplasty are in development.

INTRODUCTION

Although surgical interventions are beneficial in carefully selected patients who fail medical therapy,[1] the associated morbidity and mortality makes many patients with severe chronic obstructive pulmonary disease (COPD) reluctant to undergo surgical intervention. Furthermore, those with lower lobe predominant emphysema are generally not considered candidates for lung volume reduction surgery and, although lung transplantation is the penultimate treatment for advanced lung disease, it has limited access owing to organ availability and strict selection criteria.

This review focuses on bronchoscopic interventions that expand treatment options for patients who have failed maximal medical therapy. Procedures include those that are approved the by US Food and Drug Administration (endobronchial valve [EBV] therapy for bronchoscopic lung volume reduction) and those that are currently being developed or undergoing evaluation in multicenter clinical trials (targeted lung denervation [TLD] and bronchoscopic treatments for chronic bronchitis).

BRONCHOSCOPIC APPROACHES TO LUNG VOLUME REDUCTION

There has been intense recent investigation into less invasive bronchoscopic procedures for lung volume reduction in patient with severely hyperinflated emphysematous. This interest has resulted in US Food and Drug Administration approval of 2 different types of EBVs. Other bronchoscopic techniques currently under investigation include endobronchial placement of self-activation coils, targeted destruction and remodeling of emphysematous tissue, and airway bypass stenting.

One-Way Endobronchial Valves

EBVs have been more extensively studied than any other bronchoscopic technique for lung

Department of Thoracic Medicine and Surgery, Lewis Katz School of Medicine at Temple University, 712 Parkinson Pavilion, 3401 North Broad Street, Philadelphia, PA 19140, USA
* Corresponding author.
E-mail address: nathaniel.marchetti@tuhs.temple.edu

Clin Chest Med 41 (2020) 547–557
https://doi.org/10.1016/j.ccm.2020.06.010
0272-5231/20/© 2020 Elsevier Inc. All rights reserved.

volume reduction. EBVs are placed in the airway at the segmental or lobar level and are designed to block inspiration but permit exhalation of air and secretions. Optimal valve placement results in lobar atelectasis and a significant reduction in end-expiratory lung volumes. EBVs are placed in the most air trapped lobe owing to emphysematous destruction. There are 2 types of EBVs. The Spiration Intrabronchial Valve (Spiration, Olympus, Tokyo, Japan) system has an umbrella design, where an occlusive cover is stretched over a titanium wire frame that allows expired air and secretions to escape around the outer edges and the airway wall (**Fig. 1**). The Zephyr valve (Pulmonx Inc., Neuchâtel Switzerland) is a cylindrical device with a duckbill 1-way valve placed in a nitinol wire cage, which permits expired air and secretions to escape through the center of the valve (**Fig. 2**).

The Endobronchial Valve for Emphysema Palliation Trial (VENT) was the first prospective randomized trial to evaluate bronchoscopic lung volume reduction using the Zephyr valve.[2] The VENT trial randomized 220 patients to EBV placement compared with 101 patients treated with maximal medical therapy alone. Valves were placed unilaterally targeting the lobe with the highest percentage of emphysema in the lung with the greatest degree of heterogeneity.

At 6 months, there were only modest improvements in the forced expiratory volume in 1 second (FEV_1) (+4.3%/34.5 mL) and 6-minute walk distance (+2.5%/9.3 m) in the EBV group compared with controls. Furthermore, there were modest differences in the quality of life, dyspnea, exercise performance, and supplemental oxygen use, all favoring the EBV group. Heterogeneity of emphysema between lobes in treated lung and the presence of complete fissures were the only factors predictive of improvements in the primary end points. For heterogeneity of emphysema, those with differences of 15% or greater in

emphysema were found to have greater improvements in FEV_1 and 6-minute walk distance at 6 months. EBV patients with intact fissures had a 16.2% improvement in FEV_1 at 6 months and 17.9% at 12 months, whereas those with incomplete fissures had changes of FEV_1 of only 2.0% and 2.8% at 6 and 12 months, respectively.[2]

The EUROVENT study was also performed in 23 European sites where 111 patients were randomized to EBV and 60 to medical therapy.[3] Although the study was underpowered compared with the US VENT study, the results were similar. At 6 months, there were modest improvements in FEV_1, quality of life, and 6-minute walk distance in the EBV group compared with the control group that were either significant or nearly significant. Once again, those with complete fissures had better results with improvements in FEV_1 (16% vs 2%) when treated with EBV compared with medical therapy. The median reduction in target lobe volume reduction relative to baseline target lung volume reduction was greater in those with complete fissures compared with incomplete fissure.[3] These 2 studies suggest that if collateral ventilation is absent then placement of EBVs can improve lung function and quality of life by reducing lung volumes.

There was debate over whether to perform unilobar total lobar collapse or bilateral subtotal lobar atelectasis to achieve volume reduction and decrease the risk of pneumothorax. Eberhardt and associates[4] randomized 22 patients to unilateral treatment with the goal of total lobar occlusion or bilateral subtotal atelectasis. They found that those treated with unilateral lobar occlusion had significant improvements in FEV_1 and 6-minute walk test at 30 and 90 days compared with baseline. The subtotal lobar occlusion bilaterally treated group did not have a significant increase in FEV_1 or 6-minute walk test at 30 or 90 days.

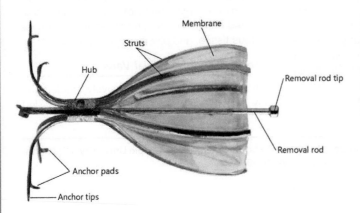

Membrane

Struts

Hub

Removal rod tip

Removal rod

Anchor pads

Anchor tips

Fig. 1. Spiration intrabronchial valve (Spiration, Olympus). Note the umbrella design with an occlusive cover over the titanium wire frame. The removal rod (the "umbrella handle") can be grasped by forceps to remove the valve while the anchors help to keep the valve in place.

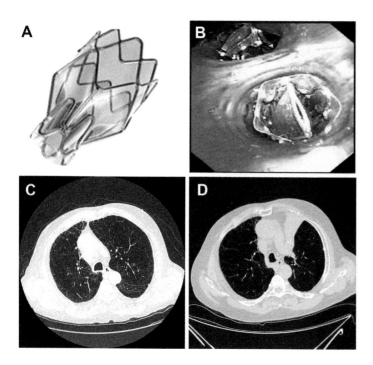

Fig. 2. Zephyr valve (Pulmonx Inc.). (*A*) Valve ex vivo. (*B*) Endobronchial view of valves with gas escaping via the center of the valves immediately after placement. (*C*) Representative high-resolution computed tomography image of severe left upper lobe emphysema. (*D*) High-resolution computed tomography image demonstrating complete left upper lobe atelectasis following EBV placement.

Additionally, the unilateral lobar occlusion group had improvements in the quality of life as measured by the St George's Respiratory Questionnaire (SGRQ) at 90 days, whereas the bilateral subtotal atelectasis arm did not. The unilateral treated group was significantly more likely to have radiologic evidence of atelectasis and volume reduction compared with the bilateral group.[4] Based on these data, future clinical trials focused on treating 1 lobe with a goal of total lobar atelectasis.

Determining whether or not an individual has intact fissures can be determined by quantitative high-resolution computed tomography (HRCT) analysis of fissure integrity (FI) or balloon occlusion of the airway and monitoring flow with the Chartis system (Pulmonx Inc.).[5,6] The Chartis system measures collateral ventilation during bronchoscopy by inserting a balloon tipped catheter into the target bronchus via the working channel of the bronchoscope to occlude the airway. The balloon tipped catheter can measure flow and pressure at its distal tip and be used as a surrogate of FI if there is no flow and pressure rises with balloon occlusion of lobe targeted for EBV treatment. **Fig. 3**A is an example of a collateral ventilation–negative patient clearly demonstrating cessation of flow and **Fig. 3**B demonstrates a patient with positive collateral ventilation, indicating that the fissure is not intact. Alternatively, FI can be measured by quantitative analysis of HRCT imaging. Some

EBV studies have used a FI of 90% or more complete as an acceptable parameter to proceed with EBV treatment.[7] Neither technique is perfect, and the sensitivity and specificity for Chartis (Pulmonx, Inc.) has been reported to be 77.8% and 73.3%, respectively, whereas QCT analysis of FI it is 83.3% and 66.7%, respectively.[6] Although it is essential to determine if there is collateral ventilation before EBV treatment it is not clear whether 1 method is better than the other or if both should be used.

Based on the VENT trial results, all subsequent EBV randomized controlled trials (RCTs) enrolled only those with intact fissures. In the TRANSFORM study, investigators compared 65 patients that had Zephyr EBVs (Pulmonx Inc.) inserted with 32 patients in the control arm. Patients were enrolled if Chartis assessment demonstrated collateral ventilation negative status. Other inclusion criteria included an FEV_1 of 15% to 45% predicted, a total lung capacity (TLC) of more than 100% predicted and a residual volume (RV) or more than 180% predicted, a heterogeneity score of greater than 10% between the targeted lobe and ipsilateral lobes, and a 6-minute walk distance between 150 and 450 m.[8] Fifty-five percent of patients treated with EBVs had a greater than 12% improved in FEV_1 compared with controls. Additionally, there were significant improvements in 6-minute walk distance, quality of life measured

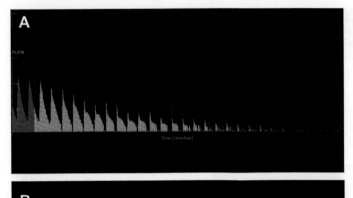

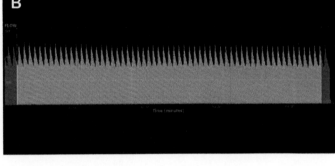

Fig. 3. Chartis (Pulmonx Inc.) assessment demonstrating (*A*) collateral ventilation negative patient (*B*) collateral ventilation positive patient.

by the SGRQ, and RV in those treated with EBVs compared with control.[8]

The *L*ung Function *I*mprovement after *B*ronchoscopic Lung Volume *R*eduction with Pulmonx Endobronchial *V*alves used in *T*reatment of *E*mphysema (LIBERATE) study recruited patients to determine the efficacy of the Zephyr valve (Pulmonx Inc.) in those with have intact fissures and at least 15% emphysema heterogeneity between lobes with more than 50% destruction in the targeted lobe.[9] Patients had an FEV_1 between 15% and 45% predicted, a TLC of greater than 100% predicted, an RV of 175% predicted or greater, and a 6-minute walk distance between 100 and 500 m following a supervised pulmonary rehabilitation program. This was the largest and longest duration of follow-up EBV trial and enrolled a total of 190 patients: 128 EBV and 62 standard care. After 1 year, more patients had improvement in FEV_1 by 15% in the EBV group compared with standard care (47.7% vs 16.8%). Additionally, quality of life, 6-minute walk distance, and dyspnea significantly improved favoring EBV. The between-group differences for FEV_1 was 0.106, 6-minute walk distance was 39.31 m, and quality of life measured by the SGRQ was −7.05. The effect was durable and at 12 months 84.2% of EBV patients achieved target lobe volume reduction of 350 mL or greater with a mean decrease of 1.14 ± 0.70 L. These data demonstrate that EBV placement in severely hyperinflated gas trapped patients with heterogeneous disease and intact fissures had meaningful clinically important improvements in lung function, quality of life, and exercise performance that were durable out to 1 year.[9]

Data also demonstrate the effectiveness of the Spiration Intrabronchial Valve (Spiration, Olympus) to perform bronchoscopic lung reduction. REACH compared the Spiration Valve System (SVS) to maximal medical therapy in a total of 107 patients. They enrolled patients with an FI of at least 90% as determined by quantitative HRCT analysis. Patients all had 15% or greater heterogeneity scores between ipsilateral lobes and similar to other trials; inclusion criteria included a FEV_1 of 45% predicted or greater, a TLC of at least 100% predicted, and an RV of at least 150%. The primary end point was change in FEV_1 at 3 months. At 3 months, the FEV_1 improved by 0.104 ± 0.178 L in the SVS group compared with 0.003 ± 0.147 L in controls. When the responder rate for FEV_1 improvement was defined as 15%, the responder rates for SVS were 49%, 48%, and 41% at 1, 3, and 6 months, respectively, compared with 22%, 13%, and 21% in controls. Quality of life significantly improved as measured by the SGRQ at 6 months in the SVS group compared with controls.[10]

The EMPROVE study using SVS (Spiration, Olympus) was a RCT which enrolled 113 patients in the SVS arm and 59 in the control arm.[11] Inclusion criteria were similar to that of the REACH study. The primary outcome for the study was the mean change in FEV_1 at 6 months compared with baseline, but data in this study were reported out to 12 months. At 6 months, the FEV_1 improved by 0.099 L in the SVS group and the FEV_1 decreased by 0.002 L in controls for a between-group difference of 0.101 L. The improvement of FEV_1 was durable out to 12 months. Secondary end points demonstrated a significant difference for the between-group differences of targeted lobar volume (−0.974 L), SGRQ (−13.0), and dyspnea as measured by the Modified Medical Research Council score (−0.6), but not the 6-minute walk distance at 6 months. Taken together, these 2 RCTs demonstrated that SVS (Spiration, Olympus) improves lung function, dyspnea, and quality of life in patients with heterogeneous emphysema that have severe airflow obstruction (FEV_1 of ≤45% predicted), hyperinflation (TLC of >100% predicted), and gas trapping (RV of >150% predicted).[11]

Endobronchial Valves for Homogeneous Emphysema

Patients with advanced homogeneous emphysema have little options after maximal medical therapy as surgical lung volume reduction surgery is contraindicated, thus leaving only lung transplantation as a less than ideal option owing to its increased morbidity, mortality, and limited availability. The use of EBVs has been studied in homogeneous disease although to a lesser degree than heterogeneous disease. One RCT used the Zephyr valve (Pulmonx Inc.) and enrolled 93 patients with severe homogeneous emphysema, an FEV_1 of 15% to 45% predicted, a TLC of greater than 100% predicted, and an RV of at least 200% predicted to either EBV placement plus standard care or to standard care alone.[12] Homogeneous emphysema was defined as a heterogeneity score of 15% or less between the target and ipsilateral nontarget lobe as determined by QCT analysis of HRCT. Additionally, patients had to have a 20% or less difference in perfusion between the right and left lungs as measured by perfusion scintigraphy. Patients were enrolled into the study if there was no evidence of collateral ventilation as measured by Chartis (Pulmonx Inc.). The mean difference in FEV_1 between groups at 3 months was 17.0% favoring the EBV group. There were significant improvements in quality of life (−9.6 points SGRQ), 6-minute walk distance (+40 m), and RV (−480 mL) in the EBV group. These data suggest that carefully selected patients with homogeneous emphysema will benefit from EBV placement.[12]

Complications Associated with Endobronchial Valve Placement

Although EBV placement is associated with less morbidity than lung volume reduction surgery there are significant complications associated with the procedure. The 2 most common complications include acute exacerbation of COPD and pneumothorax. **Table 1** lists the rates for these complications for the RCTs that enrolled patients with intact fissures. Most studies have reported a pneumothorax rate of 25% to 34%.[8–11,13,14] The REACH trial had fewer episodes of pneumothorax compared with other reports.[10] Although the reason for this finding is not clear, the investigators suggest that it may be due to conservative post-procedure care (6-day hospitalization and bed rest), less emphysema in the ipsilateral lobe relative to treatment lobe, or possibly less experience with EBV placement. Most, but not all, pneumothoraces required chest tube placement. Published guidelines suggest when valves should be removed or if surgical intervention is required.[15] The majority of pneumothoraces occur within the first few days after EBV placement and for this reason patients are usually hospitalized for 3 or 4 days after EBV placement to monitor for pneumothorax development. Mortality after EBV placement in the 2 largest trials to date is reported at 3.1%[9] and 5.3%.[11] Other reported complications include hemoptysis, valve migration/expectoration, pneumonia, and formation of granulation tissue.

Self-Activating Coils for Lung Volume Reduction

Endobronchial coils are nonocclusive coils that are placed straight bronchoscopically into subsegmental airways, and then upon release recover to a predetermined shape (**Fig. 4**A). Although not proven, the proposed mechanism for improvement is felt to be due to a combination of the coils reducing lung volume by compressing emphysematous tissue and by restoration of lung elastic recoil.[16] Lung volume reduction coils function independent of collateral ventilation and the treatment involves placement of 10 coils in each lung in 2 subsequent bronchoscopies (**Fig. 4**B).

RENEW was the largest (n = 315) multicenter RCT that compared endobronchial coils with maximal medical therapy in severe emphysema.[17] Patients were recruited with severe emphysema (homogeneous or heterogeneous), an FEV_1

Table 1
Rates of pneumothoraces and acute exacerbations of COPD in randomized controlled studies in patients with intact fissures (ie, no collateral ventilation)

	LIBERATE[8] (n = 128)	TRANSFORM[7] (n = 65)	IMPACT[11] (n = 43)	BeLieVer HIFi[12] (n = 25)	STELVIO[13] (n = 34)	REACH[9] (n = 72)	EMPROVE[10] (n = 113)	Total (n = 480)
Pneumothorax events	46	20	12	2	6	5	31	122
Patients with pneumothorax	44 (34.4%)	16 (29.2%)	12 (25.6%)	2 (8%)	6 (18%)	5 (7.5%)	0–6 mo: 32 (28.3%)	116 (24.2%)
Patients with acute exacerbation of COPD	Days 1–45: 10 (7.8%)	3 (4.65%)	10 (16.3%)	16 (64%)	4 (12%)	5 (7.6%)	0–6 mo: 19 (16.8%)	67 (14.0%)

Data from Refs.[7–13]

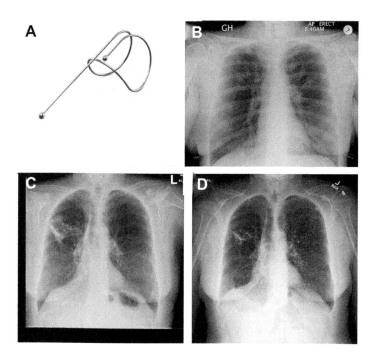

Fig. 4. Endobronchial coil (PneumRx Inc., BTG London, UK). (*A*) Ex vivo coil. (*B*) Chest radiograph after insertion of endobronchial coils placed in bilaterally upper lobes over 2 different bronchoscopic procedures. (*C*) Chest radiograph on postprocedure day 2 with right upper lobe opacity. (*D*) Chest radiograph 4 months later, after insertion of coils in left lung demonstrating resolution of coil*associated opacity, except for a band of scar tissue with associated volume loss on right.

percent predicted of at least 45%, an RV of at least 220% predicted (decreased to 175% predicted after 169 patients enrolled), and a TLC of more than 100% predicted. The lobe with the most emphysema was treated in heterogeneous emphysema patients, whereas the upper lobes were targeted in those with homogeneous disease. The primary outcome was an improvement in 6-minute walk distance at 12 months and the usual secondary outcomes of FEV_1, RV, and quality of life (SGRQ) at 12 months. The 6-minute walk distance improved 10.3 m in endobronchial coil group, whereas the control group 6-minute walk distance decreased 7.6 m for a between-group difference of 14.6 m favoring the endobronchial coil group. There were significant improvements in FEV_1, SGRQ, and RV in the coil group. Prespecified subgroup analyses demonstrated that those with an RV of at least 225% predicted and those with heterogeneous emphysema had greater improvements. There was no difference in mortality between groups, although there were more major complications in the endobronchial coil group (n = 54 [34.8%] vs n = 30 [19.1%]). The difference was largely owing to increased lower respiratory tract infections in the endobronchial coil group (18.7% vs 4.5%) and pneumothoraces in the endobronchial coil group (n = 15 [9.7%] vs n = 1 [0.6%]). A post hoc analysis of the reported pneumonia events revealed that 35% of the opacities on chest radiograph were attributable to

infections. Those opacities were due to noninfectious causes and coined coil-associated opacities (**Fig. 4**C, D). These patients tended to have better outcomes.[17] The etiology of the noninfectious opacities is not clear, but could be related to coil-induced atelectasis owing to stress forces from coils on the surrounding lung parenchyma or coil-induced inflammatory changes.

These data demonstrated a modest improvement in the 6-minute walk distance and FEV_1, but improvements in quality of life as measured by the SGRQ were more robust. However, the endobronchial coils did not gain US Food and Drug Administration approval.

Biologic Lung Reduction

This approach uses a biodegradable sclerosant gel designed to polymerize in small airways and alveolar spaces reducing lung volumes by scarring and remodeling of targeted lung regions that occurs over a period of several weeks. The Aeriseal Emphysematous Lung Sealant (ELS; Pulmonx, Inc.) used aminated polyvinyl alcohol and glutaraldehyde mixed with air to create the AeroSeal foam, which is then delivered to targeted pulmonary segments via bronchoscopy. This procedure is not affected by the presence of collateral ventilation. Early pilot studies demonstrated encouraging results, but the procedure was associated with a flulike reaction 8 to 24 hours after the procedure.[18,19] The most common adverse events were dyspnea, fever, and leukocytosis.

A multicenter RCT, the ASPIRE trial, was designed to determine the efficacy of AeriSeal treatment in severe upper lobe predominant emphysema compared with medical therapy.[20] Unfortunately, owing to financial reasons the sponsor closed the study after enrolling 95 patients, but 57 patients (34 treatment and 23 control) had efficacy data available at 3 months and 34 patients (21 treatment and 13 control) had data at 6 months. At 3 months, the median improvement in FEV_1 was 11.4% in the ELS-treated group compared with a change of −2.1% in control group. Additionally, there were improvements in SGRQ score in the ELS treated compared with control (−11 points). By 6 months, 52% of patient in the ELS group still had a response above the minimum clinically important difference for both FEV_1 and 6-minute walk distance, although only 21 patients had 6-month data available. There were 2 deaths and 3 patients had 4 episodes of respiratory failure requiring invasive mechanical ventilation in the ELS group and none in the control group.[20] Data from pilot studies and a truncated RCT demonstrate potential benefits with AeriSeal treatment, but the sclerosing agent needs refinement to be less toxic before any future studies using this technique.

Airway Bypass Tract Stent Placement

Airway bypass is a bronchoscopic technique designed for homogeneous emphysema in which airway passages are created to deflate trapped air using paclitaxel eluding-eluting stents to maintain patency of the bypass tracts (Broncus Technologies, Mountain View, CA). The Exhale Airway Stents for Emphysema (EASE) trial is a randomized, sham-controlled study designed to investigate the safety and efficacy of these stents.[21] EASE enrolled 315 patients (208 in the stent arm) with severe homogeneous emphysema that were severely gas trapped. The investigators had a coprimary end point of an increase in forced vital capacity by 12% as well as a decrease in Modified Medical Research Council dyspnea scale of 1 point. There was no difference between the sham procedure or airway bypass stenting in regard to coprimary end points. There were no differences in lung function or lung volumes at 6 or 12 months. Possible explanations included loss of stents from expectoration or occlusion from tissue debris.

Bronchoscopic Thermal Vapor Ablation

Bronchoscopic thermal vapor ablation (BTVA) uses heated water vapor to produce thermal injury in airways, resulting in an inflammatory response followed by fibrotic and atelectatic changes to induce volume reduction. The theoretic advantages of this technique are that collateral ventilation positive patients can be treated and the most diseased subsegments of the lung can be targeted allowing preservation of less diseased lung tissue, even if present in the same lobe. A pilot study of 44 patients with upper lobe predominant emphysema demonstrated a significant reduction in target lobe volume as well as significant improvements in FEV_1, 6-minute walk distance, and quality of life as measured by SGRQ.[22] A multi-center RCT (STEP-UP trial) comparing BTVA with medical therapy in 70 patients (46 treatment and 24 control) with advanced upper lobe predominant emphysema.[23] Investigators recruited patients with an FEV_1 of 20% to 45% predicted, a TLC of greater than 100% predicted, and an RV of at least 150% predicted. There was a significant improvement in FEV_1 (14.7%) and SGRQ (−9.7 points) between groups favoring BTVA, but no significant differences in 6-minute walk distance. The incidence of COPD exacerbations requiring hospitalization was 24% in the treated compared with 4% in the control group, whereas pneumonia or pneumonitis occurred in 18% of treated and 8% of controls.[23] Although early data suggest that BTVA is a promising therapy for advanced emphysema, more research is needed to maximize benefit while minimizing significant adverse events. The role of BTVA role in treating diffuse emphysema is unclear at this time, although clinical trials are planned to address these limitations.

TARGETED LUNG DENERVATION

Cholinergic sympathetic nerves provide innervation to both small and large airways providing the dominant innervation to human lung. Activation of parasympathetic nerves in airways lead to bronchoconstriction and mucus production.[24] Pharmacologic manipulation of the parasympathetic nervous system in the lung is a mainstay of COPD therapy. Tiotropium, a long-acting muscarinic antagonist, has been shown to significantly improve lung function, decrease static and dynamic hyperinflation, improve exercise performance, and decrease acute exacerbations of COPD.[25,26] TLD is a novel bronchoscopic technique that uses radiofrequency (RF) ablation to damage the parasympathetic nerves that run along the outside of the main stem bronchi. The catheter is designed with the RF electrode inside of a balloon, which allows for coolant to be circulated around and through the electrode, which prevents heating of the airway to reduce risk of airway stenosis.[27] Early studies demonstrated feasibility and an acceptable safety profile for the procedure.[27,28] Five of the first 13 patients enrolled in the AIRFLOW-1 study had impaired gastric emptying leading to a temporary cessation in the study.[28] The investigators determined that the RF ablation was damaging esophageal branches of the vagus nerve. The protocol was amended to include placement of an esophageal balloon, which permitted measurement of the distance between the RF catheter and the esophagus allowing investigators to avoid treating the airway in an area too close to the esophagus. The AIRFLOW2 study was a randomized, multicenter, sham bronchoscopy controlled, double-blind study in patients with symptomatic COPD (FEV$_1$ of 30%–60%) comparing TLD with a sham bronchoscopy to determine safety and adverse events after TLD treatment. The primary outcome was all inclusive respiratory events between 3.0 and 6.5 months after randomization and patients were followed out to 12.5 months.[29] The investigators enrolled 82 patients (67.7 ± 6.8 years, FEV$_1$ of 41.6 ± 7.3%, modified Research Council dyspnea scale of 2.2 ± 0.7) and found the TLD group had significantly fewer respiratory adverse events than those randomized to a sham procedure (32% vs 71%). Furthermore, the risk of COPD exacerbations requiring hospitalization at 12.5 months after randomization was lower in the TLD group compared with sham group. Although there was no difference in gastrointestinal adverse events between TLD and the sham bronchoscopy groups, there was a trend toward more gastrointestinal events in the TLD arm (primarily impaired gastric emptying).[29] Taken together, these early feasibility studies suggest that TLD is both feasible and safe in patients with moderate to severe COPD. The Airflow3 study plans to enroll 520 patients across multiple centers, which will compare TLD versus sham bronchoscopy at 12 centers in the United States and Europe. The primary outcome for the study is a decrease in the number of acute exacerbations of COPD.

Interventional Therapies for Chronic Bronchitis

Effective medical therapy for chronic bronchitis and mucus hypersecretion is largely nonexistent or ineffective, and most therapies are directed at clearing mucus from the airway.[30] There has been recent interest in developing bronchoscopic techniques that will damage airway epithelium and permit regeneration of a healthy epithelium with a reduced number of goblet cells. Liquid nitrogen (−196°C) can be delivered via a flexible bronchoscope as a metered cryospray (MCS) (CSA Medical, Lexington, MA), which kills airway epithelial cells as well as hyperplastic mucus producing goblet cells on contact, but leaves the extracellular matrix intact, which has been postulated to facilitate rapid regrowth of normal epithelium without inducing airway scarring. Enough liquid nitrogen is delivered to the lobar and segmental airways to cause a 10-mm circular cryoablation with a depth between 0.1 and 0.5 mm. The results of a limited number of patients undergoing this procedure have been published demonstrating feasibility, safety and proof of concept for MCS. Patients had MCS therapy and then immediately underwent lobectomy for lung cancer (n = 11, mean time from MCS to surgery was 37.3 ± 21.8 minutes) or underwent lobectomy for lung cancer at a later date (n = 5, mean time from MCS to surgery was 14 ± 1.4 days).[31] There were no device-related adverse events in either group, and the histology in those undergoing immediate resection demonstrated cryothermic changes in the airway epithelium without any damage to cartilage in 5 of the 8 available specimens. There was no evidence of airway scarring or narrowing at the site of prior MCS therapy during bronchoscopy performed immediately before resection. Histologic evaluation of these airways demonstrated complete reepithelialization at MCS treatment site when it was identifiable.[31] These limited data provide evidence that liquid nitrogen can be delivered in a safe manner to airways via flexible bronchoscopy, and pivotal multicenter studies are being planned to determine the clinical benefit of this approach.

Bronchial rheoplasty targets bronchial epithelium and goblet cell hyperplasia by using short bursts of electrical energy delivered via an endobronchial catheter. The treatment is applied to the entire airway accessible via flexible bronchoscopy and is designed to eradicate airway epithelium and goblet cells, thus permitting regeneration of a healthier epithelium with less goblet cell hyperplasia. Clinical trials using this therapy are ongoing and some preliminary data have been published but only in abstract form.[32] Investigators enrolled 31 patients that underwent bronchial rheoplasty bilaterally in 2 staged procedures. The investigators enrolled 31 patients (age of 67.6 ± 7.4 years; FEV$_1$ of 64.8 ± 20.9%) and found a reduction in goblet cell hyperplasia score in 49% of treated airways. There were also improvements in mean COPD Assessment Test (−6.4 ± 1.9) and SGRQ (−11.4 ± 4.5) scores at 6 months, and these decreases were maintained at 12 months as well.[32] There was no change in lung function. There were no unexpected adverse events related to rheoplasty, but acute exacerbations were the most common serious adverse event occurring in 2 patients.

Early pilot studies have demonstrated that these bronchoscopic procedures for chronic bronchitis are feasible and safe, but more work is required to determine if they can reduce the significant symptom burden of chronic bronchitis.

SUMMARY

Patients with advanced COPD who have disabling symptoms or poor quality of life despite maximal medical therapy have surgical and other interventional options that can dramatically improve lung function, dyspnea, and quality of life in carefully selected patients. For patients with severe emphysema, most experts suggest evaluation for bronchoscopic lung volume reduction with EBVs if they qualify. Lung volume reduction surgery can be reserved for those not eligible for EBVs owing to the presence of collateral ventilation or those that do not improve with EBVs (GOLD guidelines). Endobronchial treatment for chronic bronchitis is a promising therapy for a condition with little to no medical therapy, and is currently under investigation as part of multicenter clinical trials.

DISCLOSURE

Dr. Marchetti reports personal fees from Astrazeneca, personal fees from Realta Life Sciences, grants from Blade Therapeutics, grants from NIH, outside the submitted work.

Dr. Duffy has nothing to disclose.

Dr. Criner reports grants and personal fees from Galaxo Smith Kline, grants and personal fees from Boehringer Ingelheim, grants and personal fees from Chiesi, grants and personal fees from Mereo, personal fees from Verona, grants and personal fees from Astra Zeneca, grants and personal fees from Pulmonx, grants and personal fees from Pneumrx, personal fees from BTG, grants and personal fees from Olympus, grants and personal fees from Broncus, personal fees from EOLO, personal fees from NGM, grants and personal fees from Lungpacer, grants from Alung, grants and personal fees from Nuvaira, grants and personal fees from ResMed, grants and personal fees from Respironics, grants from Fisher Paykel, grants and personal fees from Patara, grants from Galapgos, outside the submitted work.

REFERENCES

1. Volgelmeier C., Agusti A., Anzueto A., et al Global strategy for the diagnosis, management, and prevention of chronic obstructive pulmonary disease, 2019 report. 2019.

2. Sciurba FC, Ernst A, Herth FJ, et al. A randomized study of endobronchial valves for advanced emphysema. N Engl J Med 2010;363(13):1233–44.

3. Herth FJ, Noppen M, Valipour A, et al. Efficacy predictors of lung volume reduction with zephyr valves in a European cohort. Eur Respir J 2012;39(6): 1334–42.

4. Eberhardt R, Gompelmann D, Schuhmann M, et al. Complete unilateral vs partial bilateral endoscopic lung volume reduction in patients with bilateral lung emphysema. Chest 2012;142(4):900–8.

5. Herth FJ, Eberhardt R, Gompelmann D, et al. Radiological and clinical outcomes of using Chartis to plan endobronchial valve treatment. Eur Respir J 2013; 41(2):302–8.

6. Schuhmann M, Raffy P, Yin Y, et al. Computed tomography predictors of response to endobronchial valve lung reduction treatment. comparison with chartis. Am J Respir Crit Care Med 2015;191(7): 767–74.

7. Criner GJ, Delage A, Voelker K, et al. Improving Lung Function in Severe Heterogenous Emphysema with the Spiration Valve System (EMPROVE). A Multicenter, Open-Label Randomized Controlled Clinical Trial. Am J Respir Crit Care Med 2019; 200(11):1354–62.

8. Kemp SV, Slebos DJ, Kirk A, et al. A multicenter randomized controlled trial of zephyr endobronchial valve treatment in heterogeneous emphysema (TRANSFORM). Am J Respir Crit Care Med 2017; 196(12):1535–43.

9. Criner GJ, Sue R, Wright S, et al. A multicenter randomized controlled trial of zephyr endobronchial valve treatment in heterogeneous emphysema (LIBERATE). Am J Respir Crit Care Med 2018; 198(9):1151–64.

10. Li S, Wang G, Wang C, et al. The REACH trial: a randomized controlled trial assessing the safety and effectiveness of the spiration(R) valve system in the treatment of severe emphysema. Respiration 2019;97(5):416–27.

11. Criner GJ, Delage A, Voelker K, et al. Improving lung function in severe heterogenous emphysema with the spiration valve system (EMPROVE). A multicenter, open-label randomized controlled clinical trial. Am J Respir Crit Care Med 2019;200(11): 1354–62.

12. Valipour A, Slebos DJ, Herth F, et al. Endobronchial valve therapy in patients with homogeneous emphysema. results from the IMPACT study. Am J Respir Crit Care Med 2016;194(9):1073–82.

13. Davey C, Zoumot Z, Jordan S, et al. Bronchoscopic lung volume reduction with endobronchial valves for patients with heterogeneous emphysema and intact interlobar fissures (the BeLieVeR-HIFi study): a

randomised controlled trial. Lancet 2015;386(9998): 1066–73.

14. Klooster K, ten Hacken NH, Hartman JE, et al. Endobronchial valves for emphysema without interlobar collateral ventilation. N Engl J Med 2015;373(24): 2325–35.

15. Valipour A, Slebos DJ, de Oliveira HG, et al. Expert statement: pneumothorax associated with endoscopic valve therapy for emphysema–potential mechanisms, treatment algorithm, and case examples. Respiration 2014;87(6):513–21.

16. Kontogianni K, Gerovasili V, Gompelmann D, et al. Effectiveness of endobronchial coil treatment for lung volume reduction in patients with severe heterogeneous emphysema and bilateral incomplete fissures: a six-month follow-up. Respiration 2014; 88(1):52–60.

17. Sciurba FC, Criner GJ, Strange C, et al. Effect of endobronchial coils vs usual care on exercise tolerance in patients with severe emphysema: the RENEW randomized clinical trial. JAMA 2016; 315(20):2178–89.

18. Criner GJ, Pinto-Plata V, Strange C, et al. Biologic lung volume reduction in advanced upper lobe emphysema: phase 2 results. Am J Respir Crit Care Med 2009;179(9):791–8.

19. Refaely Y, Dransfield M, Kramer MR, et al. Biologic lung volume reduction therapy for advanced homogeneous emphysema. Eur Respir J 2010;36(1): 20–7.

20. Come CE, Kramer MR, Dransfield MT, et al. A randomised trial of lung sealant versus medical therapy for advanced emphysema. Eur Respir J 2015;46(3):651–62.

21. Shah PL, Slebos DJ, Cardoso PF, et al. Bronchoscopic lung-volume reduction with exhale airway stents for emphysema (EASE trial): randomised, sham-controlled, multicentre trial. Lancet 2011; 378(9795):997–1005.

22. Snell G, Herth FJ, Hopkins P, et al. Bronchoscopic thermal vapour ablation therapy in the management of heterogeneous emphysema. Eur Respir J 2012; 39(6):1326–33.

23. Herth FJ, Valipour A, Shah PL, et al. Segmental volume reduction using thermal vapour ablation in patients with severe emphysema: 6-month results of the multicentre, parallel-group, open-label, randomised controlled STEP-UP trial. Lancet Respir Med 2016;4(3):185–93.

24. Belmonte KE. Cholinergic pathways in the lungs and anticholinergic therapy for chronic obstructive pulmonary disease. Proc Am Thorac Soc 2005;2(4): 297–304.

25. O'Donnell DE, Fluge T, Gerken F, et al. Effects of tiotropium on lung hyperinflation, dyspnoea and exercise tolerance in COPD. Eur Respir J 2004; 23(6):832–40. Available at: http://erj.ersjournals. com/cgi/content/abstract/23/6/832.

26. Vogelmeier C, Hederer B, Glaab T, et al. Tiotropium versus salmeterol for the prevention of exacerbations of COPD. N Engl J Med 2011;364(12): 1093–103.

27. Slebos DJ, Klooster K, Koegelenberg CF, et al. Targeted lung denervation for moderate to severe COPD: a pilot study. Thorax 2015;70(5):411–9.

28. Valipour A, Shah PL, Pison C, et al. Safety and dose study of targeted lung denervation in moderate/severe COPD patients. Respiration 2019;98(4): 329–39.

29. Slebos DJ, Shah PL, Herth FJF, et al. Safety and adverse events after targeted lung denervation for symptomatic moderate to severe chronic obstructive pulmonary disease (AIRFLOW). A multicenter randomized controlled clinical trial. Am J Respir Crit Care Med 2019;200(12):1477–86.

30. Kim V, Criner GJ. Chronic bronchitis and chronic obstructive pulmonary disease. Am J Respir Crit Care Med 2013;187(3):228–37.

31. Slebos DJ, Breen D, Coad J, et al. Safety and histological effect of liquid nitrogen metered spray cryotherapy in the lung. Am J Respir Crit Care Med 2017;196(10):1351–2.

32. Valipour A, Ing A, Williamson JP, et al. First-in-human results of bronchial rheoplasty: an endobronchial treatment for chronic bronchitis. May 2019.

Surgical Therapies for Chronic Obstructive Pulmonary Disease

Sean Duffy, MD, Nathaniel Marchetti, DO*, Gerard J. Criner, MD

KEYWORDS

- Lung volume reduction surgery • Lung transplantation • Bullectomy

KEY POINTS

- Lung volume reduction surgery improves lung function and quality of life in patients with severe hyperinflation and upper lobe predominant emphysema.
- Bullectomy should be considered when the bulla occupies at least one-third of the hemithorax, compresses adjacent lung tissue, and a forced expiratory volume in 1 second of 50% predicted or less.
- Lung transplantation is reserved for patients with severe chronic obstructive pulmonary disease.
- Criteria include a BODE Score of greater than 7, forced expiratory volume in 1 second and/or carbon monoxide diffusing capacity of 20% predicted or less, $Paco_2$ greater than 50 mm Hg, or presence of cor pulmonale.

INTRODUCTION

Medical therapy for chronic obstructive pulmonary disease (COPD) has improved with many options now available that improve dyspnea, reduce exacerbations, improve exercise performance, and enhance quality of life.[1] Despite these therapeutic interventions, COPD remains a leading cause of death in the world and even with maximal medical therapy patients often have disabling dyspnea and a poor quality of life. For those having disabling symptoms despite maximal medical therapy, surgical options are available to help alleviate those symptoms. Because of the morbidity associated with these procedures, careful patient selection is essential to increase the likelihood of a successful outcome. This review focuses on surgical interventions (lung volume reduction surgery [LVRS], bullectomy, and lung transplantation) available to patients with advanced COPD refractory to maximal medical therapy.

RATIONALE FOR LUNG VOLUME REDUCTION

Lung hyperinflation has been recognized as a major contributor to poor respiratory function and has been associated with increased mortality as well.[2,3] In addition to poor respiratory function, hyperinflation increases the sensation of dyspnea and causes a reduction in exercise capacity owing to distortions of the chest wall and pulmonary muscle mechanics.[4] Furthermore, hyperinflation is associated with decreased cardiac function.[5] Thus, hyperinflation has been an ever important target of therapy in patients with COPD.

HISTORY OF LUNG VOLUME REDUCTION SURGERY

LVRS was initially described in the 1950s.[6] He described the surgery as "an operation directed at restoration of a physiologic principle ... not concerned with the removal of pathologic tissue." Despite sound physiology and some promising outcomes, the surgery was never widely used or studied until the 1990s. A case series of 20 patients with severe emphysema and hyperinflation was published showing that surgical resection of 20% to 30% of each lung resulted in

a Department of Thoracic Medicine and Surgery, Lewis Katz School of Medicine at Temple University, 712 Parkinson Pavilion, 3401 North Broad Street, Philadelphia, PA 19140, USA
* Corresponding author.
E-mail address: nathaniel.marchetti@tuhs.temple.edu

Clin Chest Med 41 (2020) 559–566
https://doi.org/10.1016/j.ccm.2020.06.011

improvements in lung volume, spirometry, walk distance, and quality-of-life measures.[7] A case series of 150 patients followed, showing similar results with a 90-day surgical mortality of only 4%.[8] These studies preceded the first randomized controlled trials in LVRS, which were published in 1999[9] and 2000.[10] These trials confirmed that LVRS succeeded at improving lung function, walk distance, and quality of life in select patients, but were underpowered to show a difference in mortality.[9,10]

THE NATIONAL EMPHYSEMA TREATMENT TRIAL

The earlier studies, while confirming the potential benefits of LVRS left questions regarding patient selection and mortality, paving the way for The National Emphysema Treatment Trial (NETT).[11,12] The NETT was a randomized trial that enrolled more than 1200 subjects from 17 centers into 2 groups; maximal medical therapy versus LVRS plus maximal medical therapy. Patients in both arms were medically optimized and participated in a pulmonary rehabilitation program before baseline testing and randomization.[11,12] The patient population was meticulously characterized with lung function testing, cardiopulmonary exercise testing and lung perfusion chest imaging. Computed tomography scans were reviewed and classified by distribution of emphysema as upper lobe predominant emphysema or non-upper lobe predominant emphysema. The primary outcomes included maximal exercise capacity and mortality. Secondary outcomes included quality of life measures, 6-minute walk distance, and lung function parameters.[11,12]

The study population consisted of subjects with severe COPD (mean forced expiratory volume in 1 second [FEV$_1$] of 27% predicted) with gas trapping (mean residual volume of >220% predicted) and hyperinflation (mean total lung capacity of >125% predicted). Nearly two-thirds of patients were classified as having predominantly upper lobe emphysema.[12] Key exclusion criteria included an FEV$_1$ of greater than 45% predicted, total lung capacity of less than 100% predicted, residual volume of less than 150% predicted, lung nodule requiring follow-up, previous sternotomy, or large lung bulla. The results of NETT proved the importance of comprehensive patient characterization and proper patient selection, because the different subgroups had vastly different outcomes. Patients with upper lobe predominant emphysema and low exercise capacity, defined as less than 40 W in men and less than 25 W in women, had improved exercise capacity and a significant mortality benefit with surgical intervention.[12] Patients with upper lobe emphysema but high exercise capacity had an improvement only in their exercise capacity and symptom score, but no mortality benefit. A long-term analysis with a median follow-up of 4.3 years confirmed the mortality benefit in the upper lobe emphysema and low exercise tolerance group (**Fig. 1**) along with long-term improvements in exercise capacity and health-related quality of life in the group with upper lobe emphysema and high exercise capacity.[13] Conversely, patients with both an FEV$_1$ and carbon monoxide diffusing capacity of less than 20% predicted or FEV$_1$ and homogeneous emphysema had increased mortality (16% vs 0%) when compared with medical management.[12,14] Patients with homogeneous or non-upper lobe predominant emphysema achieved no durable benefit with LVRS (**Table 1**). Based on the mortality benefit in NETT, patients with upper lobe emphysema and low exercise capacity should be considered for LVRS. Additionally, patients with upper lobe emphysema with high exercise tolerance can be considered for LVRS based on improved symptoms and exercise capacity. Follow-up studies have also shown that a subset of these patients with low perfusion to the upper lobe have a mortality benefit with LVRS.[15] Another benefit of LVRS is a decrease in rate of acute exacerbation of COPD. An analysis of the NETT data showed a 30% decrease in the exacerbation rate for LVRS patients when compared with the control arm. The improvement in the exacerbation rate was most pronounced in patients with at least a 200 mL improvement in FEV$_1$ at 6 months after surgery.[16] A follow-up analysis confirmed that LVRS significantly improves exercise capacity and health-related quality of life up to 3 and 5 years out from surgery, respectively.[17]

Further analysis showed that LVRS improved cardiovascular function and pulmonary mechanics. Jörgensen and colleagues[18] evaluated left ventricular filling pressures and hemodynamics using a pulmonary artery catheter and echocardiography to show that patients undergoing LVRS for relief of hyperinflation had significant improvements in end-diastolic filling, left ventricular function, and cardiac index. Lammi and colleagues[19] showed that noninvasive surrogates for stroke volume such as pulse pressure and O$_2$ pulse were increased at 6 months postoperatively in patients who had undergone LVRS. LVRS also improves respiratory muscle function and dynamic hyperinflation. Before NETT, 1 study showed an improvement in end-expiratory lung volume during exercise in patients who had undergone LVRS at least 3 months prior.[20] Criner and colleagues[21] found that LVRS resulted in

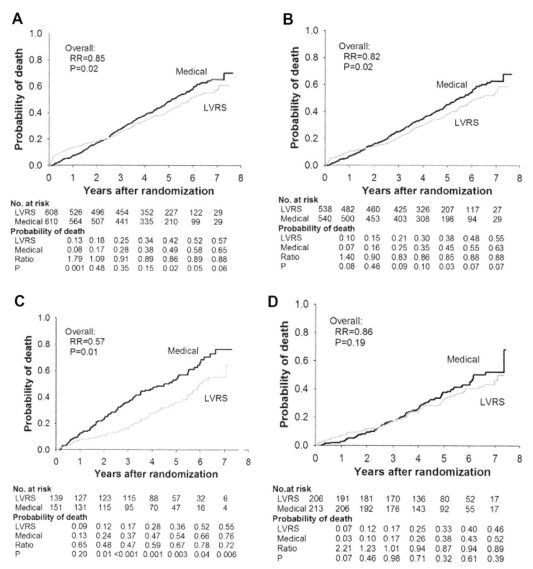

Fig. 1. Kaplan–Meier estimates of the cumulative probability of death as a function of years after randomization to LVRS. The overall relative risk (RR) and P value represent the 4.3 years median follow-up. Shown below each plot is the number of subjects at risk in each arm, probability of death in each arm and the RR (LVRS:Medical) for each year and the P value for difference in the probability. (A) All patients (n = 1218.) (B) Non–high-risk patients (n = 1078). (C) Upper lobe predominant and low baseline exercise performance (n = 290). (D) Upper lobe predominant and high exercise capacity (n = 419). (From Naunheim KS, Wood DE, Mohsenifar Z, et al. Long-term follow-up of patients receiving lung-volume-reduction surgery versus medical therapy for severe emphysema by the National Emphysema Treatment Trial research group. Ann Thorac Surg. 2006;82(2):431-443; with permission.)

deeper, slower breathing with decreased dead space and improved ventilation during exercise. A further analysis of the NETT population shows that patients who have undergone LVRS use less supplemental oxygen. Resting Pao_2 was found to be significantly higher in the LVRS cohort 2 years after surgery when compared with medical management alone.[22]

LUNG VOLUME REDUCTION SURGERY: CURRENT STATE

Despite clear benefits in carefully selected patients, LVRS has not been used as a mainstay of therapy in the population with emphysema. In fact, LVRS was only performed about 3300 times in the United States from 2000 to 2010 with

Table 1
Patients with homogeneous or non-upper lobe predominant emphysema*

	Mortality	Exercise Capacity	Symptoms
Upper lobe predominant emphysema, low exercise	Improved	Improved	Improved
Upper lobe predominant emphysema, high exercise	No change	Improved	Improved
Non-upper lobe predominant emphysema, low exercise	No change	No change	No change
Non-upper lobe predominant emphysema, high exercise	Worsened	No change	No change

* There were some short-term improvements in exercise capacity in this group, but they were not sustained in the long term.

Data from Fishman A, Martinez F, Naunheim K, et al. A randomized trial comparing lung-volume-reduction surgery with medical therapy for severe emphysema. *N Engl J Med*. 2003;348(21):2059-2073.

numbers decreasing in the latter part of the decade.[23] Although still relatively few, in 2013 numbers had increased with 605 surgeries performed, nearly doubling the total from 2007.[24] The relatively low number of lung volume reduction surgeries is certainly due in part to the emergence of less invasive and bronchoscopic techniques of achieving lung volume reduction, along with the perceived risk of perioperative morbidity and mortality. There has also been concern that LVRS may preclude patients from undergoing lung transplantation. An analysis of patients undergoing lung transplantation after LVRS showed no significant difference in 5-year mortality as compared with patients who did not have prior LVRS. There was potential for increased postoperative bleeding and renal injury. Prior LVRS must be taken into consideration preoperatively, but it should not be a contraindication to lung transplantation.[25] With the caveat that LVRS has proven more costly than medical management[26] and should only be performed in experienced centers, the GOLD guidelines maintain that LVRS is a potential option for patients with upper lobe emphysema and low exercise tolerance.[1]

BULLECTOMY

A bulla is defined as an airspace in the lung with a diameter of greater than 1 cm. Most bullae are clinically insignificant and not amenable to surgery. A giant bulla is an air space in the lung that occupies about 30% or more of the hemithorax. Giant bullae are rare and typically associated with cigarette smoking. Additionally, marijuana smoking,[27] intravenous drug use,[28] and human immunodeficiency virus infection[29] have all been linked to the development of giant bullae.

The clinical effect of bullous lung disease can vary widely. Some patients have relatively normal lung function and mild dyspnea, whereas others are severely limited in their daily life.[30] The clinical

effect largely depends on the degree of hyperinflation and the extent of compression of normal lung tissue adjacent to the bulla. Surgical resection is reserved for those patients with considerable impairment and the best chance of improved lung function postoperatively. The majority of published outcomes data comes from case series. Snider[30] published a review of 22 articles ranging from 1950 to 1996 analyzing more than 450 bullectomy cases performed mainly for persistent dyspnea. The review found that bullectomy was most successful in patients with an FEV_1 of less than 50% predicted, compressed adjacent lung tissue, and bullae covering more than one-third of the hemithorax.[30] These criteria have since become the foundation for patient selection in bullectomy cases. **Fig. 2** is a chest radiograph and computed tomography scan of a patient meeting these criteria preoperatively and postoperatively.

Subsequent case series studied the long-term outcomes of patients undergoing bullectomy. In a single-center review of cases between 1994 and 2002, bullectomy was performed on 43 patients with giant bullae, severe obstruction, and evidence of adjacent lung compression. Postoperative testing revealed clinically significant improvement in FEV_1 at 6 months and 3 years compared with baseline. More than 80% of patients had maintained significant improvement in FEV_1 at 3 years. Additionally, patients were found to have improved 6-minute walk distance, decreased gas trapping, and improved oxygenation.[31] An additional study of 41 patients undergoing bullectomy separated the patients into 2 groups based on the presence or absence of diffuse emphysema on computed tomography scan. This study similarly showed durable improvement in FEV_1 as well as dyspnea for the entire cohort 5 years postoperatively. FEV_1 was noted to improve for the first 2 years after surgery, then begin to decline in year 3 and beyond. There was a 12% mortality rate at 5 years in the entire

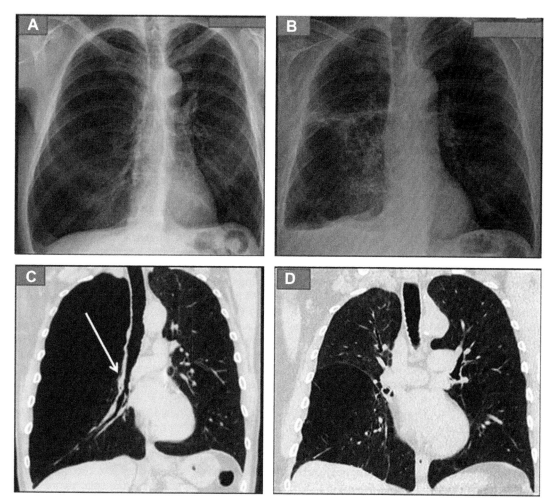

Fig. 2. (*A*) Preoperative chest radiograph of a large right-sided bulla occupying more than 50% of the hemi-thorax and (*B*) postoperative chest radiograph after bullectomy in the same patient. (*C*) Coronal computed tomography image of giant bulla showing compressed lung (*arrow*) in the same patient preoperatively. (*D*) Coronal computed tomography image of the chest after right-sided bullectomy showing reexpansion of the compressed lung.

cohort. All deaths occurred in the group with diffuse emphysema.[32] In each study, the most common complication was prolonged air leak lasting more than 7 days.[31,32] Bullectomy has also been shown to improve diaphragm function and in some cases cardiac output. In a smaller case series, O'Donnell and colleagues[33] showed a decrease in exertional dyspnea owing to improvement in dynamic hyperinflation and respiratory frequency. Additional studies have shown improvements in diaphragm muscle strength[34] and even cardiac output in cases where the bulla causes mediastinal shift.[35] In summary, bullectomy has demonstrated symptomatic benefit, improvement in lung function, and improved cardiopulmonary mechanics in patients with giant bulla showing evidence of compressed adjacent lung tissue.

LUNG TRANSPLANTATION IN CHRONIC OBSTRUCTIVE PULMONARY DISEASE

Lung transplantation was first performed and published as a case report in 1963.[36] Since then, more than 50,000 lung transplantations[37] have been performed with more than 2700 lung transplantations performed in the United States in 2019[38] and more than 2000 lung transplants performed in Europe in 2016.[39] Between 1995 and 2012, COPD was the most common indication for lung transplantation worldwide, accounting for more than 39% of the total lung transplant volume.[37] Outcomes have improved over the last 25 years and the current median survival is about 5.6 years.[40]

Transplantation should be carefully considered in any patient with end-stage lung disease. Generally, patients should be considered for lung transplantation if they have a high risk (>50%) of death within 2 years, but are also highly likely (>80%) to survive the postoperative period and 5 years after successful transplantation.[41] Indications specific to COPD include a body mass index, obstruction (FEV_1), dyspnea and exercise (BODE) score of more than 7, an FEV_1 of less than 20% predicted, carbon monoxide diffusing capacity of less than 20% predicted, Pco_2 of greater than 50, and/or the presence of cor pulmonale.[41] Common absolute contraindications to lung transplantation include malignancy within 5 years or 2 years for nonmelanoma skin cancer, cigarette smoking within 6 months, a body mass index of greater than 35, uncorrectable organ dysfunction, and functional limitation preventing rehabilitation after transplantation.[41]

Disease progression in late-stage COPD can be difficult to predict when compared with pulmonary fibrosis and other common indications for transplant. The BODE score is the most well-established predictor of 4-year mortality in COPD. The BODE score is an aggregate score of those 4 factors based on severity of abnormality. A BODE score of 7 or greater confers a mortality risk of about 80% at 4 years.[42] A recent retrospective analysis showed that transplant candidates are likely to outlive their BODE-predicted mortality. Reed and colleagues[43] compared mortality rates between lung transplant candidates in the BODE fourth quartile and the corresponding group in the BODE validation cohort. They found that the median survival was 59 months in the transplant candidates and 37 months in the BODE validation cohort.[43] Respiratory failure made up a higher percentage of deaths in the transplant cohort (73%) than the BODE validation cohort (61%). This factor was likely a result of the transplant evaluation process selecting out patients with significant comorbid disease.[43] Thus, survival benefit remains a controversial end point in patients undergoing lung transplant for native COPD. A retrospective analysis of more than 13,000 lung transplant candidates from 2005 to 2011 showed that lung transplantation conferred a 3-year survival benefit to 56% of patients transplanted for obstructive lung disease as compared with 98% of patients transplanted for restrictive lung disease.[44] Single versus double lung transplant in COPD is another important factor in post-transplant survival. A retrospective review analyzed data from more than 9000 transplant recipients and found that patients receiving a double lung transplant had a higher median survival than patients receiving a single lung transplant (6.4 years vs 4.9 years). A further analysis showed that the survival benefit held true only in recipients less than 60 years of age.[45]

Quality of life after transplant does improve considerably in patients transplanted for COPD. A recent review showed that transplant recipients had a 48-point improvement in the St. George's Respiratory Questionnaire (minimum clinically important difference = 4), a validated tool used to assess health related quality of life at 1 year after transplantation.[46] In comparison, patients undergoing LVRS experienced a 10- to 12-point improvement in the St. George's Respiratory Questionnaire.[12] In patients who are appropriate for both LVRS and lung transplantation, LVRS should be considered on a case-by-case basis because it may impart a mortality benefit and could postpone or prevent the need for future transplant. In summary, lung transplantation in severe COPD offers considerable quality-of-life benefit in carefully selected patients when compared with other surgical interventions

Table 2
Common indications for surgical intervention in advanced emphysema

LVRS	Bullectomy	Lung Transplantation
Limitation in exercise tolerance	Bulla >one-third hemithorax	BODE >7
Upper lobe predominant emphysema	FEV_1 <50% predicted	FEV_1 <20% predicted
TLC >100% predicted	Compressed adjacent lung tissue	D_LCO <20% predicted
RV >150% predicted	Limitation in exercise tolerance	P_aco_2 >50 mm Hg

Abbreviations: D_LCO, carbon monoxide diffusing capacity; RV, residual volume; TLC, total lung capacity.

available in this population. Transplantation should be offered in appropriate patients, especially if they are too ill or not appropriate for less morbid interventions.

SUMMARY

Surgical intervention in advanced emphysema can offer considerable improvement to a patient's quality of life and in some cases even confer a mortality benefit. The most crucial aspect of surgical intervention in COPD is proper and meticulous patient selection. **Table 2** summarizes common indications for LVRS, bullectomy, and lung transplantation. Before surgery is offered, patients must fail optimal medical therapy and should participate in a pulmonary rehabilitation program. Of the surgical options available, LVRS provides the most well-established mortality benefit with proper patient selection, whereas bullectomy has been shown to improve lung function and dyspnea in patient with giant bullae. Finally, lung transplantation offers a profound improvement in quality of life, especially in patients who are too ill or not candidates for other interventions.

DISCLOSURE

Dr. Marchetti reports personal fees from Astrazeneca, personal fees from Realta Life Sciences, grants from Blade Therapeutics, grants from NIH, outside the submitted work.

Dr. Duffy has nothing to disclose.

Dr. Criner reports grants and personal fees from Galaxo Smith Kline, grants and personal fees from Boehringer Ingelheim, grants and personal fees from Chiesi, grants and personal fees from Mereo, personal fees from Verona, grants and personal fees from Astra Zeneca, grants and personal fees from Pulmonx, grants and personal fees from Pneumrx, personal fees from BTG, grants and personal fees from Olympus, grants and personal fees from Broncus, personal fees from EOLO, personal fees from NGM, grants and personal fees from Lungpacer, grants from Alung, grants and personal fees from Nuvaira, grants and personal fees from ResMed, grants and personal fees from Respironics, grants from Fisher Paykel, grants and personal fees from Patara, grants from Galapgos, outside the submitted work.

REFERENCES

1. Volgelmeier C., Agusti A., Anzueto A., et al Global strategy for the diagnosis, management, and prevention of chronic obstructive pulmonary disease, 2020 report.

2. Casanova C, Cote C, de Torres JP, et al. Inspiratory-to-total lung capacity ratio predicts mortality in patients with chronic obstructive pulmonary disease. Am J Respir Crit Care Med 2005;171(6):591–7.

3. O'Donnell DE, Revill SM, Webb KA. Dynamic hyperinflation and exercise intolerance in chronic obstructive pulmonary disease. Am J Respir Crit Care Med 2001;164(5):770–7.

4. O'Donnell DE, Hamilton AL, Webb KA. Sensory-mechanical relationships during high-intensity, constant-work-rate exercise in COPD. J Appl Physiol (1985) 2006;101(4):1025–35.

5. Watz H, Waschki B, Meyer T, et al. Decreasing cardiac chamber sizes and associated heart dysfunction in COPD: role of hyperinflation. Chest 2010;138(1):32–8.

6. Brantigan OC, Mueller E, Kress MB. A surgical approach to pulmonary emphysema. Am Rev Respir Dis 1959;80(1, Part 2):194–206.

7. Cooper JD, Trulock EP, Triantafillou AN, et al. Bilateral pneumectomy (volume reduction) for chronic obstructive pulmonary disease. J Thorac Cardiovasc Surg 1995;109(1):106–19. Available at: https://www.sciencedirect.com/science/article/pii/S0022522395704264.

8. Cooper JD, Patterson GA, Sundaresan RS, et al. Results of 150 consecutive bilateral lung volume reduction procedures in patients with severe emphysema. J Thorac Cardiovasc Surg 1996; 112(5):1319–30. Available at: https://www.sciencedirect.com/science/article/pii/S0022522396701472.

9. Criner GJ, Cordova FC, Furukawa S, et al. Prospective randomized trial comparing bilateral lung volume reduction surgery to pulmonary rehabilitation in severe chronic obstructive pulmonary disease. Am J Respir Crit Care Med 1999;160(6):2018–27.

10. Geddes D. Effect of lung-volume-reduction surgery in patients with severe emphysema. JAMA 2001;285(2):149.

11. Rationale and design of the National Emphysema Treatment Trial: a prospective randomized trial of lung volume reduction surgery. The National Emphysema Treatment Trial research group. Chest 1999;116(6):1750–61.

12. Fishman A, Martinez F, Naunheim K, et al. A randomized trial comparing lung-volume-reduction surgery with medical therapy for severe emphysema. N Engl J Med 2003;348(21):2059–73.

13. Naunheim KS, Wood DE, Mohsenifar Z, et al. Long-term follow-up of patients receiving lung-volume-reduction surgery versus medical therapy for severe emphysema by the National Emphysema Treatment Trial research group. Ann Thorac Surg 2006;82(2):431–43.

14. National Emphysema Treatment Trial Research Group. Patients at high risk of death after lung-volume-reduction surgery. N Engl J Med 2001;345(15):1075–83.

15. Chandra D, Lipson DA, Hoffman EA, et al. Perfusion scintigraphy and patient selection for lung volume reduction surgery. Am J Respir Crit Care Med 2010;182(7):937–46.

16. Washko GR, Fan VS, Ramsey SD, et al. The effect of lung volume reduction surgery on chronic obstructive pulmonary disease exacerbations. Am J Respir Crit Care Med 2008;177(2):164–9.

17. Criner GJ, Cordova F, Sternberg AL, et al. The National Emphysema Treatment Trial (NETT) part II: lessons learned about lung volume reduction surgery. Am J Respir Crit Care Med 2011;184(8):881–93.

18. Jörgensen K, Houltz E, Westfelt U, et al. Effects of lung volume reduction surgery on left ventricular diastolic filling and dimensions in patients with severe emphysema. Chest 2003;124(5):1863–70.

19. Lammi MR, Ciccolella D, Marchetti N, et al. Increased oxygen pulse after lung volume reduction surgery is associated with reduced dynamic hyperinflation. Eur Respir J 2012;40(4):837–43.

20. Martinez FJ, de Oca MM, Whyte RI, et al. Lung-volume reduction improves dyspnea, dynamic hyperinflation, and respiratory muscle function. Am J Respir Crit Care Med 1997;155(6):1984–90.

21. Criner GJ, Belt P, Sternberg AL, et al. Effects of lung volume reduction surgery on gas exchange and breathing pattern during maximum exercise. Chest 2009;135(5):1268–79.

22. Snyder ML, Goss CH, Neradilek B, et al. Changes in arterial oxygenation and self-reported oxygen use after lung volume reduction surgery. Am J Respir Crit Care Med 2008;178(4):339–45.

23. Ahmad S, Taneja A, Kurman J, et al. National trends in lung volume reduction surgery in the United States: 2000 to 2010. Chest 2014;146(6):e228–9.

24. Attaway AH, Hatipoglu U, Murthy S, et al. Lung volume reduction surgery in the United States from 2007 to 2013: increasing volumes and reason for caution. Chest 2019;155(5):1080–1.

25. Shigemura N, Gilbert S, Bhama JK, et al. Lung transplantation after lung volume reduction surgery. Transplantation 2013;96(4):421–5.

26. Ramsey SD, Shroyer AL, Sullivan SD, et al. Updated evaluation of the cost-effectiveness of lung volume reduction surgery. Chest 2007;131(3):823–32.

27. Johnson MK, Smith RP, Morrison D, et al. Large lung bullae in marijuana smokers. Thorax 2000;55(4):340–2.

28. Goldstein DS, Karpel JP, Appel D, et al. Bullous pulmonary damage in users of intravenous drugs. Chest 1986;89(2):266–9.

29. Diaz PT, Clanton TL, Pacht ER. Emphysema-like pulmonary disease associated with human immunodeficiency virus infection. Ann Intern Med 1992;116(2):124–8.

30. Snider GL. Health-care technology assessment of surgical procedures: the case of reduction pneumoplasty for emphysema. Am J Respir Crit Care Med 1996;153(4 Pt 1):1208–13.

31. Schipper PH, Meyers BF, Battafarano RJ, et al. Outcomes after resection of giant emphysematous bullae. Ann Thorac Surg 2004;78(3):976–82.

32. Palla A, Desideri M, Rossi G, et al. Elective surgery for giant bullous emphysema: a 5-year clinical and functional follow-up. Chest 2005;128(4):2043–50.

33. O'Donnell DE, Webb KA, Bertley JC, et al. Mechanisms of relief of exertional breathlessness following unilateral bullectomy and lung volume reduction surgery in emphysema. Chest 1996;110(1):18–27.

34. Travaline JM, Addonizio VP, Criner GJ. Effect of bullectomy on diaphragm strength. Am J Respir Crit Care Med 1995;152(5 Pt 1):1697–701.

35. Marchetti N, Criner KT, Keresztury MF, et al. The acute and chronic effects of bullectomy on cardiovascular function at rest and during exercise. J Thorac Cardiovasc Surg 2008;135(1):205–6, 206.e1.

36. Hardy JD, Webb WR, Dalton ML Jr, et al. Lung homotransplantation in man. JAMA 1963;186:1065–74.

37. Yusen RD, Edwards LB, Kucheryavaya AY, et al. The registry of the international society for heart and lung transplantation: thirty-first adult lung and heart-lung transplant report–2014; focus theme: retransplantation. J Heart Lung Transplant 2014;33(10):1009–24.

38. UNOS. National data report. united network of organ sharing. UNOS Web site. 2020. Available at: https://optn.transplant.hrsa.gov/data/view-data-reports/national-data/. Accessed January 15, 2020.

39. Hofsteter E, Henig NR, Boerner G. ISHLT registry data and country registries: comparison of reported European lung transplant activities in 2016. European Respiratory Journal 2019; 54: Suppl. 63, PA3367.

40. Whitson BA, Hayes D. Indications and outcomes in adult lung transplantation. J Thorac Dis 2014;6(8):1018–23.

41. Weill D, Benden C, Corris PA, et al. A consensus document for the selection of lung transplant candidates: 2014–an update from the pulmonary transplantation council of the international society for heart and lung transplantation. J Heart Lung Transplant 2015;34(1):1–15.

42. Celli BR, Cote CG, Marin JM, et al. The body-mass index, airflow obstruction, dyspnea, and exercise capacity index in chronic obstructive pulmonary disease. N Engl J Med 2004;350(10):1005–12.

43. Reed RM, Cabral HJ, Dransfield MT, et al. Survival of lung transplant candidates with COPD: BODE score reconsidered. Chest 2018;153(3):697–701.

44. Vock DM, Durheim MT, Tsuang WM, et al. Survival benefit of lung transplantation in the modern era of lung allocation. Ann Am Thorac Soc 2017;14(2):172–81.

45. Thabut G, Christie JD, Ravaud P, et al. Survival after bilateral versus single lung transplantation for patients with chronic obstructive pulmonary disease: a retrospective analysis of registry data. Lancet 2008;371(9614):744–51.

46. Thabut G, Mal H. Outcomes after lung transplantation. J Thorac Dis 2017;9(8):2684–91.

Moving?

Make sure your subscription moves with you!

To notify us of your new address, find your **Clinics Account Number** (located on your mailing label above your name), and contact customer service at:

Email: **journalscustomerservice-usa@elsevier.com**

800-654-2452 (subscribers in the U.S. & Canada)
314-447-8871 (subscribers outside of the U.S. & Canada)

Fax number: 314-447-8029

Elsevier Health Sciences Division
Subscription Customer Service
3251 Riverport Lane
Maryland Heights, MO 63043

Moving?

Make sure your subscription moves with you!

To notify us of your new address, find your Clinics Account number (located on your mailing label above your name), and contact customer service at:

Email: journalscustomerservice-usa@elsevier.com

800-654-2452 (subscribers in the U.S. & Canada)
314-447-8871 (subscribers outside of the U.S. & Canada)

Fax number: 314-447-8029

Elsevier Health Sciences Division
Subscription Customer Service
3251 Riverport Lane
Maryland Heights, MO 63043

To ensure uninterrupted delivery of your subscription, please notify us at least 4 weeks in advance of move.

Printed and bound by CPI Group (UK) Ltd, Croydon, CR0 4YY

08/05/2025

01864746-0011